OXFORD MEDICAL PUBLICATIONS

Cardiovascular Magnetic Resonance

Oxford Specialist Handbooks published and forthcoming

General Oxford Specialist Handbooks
A Resuscitation Room Guide
Addiction Medicine
Hypertension
Perioperative Medicine, Second Edition
Post-Operative Complications, Second Edition
Pulmonary Hypertension
Renal Transplantation

Oxford Specialist Handbooks in Anaesthesia
Cardiac Anaesthesia
Day Case Surgery
General Thoracic Anaesthesia
Neuroanaethesia
Obstetric Anaesthesia
Paediatric Anaesthesia
Regional Anaesthesia, Stimulation and Ultrasound Techniques

Oxford Specialist Handbooks in Cardiology
Adult Congenital Heart Disease
Cardiac Catheterization and Coronary Intervention
Cardiac Electrophysiology
Cardiovascular Magnetic Resonance
Echocardiography
Fetal Cardiology
Heart Failure
Nuclear Cardiology
Pacemakers and ICDs
Valvular Heart Disease

Oxford Specialist Handbooks in Critical Care
Advanced Respiratory Critical Care

Oxford Specialist Handbooks in End of Life Care
End of Life Care in Dementia
End of Life Care in Nephrology
End of Life in the Intensive Care Unit

Oxford Specialist Handbooks in Neurology
Epilepsy
Parkinson's Disease and Other Movement Disorders
Stroke Medicine

Oxford Specialist Handbooks in Paediatrics
Paediatric Dermatology
Paediatric Endocrinology and Diabetes
Paediatric Gastroenterology, Hepatology, and Nutrition
Paediatric Haematology and Oncology
Paediatric Intensive Care
Paediatric Nephrology
Paediatric Neurology
Paediatric Palliative Care
Paediatric Radiology
Paediatric Respiratory Medicine

Oxford Specialist Handbooks in Psychiatry
Child and Adolescent Psychiatry
Old Age Psychiatry

Oxford Specialist Handbooks in Radiology
Interventional Radiology
Musculoskeletal Imaging
Pulmonary Imaging

Oxford Specialist Handbooks in Surgery
Cardiothoracic Surgery
Colorectal Surgery
Hand Surgery
Liver and Pancreatobiliary Surgery
Operative Surgery, Second Edition
Oral Maxillofacial Surgery
Otolaryngology and Head and Neck Surgery
Paediatric Surgery
Plastic and Reconstructive Surgery
Surgical Oncology
Urological Surgery
Vascular Surgery

Oxford Specialist Handbooks in Cardiology

Cardiovascular Magnetic Resonance

Edited by

Saul G. Myerson

Consultant Cardiologist,
Honorary Senior Clinical Lecturer,
University of Oxford Centre for
Clinical Magnetic Resonance Research,
John Radcliffe Hospital, Oxford, UK

Jane Francis

Chief Technologist,
University of Oxford Centre for
Clinical Magnetic Resonance Research,
Oxford, UK

and

Stefan Neubauer

Professor of Cardiovascular Medicine,
Clinical Director,
University of Oxford Centre for
Clinical Magnetic Resonance Research,
Oxford, UK

OXFORD
UNIVERSITY PRESS

OXFORD
UNIVERSITY PRESS

Great Clarendon Street, Oxford, OX2 6DP,
United Kingdom

Oxford University Press is a department of the University of Oxford.
It furthers the University's objective of excellence in research, scholarship, and education by publishing worldwide. Oxford is a registered trade mark of Oxford University Press in the UK and in certain other countries

First Edition published in paperback 2013

Published in the United States of America by Oxford University Press
198 Madison Avenue, New York, NY 10016, United States of America

British Library Cataloguing in Publication Data
Data available

Library of Congress Cataloging in Publication Data
Data available

ISBN 978–0–19–968292–8

Foreword

Cardiovascular magnetic resonance (CMR) is fast becoming the gold standard for visualizing the heart and large arteries. This book, one of a series published by Oxford University Press, is written by established experts in the field, from internationally renowned CMR centres, and will appeal both to those who want to learn more about this technique and those who are already expert. Cardiologists have had excellent diagnostic imaging tools at their disposal for decades, though in recent years CMR has provided a much more accurate and refined look at the anatomy, function, and in particular, the tissue characteristics of the myocardium, such as fibrosis and oedema – aspects which have previously been inaccessible. As a result, this relatively new imaging modality has rapidly become an important part of diagnostic cardiac imaging. There is still, however, a shortfall in training opportunities, and this handbook should play an important role, particularly with its focus on the practical aspects of acquiring and interpreting images. Established practitioners will also find its quick reference and practical format an invaluable aide-mémoire.

Chapters that particularly caught my eye, reflecting my own interests, included the first chapter explaining the concept of CMR with clarity and skill; the chapters on ventricular function, and in ischaemic heart disease including myocardial viability, and a challenging final chapter on 'new horizons' for CMR. There are many areas where the book makes timely contributions. For example, an exact assessment of myocardial infarct size is rapidly becoming more and more important as the new therapeutic concept of postconditioning takes hold. Current therapy is moving towards a situation where prompt myocardial reperfusion is no longer sufficient. Rather, lethal reperfusion-induced cell necrosis must also be limited. To meet these requirements, CMR will certainly be used, and its potential and practical application is well explained here. When combined with myocardial perfusion imaging, a comprehensive assessment in ischaemic heart disease can be obtained – CMR acquires a dynamic sequence of images during the passage of the contrast medium through the heart, with excellent sensitivity and good specificity for detecting myocardial ischaemia. Its diagnostic potential is at least equal to that of nuclear perfusion imaging and is likely to become an important mainstream clinical test. In the future, using the blood oxygenation level-dependent (BOLD) effect, CMR may even potentially assess myocardial tissue oxygenation without the need for a contrast agent.

Although CMR is already the most versatile of all cardiovascular imaging techniques, it is likely to see further major developments and the authors conclude that 'In future, targeted molecular imaging may accelerate and re-define diagnosis, provide more precise disease characterization, enable specific treatments to be targeted in individual patients, enable drug delivery to the site of pathology and monitor responses to treatment'.

What more can we wish for? There has probably never been a more interesting time to become a cardiac imager nor for those who want to learn about CMR!

Professor Lionel H Opie, MD, DPhil (Oxon), DSc, FRCP
Director, Hatter Cardiovascular Research Institute,
Department of Medicine, University of Cape Town
Honorary Professor, Department of Medicine,
University College London

Preface

Cardiovascular Magnetic Resonance (CMR) has become an important imaging modality in clinical cardiology. Recent developments in magnet and coil design, imaging sequences and image post-processing now allow imaging of cardiac anatomy, function, perfusion and viability with superb resolution, providing clinicians with unprecedented detail for the evaluation of cardiovascular disease. The rapidly growing interest from cardiology and radiology centres around the world is testimony to this. CMR is a complex imaging modality however, with many aspects to master: MR theory, image acquisition and analysis, interpretation and reporting. A number of outstanding text books on CMR have been published in recent years, but while these books provide scholarly and comprehensive information on the state of the field, no previous book has focused on the practical aspects of CMR scanning in daily practice.

Cardiovascular Magnetic Resonance (Oxford Specialist Handbook) is designed as a practical guide on performing, analysing and interpreting CMR scans. It is not meant as a comprehensive text book, but covers all major disease areas in sufficient detail. It is aimed at all CMR users, particularly those new to CMR, though we hope that even the advanced user will find useful tips and tricks. The format is designed to be easily accessible and is laid out in easy to navigate sections, as with other handbooks. It is meant as a quick-reference guide to live near the MR console and case viewing station, or on the office shelf.

The book has three main sections: understanding CMR (the physics and technical aspects), practical aspects of scan acquisition (including patient safety and preparation, scan protocols, optimal image acquisition and standard views), and integrated pathology (what imaging to use for each major cardiology diagnoses, and how to interpret the images). Each chapter is focussed on the clinical context, and examples of typical CMR reports are presented for the most common CMR indications. The book is kept as generally applicable as possible, including all MR scanner manufacturers, though where technical aspects are specific to individual vendors, this has been noted.

We hope that you will find *Cardiovascular Magnetic Resonance* an enjoyable and valuable tool for your CMR practice, and provide you with as much satisfaction as we have enjoyed!

Saul G. Myerson
Jane Francis
Stefan Neubauer
Editors

Acknowledgement

The editors are most grateful to Dr Carmel Hayes, Siemens Healthcare, for her detailed, competent and excellent advice on all chapters of the book, which has provided an MR system manufacturer perspective. The book is not vendor-specific however, and is applicable to all MR system manufacturers.

Contents

Detailed contents

Contributors

Hassan Abdel-Aty
Consultant Radiologist
Director, Fellowship Training Program
Franz-Volhard-Klinik, Charité Campus, Berlin Buch, Germany
(Chapter 9 – Cardiac masses and tumours)

Robin Choudhury
Welcome Trust Clinical Fellow, University of Oxford
Honorary Consultant Cardiologist, John Radcliffe Hospital, Oxford, UK
(Chapter 14 – Carotid and aortic vessel wall imaging)

Colin Ferrett
Consultant Radiologist
John Radcliffe Hospital, Oxford, UK
(Chapter 17 – Extracardiac findings)

Jane Francis
Chief Technologist
University of Oxford Centre for Clinical Magnetic Resonance Research Oxford, UK
(Chapter 1 – Artefacts, Chapter 2 – Scan setup and optimization, Chapter 3 – Image acquisition and standard views, Chapter 17 – Extracardiac findings)

Matthias Friedrich
Associate Professor, Department of Cardiac Sciences and Radiology
Director, Stephenson Cardiovascular MR Centre, Calgary, Canada
(Chapter 8 – Myocardial inflammation and infiltration, Chapter 11 – Pericardial disease)

Christoph Herborn
Associate Professor of Radiology & Director of MRI
University Medical Center Hamburg-Eppendorf, Germany
(Chapter 14 – Peripheral arteries)

Lucy Hudsmith
Specialist Registrar
John Radcliffe Hospital, Oxford, UK
(Chapter 12 – Congenital heart disease)

Rod Jones
Senior Radiographer
Centre for CMR, UCL Institute of Child Health, London, UK
(Chapter 2 – CMR in young children, General anaesthesia and CMR)

Theodoros Karamitsos
Honorary Consultant Cardiologist
John Radcliffe Hospital, Oxford, UK
(Chapter 3 – Perfusion imaging, Chapter 4 – Image processing, Chapter 6 – Ischaemic heart disease)

Kraig Kissinger
Senior Cardiac MR Technologist
Beth Israel Deaconess Medical Center, Boston, USA
(Chapter 15 – Coronary MRI)

Warren Manning
Section Chief, Non-Invasive Cardiac Imaging
Associate Professor of Medicine & Radiology, Harvard Medical School
Beth Israel Deaconess Medical Center, Boston, USA
(Chapter 15 – Coronary MRI)

Oliver Mohrs
Associate Professor of Radiology
University of Heidelberg, Germany
(Chapter 14 – Peripheral arteries)

Vivek Muthurangu
Senior Clinical Research Fellow
Centre for CMR, UCL Institute of Child Health, London, UK
(Chapter 2 – CMR in young children, General anaesthesia and CMR)

Saul Myerson
Consultant Cardiologist
Honorary Senior Clinical Lecturer, University of Oxford
John Radcliffe Hospital, Oxford, UK
(Chapter 2 – Scan setup and optimization, Chapter 3 – Planning an unusual image plane, Flow imaging, Chapter 4 – Image processing, Chapter 9 – Tumours and masses, Chapter 10 – Valve disease, Chapter 12 – Congenital heart disease, Chapter 13 – Aortic disease, Chapter 16 – Systemic and pulmonary veins)

Stefan Neubauer
Professor of Cardiovascular Medicine
Clinical Director, University of Oxford Centre for Clinical Magnetic Resonance Research, Oxford, UK
(Chapter 6 – Ischaemic heart disease, Chapter 18 – New horizons for CMR)

Wendy Norman
Superintendent Radiographer
Centre for CMR, UCL Institute of Child Health, London, UK
(Chapter 2 – CMR in young children, General anaesthesia and CMR)

Steffen Petersen
Clinical Lecturer in Cardiovascular Medicine
University of Oxford, UK
(Chapter 5 – Ventricular function assessment, Chapter 7 – Inheritable cardiomyopathies)

Matthew Robson
Head of Cardiac MR Physics
University of Oxford Centre for Clinical Magnetic Resonance Research, UK
(Chapter 1 – Understanding CMR)

Jeannette Schulz-Menger
Professor of Cardiology
Franz-Volhard-Klinik, Charité Campus, Berlin Buch, Germany
(Chapter 9 – Tumours and masses)

Oliver Strohm
Deputy-Director,
Stephenson Cardiovascular MR Centre, Calgary, Canada
(Chapter 8 – Myocardial inflammation and infiltration, Chapter 11 – Pericardial disease)

Andrew Taylor
Consultant Radiologist
Centre for CMR, UCL Institute of Child Health, London, UK
(Chapter 2 – CMR in young children, General anaesthesia and CMR)

Sara Thorne
Consultant Cardiologist in Adult Congenital Heart Disease
Queen Elizabeth Hospital, Birmingham, UK
(Chapter 12 – Congenital heart disease)

Damian Tyler
University Research Lecturer
Department of Physiology, Anatomy and Genetics, Oxford, UK
(Chapter 1 – Understanding CMR)

Ralf Wassmuth
Franz-Volhard-Klinik, Charité Campus, Berlin Buch, Germany
(Chapter 9 – Tumours and masses)

Symbols and abbreviations

~	approximately
Δ	differential diagnosis
ω	Larmor frequency
γ	gyromagnetic ratio
→	leading to
📖	reference
↑	increased /increasing
↓	decreased/decreasing
🖱	website
►	important
>>	much greater than
1°	primary
2°	secondary
B_o	main magnetic field
AF	atrial fibrillation
AHA	American Heart Association
Ao	aorta
AoV	aortic valve
AP	anteroposterior
AR	aortic regurgitation
ARVC	arrhythmogenic right ventricular cardiomyopathy
AS	aortic stenosis
ASD	atrial septal defect
ASTM	American Society for Testing and Materials
ATP	adenosine triphosphate
AV	atrioventricular
AVM	arteriovenous malformation
AVSD	atrioventricular septal defect
BFFE	balanced fast field echo
BMD	Becker muscular dystrophy
BMI	body mass index
BOLD	blood oxygenation level dependent
BP	blood pressure
BT	Blalock-Taussig
CAD	coronary artery disease
CBD	common bile duct

ccTGA	congenitally corrected transposition of the great arteries
CE	contrast-enhanced
CE-MRA	contrast-enhanced MR angiography
CHD	congenital heart disease
CMR	cardiovascular magnetic resonance
CNR	contrast-to-noise ratio
COPD	chronic obstructive pulmonary disease
CT	computed tomography
CXR	chest X-ray
DA	descending aorta
DCM	dilated cardiomyopathy
DMD	Duchenne muscular dystrophy
DSA	digital subtraction angiography
DTPA	diethylene-triamine penta-acetate
ECG	electrocardiogram
eGFR	estimated glomerular filtration rate
EPI	echo-planar imaging
FDA	Food and Drug Administration (USA)
FID	free induction decay
FIESTA	fast imaging employing steady state acquisition
True FISP	True fast imaging with steady state precession
FLASH	Fast Low Angle Shot
FMD	fibromuscular dysplasia
FOV	field of view
FT	Fourier transformation
GA	general anaesthesia
Gd	gadolinium
GE	General Electric
GFR	glomerular filtration rate
GRE	gradient echo
HASTE	Half-Fourier Acquisition Single Shot Turbo Spin Echo
HCM	hypertrophic cardiomyopathy
HLA	horizontal long axis
ICD	implantable cardioverter-defibrillator
IHD	ischaemic heart disease
IR	inversion recovery
IV	intravenous
IVC	inferior vena cava
JVP	jugular venous pressure
LA	left atrium

LAA	left atrial appendage
LBBB	left bundle branch block
LAD	left anterior descending
LCx	left circumflex
LGE	late gadolinium enhancement
LLPV	left lower pulmonary vein
LMS	left main stem
LNVC	left ventricular non-compaction
LPA	left pulmonary artery
LSA	left subclavian artery
LUPV	left upper pulmonary vein
LV	left ventricular
LVEDV	left ventricular end diastolic volume
LVH	left ventricular hypertrophy
LVNC	left ventricular non-compaction
LVOT	left ventricular outflow tract
MAPCA	major aorto-pulmonary collateral arteries
MCDT	multi-cystic degeneration of the thyroid
MD	muscular dystrophy
MDRD	modification of diet in renal disease
MI	myocardial infarction
MIP	maximal intensity projection
MR	magnetic resonance
MRA	magnetic resonance angiography
MRCP	magnetic resonance cholangio-pancreatography
MRI	magnetic resonance imaging
MRS	MR spectroscopy
MS	mitral stenosis
MV	mitral valve
NEX	number of acquisitions
NSF	nephrogenic systemic fibrosis
PA	pulmonary artery
PC	phase-contrast
PCr	phosphocreatine
PD	proton density
PDA	patent ductus arteriosus
PEEP	positive end-expiratory pressure
PFO	patent foramen ovale
PNS	peripheral nerve stimulation
PPG	peripheral pulse gating

PR	pulmonary regurgitation
PS	pulmonary stenosis
PSIR	phase sensitive inversion recovery
PV	pulmonary valve
PVOD	peripheral vascular occlusive disease
RA	right atrium
RARE	rapid acquisition relaxation enhancement
RBBB	right bundle branch block
RCA	right coronary artery
RF	radiofrequency
RLPV	right lower pulmonary vein
RPA	right pulmonary artery
RUPV	right upper pulmonary vein
RV	right ventricle
RVOT	right ventricular outflow tract
SA	short axis
SAM	systolic anterior motion
SAR	specific absorption rate
SI	signal intensity
SNR	signal to noise ratio
SPECT	single photon emission computed tomography
SpO_2	O_2 partial pressure
SSFP	steady state free precession
SS-FSE	Single-Shot Fast Spin Echo
SVC	superior vena cava
T1	longitudinal relaxation time
T1-WI	T1-weighted imaging
T2	transverse relaxation time
T2-WI	T2-weighted imaging
TAPVD	total anomalous pulmonary venous drainage
TE	echo time
TGA	transposition of the great arteries
TI	inversion time
TOE	transoesophageal echocardiography
ToF	tetralogy of Fallot
TOF	time-of-flight
TR	repetition time
TR	tricuspid regurgitation
TSE	turbo spin echo
TSR	saturation recovery time

TV	tricuspid valve
UTE	ultrashort echo time
VF	ventricular fibrillation
VLA	vertical long axis
VSD	ventricular septal defect
VT	ventricular tachycardia
WHO	World Health Organization

Chapter 1

Understanding cardiovascular magnetic resonance

The principles of magnetic resonance

Summary: magnetic resonance 'in a nutshell'

Magnetic resonance imaging (MRI) uses hydrogen atoms in the body to generate an image. When hydrogen atoms are placed in a strong magnetic field, they align themselves in the direction of the field. A radiofrequency (RF) pulse ('radio-wave') is then applied, which delivers energy to the atoms and causes some to align in a different direction. When the RF pulse is removed, the atoms return to their resting state, releasing the energy and emitting a signal as they do so. This signal is picked up and turned into an image.

Properties of atomic nuclei

The signal used in MRI is emitted from the protons (hydrogen atoms) of the water and fat molecules in the human body. These protons have the nuclear property of *spin* (in common with the nuclei of other atoms), which causes them to act like tiny bar magnets. When placed in an external magnetic field, these 'spins' either align with the magnetic field (spin up) or against it (spin down).

It takes more energy for a proton to align against the magnetic field than with it, which leads to two groups of spins with different *energy levels*, with more spins in the 'spin up' (low energy) than the 'spin down' state. The difference between energy levels is proportional to the magnetic field strength, but at field strengths and temperatures commonly used for MRI, the difference is small (Fig. 1.1). This small difference in energy levels leads to the low signal generated, which requires sensitive receiver coils and significant amplification to be used to form an image.

The ratio of spins in the two different energy levels is described by the *Boltzmann distribution*, as shown by equation 1:

$$Spin^{up}/Spin^{down} = e^{\Delta E/k_B T} \quad [1]$$

where ΔE is the energy difference between the two levels, k_B is the Boltzmann constant, and T is the temperature.

Precession and the Larmor equation

When spins are placed in a magnetic field, as well as aligning with the field, they rotate (precess) around their own axis and around the magnetic field. This is similar to the motion of a gyroscope as it rotates about its own axis and also around the gravitational field of the earth (Fig. 1.2). The frequency with which spins precess is proportional to the size of the magnetic field and is known as the Larmor frequency (equation 2):

$$\omega = \gamma \cdot B_0 \quad [2]$$

where ω is the Larmor frequency, γ is the gyromagnetic ratio (a nucleus specific constant) and B_0 is the main magnetic field strength. Table 1.1 gives some examples of different nuclei, their gyromagnetic ratios, and their Larmor frequencies at the main clinical field strengths of 1.5 and 3.0T.

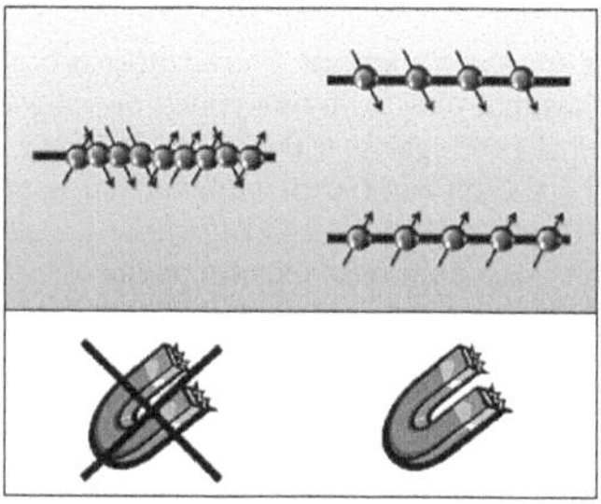

Fig. 1.1 The Boltzmann distribution, demonstrating the distribution of spins in the 'spin up' and 'spin down' states when the sample is placed into a magnetic field. At routinely used magnetic field strengths and physiological temperatures, the difference in the two populations is very small.

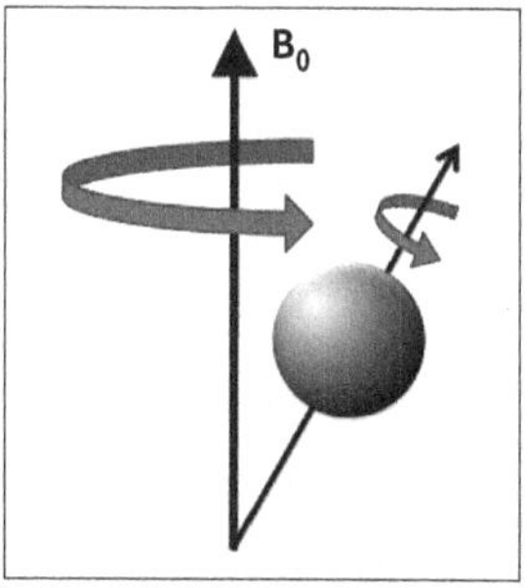

Fig. 1.2 Spin precession: when placed in a magnetic field, spins precess about the applied magnetic field, as well as about their own axis. The frequency of precession is proportional to the magnetic field strength and is described by the Larmor equation.

Table 1.1 MR active nuclei and their Larmor frequencies at the clinical field strengths of 1.5 and 3.0T (to 1 decimal place)

Nuclei	**γ (MHz/T)**	**ω: 1.5T (MHz)**	**ω: 3.0T (MHz)**
Protons (^{1}H)	42.6	63.9	127.7
Carbon (^{13}C)	10.7	16.1	32.1
Sodium (^{23}Na)	11.3	16.9	33.8
Phosphorus (^{31}P)	17.2	25.9	51.7

Magnetization

When all the spins in a sample are considered, their precession around the magnetic field means that they form two cones, one aligned with the magnetic field and one aligned against it (Fig. 1.3). Opposing spins cancel one another out, leaving a small number of 'unpaired' spins precessing around the applied magnetic field. The effect from these unpaired spins can be added together to create a net *magnetization vector*, which is aligned along the direction of the applied magnetic field (Fig. 1.3).

The effect of a radiofrequency pulse

The collection of spins can be 'excited' by the application of a short burst (a pulse) of RF energy, also known as radio-waves. The frequency of the RF pulses must be the same as the Larmor frequency; this is the *resonance* condition of MRI. The effect of RF pulses can be thought of in two ways (Fig. 1.4):

Quantum theory

The energy in the RF pulses allows some of the spins in the lower energy state ('spin up') to move to the higher energy state ('spin down').

Classical theory

The energy in the RF pulses causes the magnetization vector to rotate perpendicularly about the magnetic field. The angle of this rotation will depend on the amplitude and duration of the applied RF pulse (e.g. a 90° or 180° pulse).

Signal generation and 'relaxation'

Following excitation by an RF pulse, the hydrogen atoms try to return back to their original (equilibrium) state, with some of the spins in the 'spin down' orientation reverting to the 'spin up' orientation. This releases some of the energy delivered by the RF pulse, which is emitted as a small signal. After considerable amplification and processing, this signal can be used to form images. The signal, known as the *free induction decay (FID)*, oscillates at the Larmor frequency (Fig. 1.5a – red line) and decays with a characteristic time (Fig. 1.5a – blue line) known as the *transverse relaxation time* or T_2.

Transverse relaxation (the spin-spin relaxation time)

The T_2 time is a fundamental property of the tissue. However, the signal will decay at a faster rate if the magnetic field is not constant (homogeneous) over the sample. This faster decay time (Fig. 1.5b) is called T_2^* and it can be lengthened by improving the homogeneity of the magnetic field using a process called shimming.

Longitudinal relaxation (the spin-lattice relaxation time)

The recovery of the magnetization vector back to its original position also occurs with a characteristic time, known as the *longitudinal relaxation time* (T_1). An example of the pattern of this recovery following a 180° pulse is shown in Fig. 1.5b.

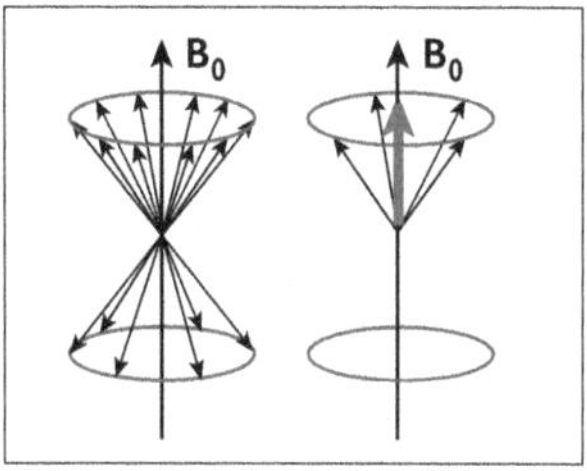

Fig. 1.3 The precession of spins forms two cones around the applied magnetic field. Cancellation of opposing spins leaves a small number of 'unpaired' spins, which creates a net magnetization vector aligned with the magnetic field (purple arrow).

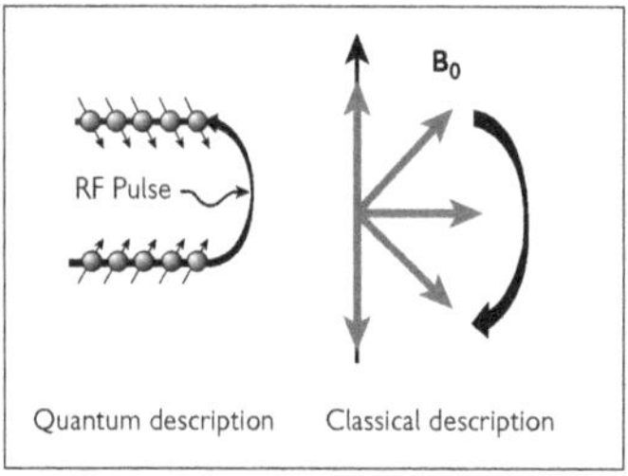

Fig. 1.4 RF pulse energy effects. *Quantum description* allows spins in the lower energy state ('spin up') to attain the higher energy state ('spin down'). *Classical description* causes the magnetization vector to rotate perpendicularly about the magnetic field. This example shows a 180° rotation.

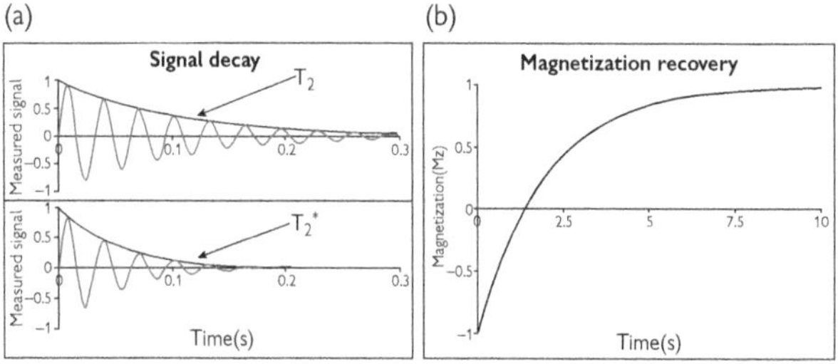

Fig. 1.5 (a) *Top*: the measured signal (purple line) oscillates at the Larmor frequency and decays with a characteristic time, T_2 (blue line). *Bottom*: due to variations in the magnetic field, the decay is faster than it should be and decays with a time, T_2^*. (b) The longitudinal relaxation time, T_1, describes the recovery of the magnetization following a 180° pulse. All relaxation processes have an exponential form.

Components of a scanner

Magnet

To obtain magnetic field strengths high enough for MRI, a superconducting magnet is needed, which requires cooling the wires in the magnet to extremely low temperatures (–269°C) using liquid helium. These wires are wound in rings, with computer-optimized distributions to maximize field uniformity and minimize fringe fields. Once in service, the magnet is always 'on', i.e. at full field strength, even when the scanning console is switched off or during a power-cut.

Cryocooler/compressor

To keep the helium cold and liquid it is continually chilled with a compressor (the 'chiller'), which makes a 'thumping' noise. This reduces helium consumption (and the need to top-up), in some cases to zero.

Magnetic resonance gradient system

The gradient system is vital for spatial differentiation. Gradients in the magnetic field are required to image the patient and these gradients are generated in three orthogonal directions. Rapid switching of the gradients (~100μs) is also needed to achieve the best image quality within practical breath-holds. There are two components:

- ***Gradient coil***: lies concentrically within the magnet bore (Fig. 1.6). It is the source of the noise and vibration of the MRI system. Generally, these are water cooled.
- ***Gradient amplifiers***: sit outside, in the equipment room. Drive the current through the gradient coils (100s of amps, with high voltages ~2kV).

Radiofrequency system

- ***RF transmit coil:*** used to excite the nuclei. Generally, and for all cardiac examinations, this is built into the bore-tube and is not visible. Locally there are large electric fields around these coils, which can be the source of RF burns if metallic objects are placed within the bore.
- ***RF amplifier:*** sited in the equipment room; drives the RF transmit coil.
- ***RF receiver coils:*** receive the signal from the patient and are critical to high quality scanning. For the best signal, these should be close to the area being scanned. Coil selection is also important as a coil with elements that are too large will have low signal to noise, a coil that is too small will not 'see' very far into the patient. Phased-array coils overcome this compromise – these consist of several small coils that are operated together, but that receive signals independently. For most cardiac applications they have become the standard.

Patient bed

This allows the patient to be positioned precisely in the centre of the MRI system. Moving the patient so that the region of interest is exactly in the centre will yield the best image quality, and some systems move the table during an examination to increase body coverage (up to whole body scanning).

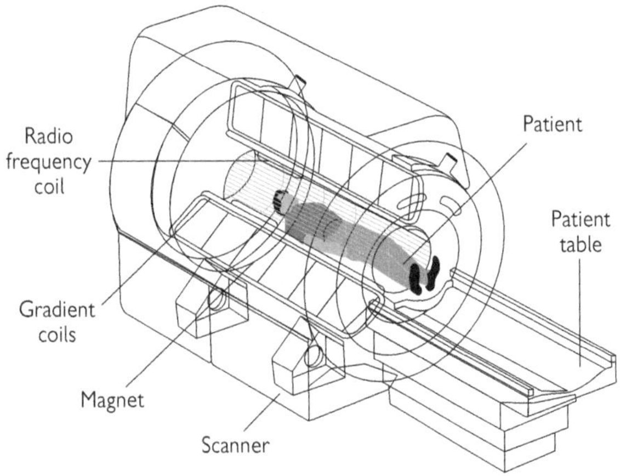

Fig. 1.6 Cut away diagram of the components of a scanner.

Image generation

Summary of the process

To generate an image:

- The hydrogen nuclei in a particular image slice are excited by a RF pulse.
- The signal from the spins in the slice is extracted.
- Repeated excitations are usually required to obtain data from the whole slice.
- The signal data are processed and turned into an image.

Exciting a single region of interest

To generate an image, it is necessary to identify the signal from each point in the image. If all the hydrogen nuclei in the body were 'excited' at the same time, the signal produced would be impossible to localize to one area. Therefore, only one 'slice' or thin 'slab' is usually excited at a time. To achieve this, the magnetic field needs to be subtly altered to allow the excitation to be applied selectively:

Magnetic field gradients

Magnetic field gradients, created by the gradient coils, are superimposed on the main magnetic field and vary the magnetic field in different directions (Fig. 1.7). There are three different gradient coils:

- The 'Z' gradient varies the magnetic field along the bore of the magnet.
- The 'X' gradient varies the magnetic field across the bore.
- The 'Y' gradient varies the magnetic field up and down in the bore.

Slice selection

To excite only the spins in the slice (or volume in 3D imaging) of interest, a magnetic field gradient is applied at the same time as the RF pulse, which excites the spins.

- The gradient, applied perpendicularly to the slice of interest, changes the magnetic field along the direction of the gradient (Fig. 1.8).
- As the frequency of precession is proportional to the magnetic field strength (the Larmor equation) the Larmor frequency of the spins increases as the magnetic field increases along the gradient.
- The applied RF pulse is designed to contain only the small range of frequencies (i.e. it has a narrow bandwidth) that are found within the slice of interest. This is achieved by changing the shape and length of the RF pulse.
- The combination of the gradient and the limited frequencies in the RF pulse means that only the spins in the slice of interest are excited and contribute to the image produced. The spins outside the image slice are not excited and so do not produce any signal.

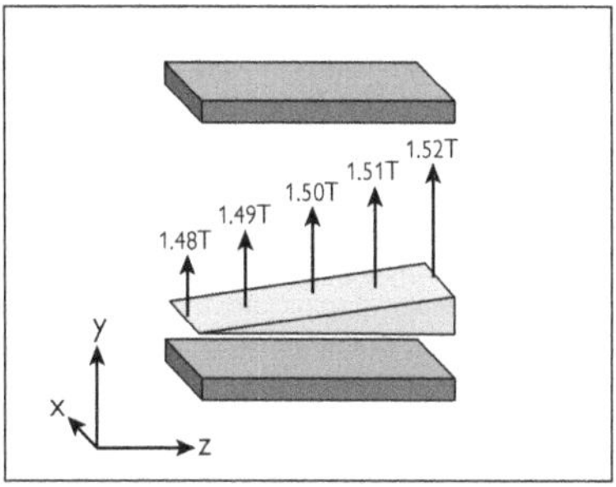

Fig. 1.7 Magnetic field gradients yield different field strengths and, hence, resonant frequencies along the sample.

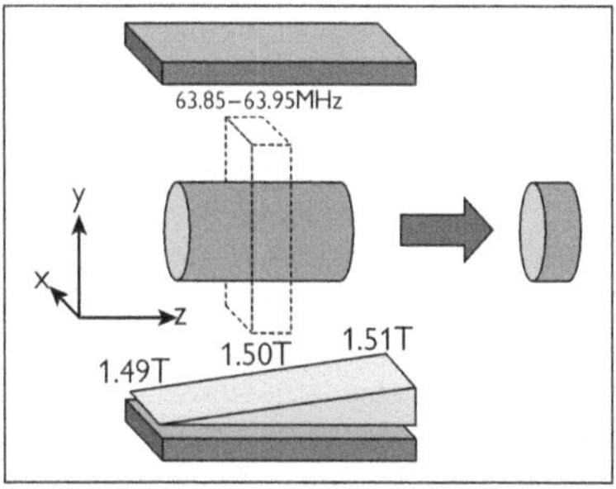

Fig. 1.8 Slice selection using an RF pulse with a frequency centred at 63.90MHz and a bandwidth of 0.1MHz.

Extracting the signal from the image slice

Following excitation of the spins, several steps are necessary to identify their position within the slice. The signals emitted have a frequency and phase, and these can be used for localization:

Frequency encoding

Used to localize the position in one direction/axis of the image slice. The frequency encoding magnetic field gradient is turned on just before the signal is acquired. As the frequency of spins (and thus the signal) is determined by the magnetic field at each point, applying a gradient alters the signal frequency, depending on the position of the spin within the image slice.

Phase encoding

Used to localize the signal in the other direction of the image. A third, phase encoding series of gradients are applied before the frequency encoding gradients. Rather than changing the frequency of the signal, the phase of the signal is altered and this too depends on the position of spins in the image. A series of acquisitions, each with a different phase encoding gradient, are therefore used to encode the image in the second dimension.

Repeated signal acquisitions

The above steps are repeated multiple times with different magnetic gradients to generate a series of signals forming the whole image, usually over several cardiac cycles. Several excitations are usually required and a short delay is required between each to allow the spins to return to their equilibrium state before re-excitation. The time between successive excitations is called the *repetition time*, or TR for short.

Generating images from the signal data

Fourier transformation

The complex signal produced contains many frequencies and phases, and a sophisticated mathematical process is required to extract the individual components and create an image. This process is called Fourier transformation (FT, Fig. 1.9), named after the mathematician who first described the mathematical model.

K-space

The collected data is put into a grid (called a *matrix*), known as K-space. For a single image, the matrix is a 2D grid, which undergoes a 2D Fourier transform to generate the final image (Fig. 1.10).

- The data in the centre of K-space generates the main contrast in the image. If only the centre of K-space data is acquired, the image formed is high in signal, but of low resolution (blurred).
- The data at the edge of K-space generates the structure and edges in the image. If only the edge of K-space data is acquired, the image is low in signal, but shows the fine detail (high resolution).

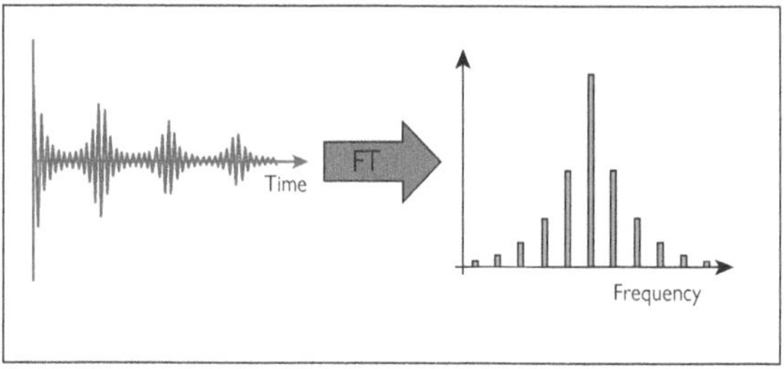

Fig. 1.9 Fourier transformation, showing an example of free induction decay, which has been Fourier transformed to reveal the different frequencies contained within it.

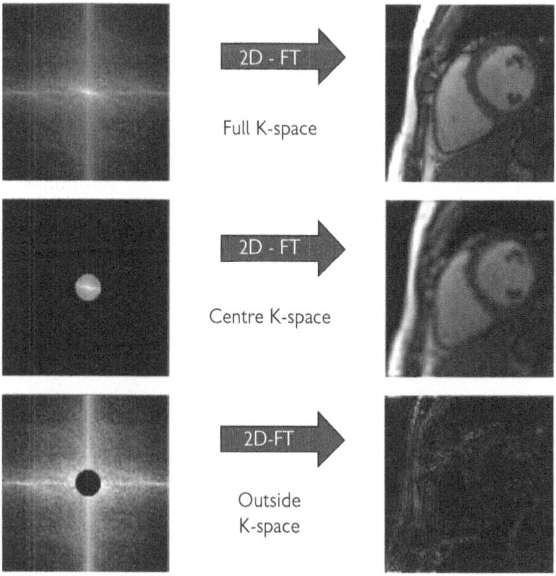

Fig. 1.10 K-space representation (left), showing an image produced from the whole of K-space (top). If only the centre of K-space is used for image generation, the image has high contrast, but is blurred (middle). If only the periphery of K-space is used, the image is sharp, but lacks contrast (bottom).

Other aspects of image generation

Image 'sequences'

There are, in fact, many possible ways of controlling the above sequence of events, with different timings, radiofrequency pulses, and gradients, to generate different types of image. Each image 'recipe' (producing a particular type of image) is programmed into the scanner and is termed a '*sequence*'. A typical imaging session may use several different sequences, depending on the type of images required.

Imaging time

Although generating an image involves many complex processes, the time taken can be relatively short (<1 second in some cases) as the processes are highly computerized. Higher quality images, and those with multiple images (e.g. cine imaging) take longer to acquire (e.g. 8–12s for a standard cine sequence).

Image resolution

Image resolution is limited by the signal produced from a single region of interest. Although, in theory, by applying a strong enough gradient, very small points might be imaged individually, the signal generated from such a small area of tissue would not be strong enough to generate a useful image. For this reason, each image 'slice' is, in fact, a thin 3D slab of typically 5–7mm thickness. This creates voxels, or 3D pixels, each the depth of the slab and with an in-plane resolution dependent on the sequence used and parameters chosen, but typically 1–2mm square (Fig. 1.11).

This means that the voxels of an image have a certain volume and are usually a few millimetres deep. If a voxel contains two or more tissue types within it, an average of all the signals is obtained, creating blurring between boundaries or *partial volume effects* in the image as a whole (Fig. 1.11).

The noise of a scanner

Imaging requires rapid switching of the gradients for image generation and optimal image quality, and this generates the noise of an MR scanner. The gradient coils themselves distort slightly as current pulses through them, which creates a noise (in the same way as a loudspeaker). The switching occurs typically several hundred times a second, generating the noise. The pitch and volume vary depending on the sequence used.

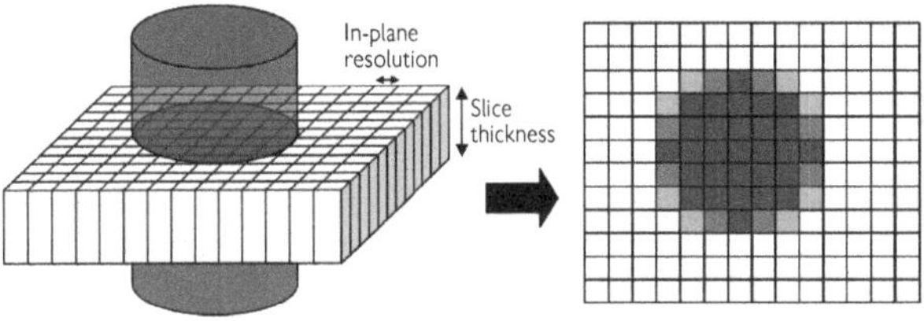

Fig. 1.11 Representation of an image slice through a vessel, demonstrating the multiple voxels contained within it (left) and the resultant image (right). Voxels that contain only part of the vessel within them have an intensity that represents an average of all the tissue signals within the voxel, in this case, a lighter grey colour.

Magnetic field around a scanner

Effect of distance

The strong magnetic fields used in MRI scanners generate safety issues from:

- Movement, especially twisting, can cause damage or failure of medical implants. Pacemakers and programmable stimulators are sensitive to very low magnetic fields.
- Metal objects (e.g. wheelchairs, crutches, scissors, oxygen cylinders) can be drawn towards the scanner by the magnetic field, causing injury to patients or operators who are inside or near the scanner.

Scanners are therefore designed with the magnetic field outside the scanner as small as possible, while keeping the magnetic field in the centre of the bore as strong as possible. This 'shielding' of the magnetic field outside the scanner means that the magnetic field drops off very quickly as you move away from the scanner. It is therefore very important to ensure that patients with incompatible implants or loose metal objects are not allowed near the scanner. A typical MR department warning sign is shown in Fig. 1.12.

Importance of a homogeneous field

It is very important that the magnetic field in the scanner is as constant (spatially and temporally homogeneous) as possible. This is because variations in the magnetic field cause the spins in different positions to precess at different frequencies, just like with frequency encoding. This causes the spins to *dephase*, reducing the signal level and also reducing the accuracy of the image localization, blurring the image.

Inhomogeneities in the magnetic field occur when a patient enters the magnet. These are overcome by 'shimming', where a set of coils, similar to the gradient coils, are used to modify the magnetic field in different directions, minimizing the variations. Shimming is particularly difficult in the heart because of cardiac motion, blood flow, and the strong inhomogeneities caused by the air-tissue interface around the heart from the lungs.

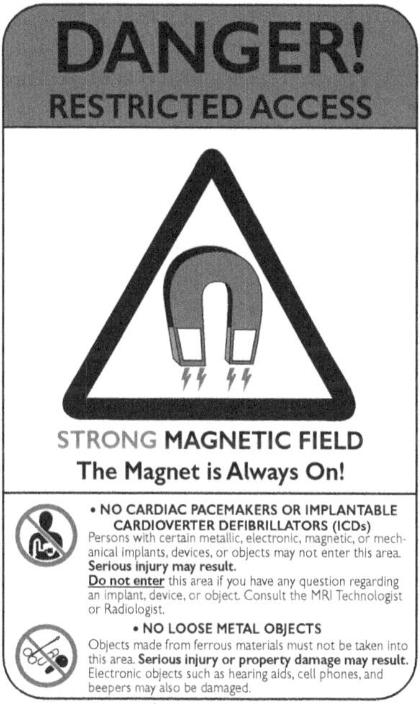
DANGER!
RESTRICTED ACCESS
STRONG MAGNETIC FIELD
The Magnet is Always On!
• NO CARDIAC PACEMAKERS OR IMPLANTABLE CARDIOVERTER DEFIBRILLATORS (ICDs)
Persons with certain metallic, electronic, magnetic, or mechanical implants, devices, or objects may not enter this area.
Serious injury may result.
Do not enter this area if you have any question regarding an implant, device, or object. Consult the MRI Technologist or Radiologist.
• NO LOOSE METAL OBJECTS
Objects made from ferrous materials must not be taken into this area. Serious injury or property damage may result.
Electronic objects such as hearing aids, cell phones, and beepers may also be damaged.

Fig. 1.12 A typical warning sign in an MR department.

Technical challenges of cardiac imaging

Cardiac magnetic resonance (CMR) has to overcome inherent difficulties due to the motion and the position of the heart in the thorax.

Motion

The rapid motion of the heart and the abdominal movement from breathing create difficulties in localizing the signals for cardiac imaging. To generate clear images free from blurring or motion artefacts, it is necessary to 'freeze' this motion, whilst the images are acquired. This is achieved by a combination of techniques:

- Respiratory motion is overcome by holding the breath or using 'navigator' sequences to limit acquisitions to certain periods of the respiratory cycle.
- Cardiac motion is 'frozen' by gating image acquisition to specific parts of the cardiac cycle, usually using the electrocardiogram (ECG) signal (Fig. 1.13).

The effects of motion are further reduced by acquiring images very quickly. Improvements in scanners, such as faster gradients and the development of rapid imaging techniques, such as parallel imaging, all help to reduce the effects of motion and improve image quality.

Many cardiac sequences involve 'cine' imaging to capture the cardiac motion. Regional and global function are important clinical assessments.

Variable planes

The variable orientation of the heart within the chest makes localization of the images unpredictable. Standard imaging planes relative to the whole body (transverse, sagittal, coronal) can be acquired, but the majority of cardiac images use the cardiac axes, which need to be identified in each individual patient.

Nevertheless, the power of MRI to create images at any angle means that views of the heart, which are difficult or impossible to achieve with other techniques can be acquired.

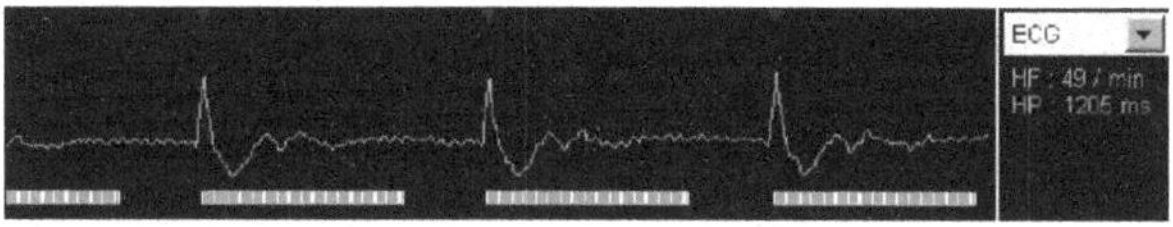

Fig. 1.13 Example of an ECG triggered sequence. The light bars on the ECG (top) represent imaging during the first three-quarters of each cardiac cycle. The resultant frames of the cine are shown below, from end-diastole to end-systole and back again.

Types of cardiac imaging

Cardiac imaging fits into two distinct groups:

'Static' images

Acquired at a single part of the cardiac cycle, which use the contrast in the image to diagnose disease.

'Cine' sequences

Involving a series of images acquired through the cardiac cycle to record cardiac motion or blood flow.

Static magnetic resonance sequences

Static images are useful for visualizing different tissues in the field of interest. They rely on the different signal received from different tissues to generate a 'contrast' between tissue types.

Tissue contrast

The magnetic resonance characteristics of protons varies between tissues, depending on the configuration of the atoms within the tissue. These inherent differences can be exploited to generate differing signal from separate tissues, which is central to static imaging. The following are important magnetic resonance characteristics utilized in static imaging.

T_1: the spin-lattice relaxation time

The spin-lattice relaxation time is determined by how rapidly protons can re-equilibrate their spins with their environment. In fat, for example, the T_1 is very short (~200ms), while in free water the T_1 is very long (>2s). By imaging with short repetition times and a large change in the net magnetization vector (flip-angle), we can emphasize the effects of T_1 with suppression of signal from tissues with a long T_1 (e.g. the water in blood). In this way, water appears dark (low signal), while fat appears bright (high signal).

Methods, which emphasize T_1 differences include:

- T_1-weighted fast-spin-echo, with a short repetition time, or TR.
- Saturation recovery.
- Inversion recovery.

T_2: the spin-spin relaxation time

The spin-spin relaxation time is determined by how rapidly the signal decays after an RF excitation pulse. For structures where water is bound tightly to large molecules (e.g. collagen), this can be incredibly short (0.4ms), and when the water is free (e.g. cerebrospinal fluid) it is very long (>100ms). By waiting a long time between excitation and acquisition (the echo time, or TE) we emphasize tissues with a long T_2 (see Fig. 1.14).

Methods that emphasize T_2 differences include:

- T_2-weighted fast-spin-echo, with a long echo time, or TE.
- T_2-prepared sequences (such as T_2-prepared SSFP).

T_2*(T_2 'star'): spin dephasing

The rate of spin dephasing is characterized by the T_2^*. The total signal from a *region* decays with time because it contains spins with different resonant frequencies, owing to significant differences in the magnetic field within the voxel, and is not a characteristic of an individual spin.

- T_2^* is short in environments that are high in iron (which is highly ferromagnetic and hence has large magnetic field variations in its vicinity). T_2^* imaging therefore finds a clinical role in the imaging of iron-overload, and experimentally in blood oxygenation measurements.
- Methods that emphasize T_2^* use gradient echo sequences with a long TE (often using a range of TEs to quantify this parameter).

Echo time

The time between excitation of the protons and acquisition of the data is called the echo time, or TE for short. In a spin-echo or fast spin-echo sequence long TE (>50ms) will lead to T_2-weighting of an image. In a gradient echo long TE (>10ms) will lead to T_2^* weighting of an image.

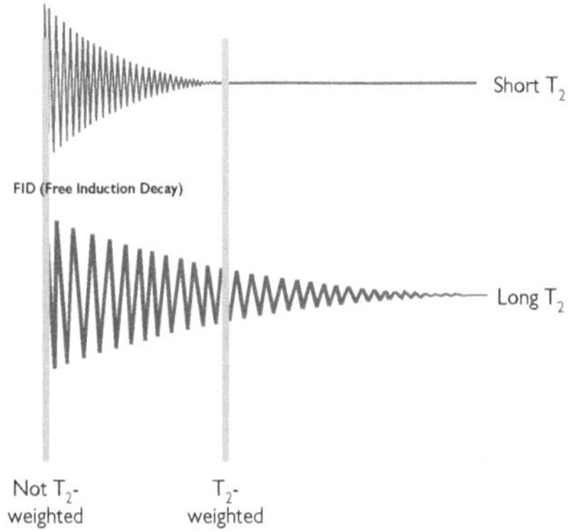

Fig. 1.14 The decay of signal with short and long T_2: by selecting a long TE we can be sensitive to the T_2 decay (T_2 weighted) or by choosing a short TE, insensitive to this decay. Vertical grey bars indicate timing of acquisition.

Spin echo acquisition

- This approach yields high quality images at a single time point in the cardiac cycle, and is often combined with dark-blood preparation pulses to minimize the signal from blood, and provide high quality images of the myocardium or vascular wall (Fig. 1.15).
- Spin echo uses an additional RF pulse that rephases the spins, and reduces signal loss due to spin dephasing (T_2*).
- Spin-echo sequences take a long time to acquire, and most cardiac imaging uses fast-spin-echo or turbo-spin-echo methods, involving a rapid series of these pulses, to shorten the scan enough to be acquired in a single breath-hold.
- A transverse stack of images through the torso can also be collected without breath-holding using a single-shot Fast Spin Echo method to yield a quick examination of the gross anatomy. The sequence is termed Half-Fourier Acquisition Single Shot Turbo Spin Echo (HASTE), or Single-Shot Fast Spin Echo (SS-FSE).

Inversion recovery

This sequence exploits the differing T_1 relaxation properties of tissues. An RF pulse is applied to invert the magnetization of the spins, which then return to their equilibrium state at rates dependent on their T_1. Imaging before the spins have completely 'recovered' to their equilibrium state can emphasize the differences in T_1 relaxation. The time between the inversion pulse and image acquisition is the *inversion time*, or TI.

Late enhancement imaging following gadolinium contrast

- Utilizes the T_1-dependent inversion recovery technique, combined with gadolinium contrast, which significantly shortens the T_1.
- Gadolinium, being a small molecule, is able to penetrate the interstitial space in the myocardium, although normally this is a tiny proportion of the myocardial tissue and would be difficult to detect with CMR. In certain conditions, however, the interstitial space is expanded (e.g. inflammation, infiltration, or the breakdown of cell membranes following infarction), and enough gadolinium is present to be detected.
- Gadolinium 'washes out' of the capillary bed in tissues quickly (within minutes), but takes longer to enter and wash out from the interstitial space (10–30min). This creates a 'window of opportunity' to image the gadolinium and exploit the difference with normal myocardium, from which the gadolinium has 'washed out'.
- The sequence is optimized to highlight gadolinium in the interstitial space. When spins return from their inverted magnetization to their equilibrium state, they pass through a point when the net magnetization vector (and thus the signal) is zero, the timing of which depends on the T_1. An inversion time is chosen at the zero, or 'null', point for normal myocardium, which appears black due to low signal. If significant amounts of gadolinium are present within an expanded interstitium, this appears much brighter, due to the greatly different T_1. and is sometimes described as 'hyper-enhancement' (Figs 1.16–1.17).

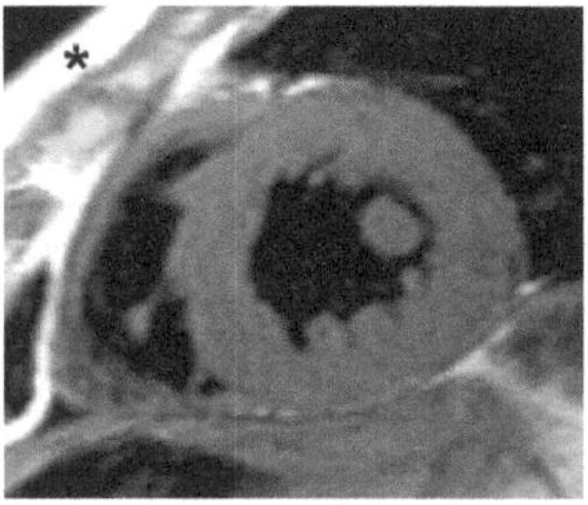

Fig. 1.15 T_1-weighted turbo spin-echo image with black-blood preparation, in the mid-ventricular short axis plane. Note the extremely low signal (black) of the blood pool, the intermediate signal (mid-grey) of the myocardium and the very high signal (white) of the subcutaneous fat (asterisk).

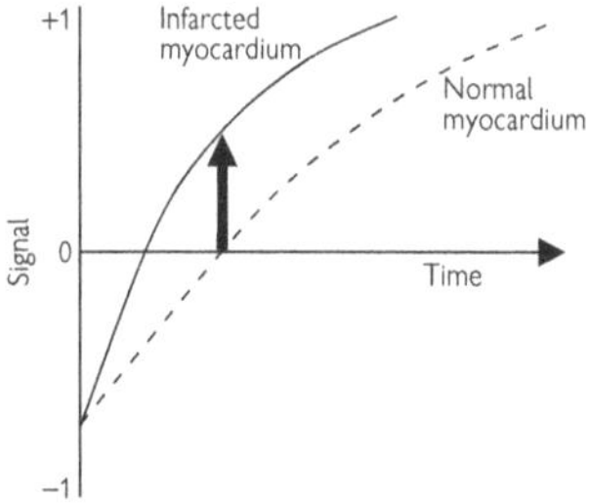

Fig. 1.16 Signal differences in late enhancement inversion recovery imaging. Tissues with a shorter T_1 (e.g. containing gadolinium) have a faster recovery time. At 10min post-contrast injection, infarcted tissue contains gadolinium, while it has 'washed out' from normal myocardium. If an inversion time is chosen to coincide with the signal from normal myocardium passing the point of zero signal (the 'null' point), signal from gadolinium-containing tissue (in this case infarcted myocardium) has a very much higher signal than normal myocardium (arrowed).

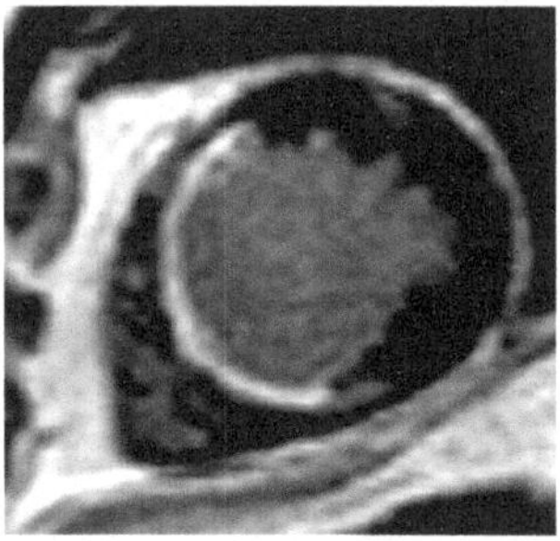

Fig. 1.17 Late enhancement image following gadolinium in the mid-ventricular short axis plane, showing a septal myocardial infarction. Note the dark (nulled) myocardium, the bright (enhanced) infarcted sections of the septum, and the mid-grey blood pool.

Saturation recovery

By applying a specific RF pulse followed by a 'crusher' gradient any net magnetization from the system can be completely obliterated. Recovery of signal is T_1-dependent, so if imaging occurs a short time afterwards, tissues with short T_1 will be emphasized (see Fig. 1.18). This approach is similar to inversion recovery, but has the advantage of speed, as the saturation recovery time (T_{SR}) can be very short and, thus, it can be used for first pass perfusion imaging (Fig. 1.19).

Fat-saturation

Fat yields high signal in CMR, but can obscure tissues of interest. The signal from fat can be suppressed, however, by first applying an excitation pulse at the frequency of fat resonance, which is sufficiently different from water resonance to affect the water signal only slightly. The fat signal is effectively saturated, making it 'invisible' before the image excitation pulse is applied. Fat-suppression requires good uniformity of the magnetic field (i.e. good shimming) to correctly suppress the fat without affecting the water.

Dark-blood preparation

It is often useful to see tissues without the signal from blood. Imaging the vessel wall is one example where having 'dark' blood emphasizes the lumen-wall boundary (e.g. plaque imaging). It is also useful for emphasizing the blood-myocardium boundary with the *F*ast *L*ow *A*ngle *SH*ot (FLASH) sequence (especially at 3T). The method relies on flowing blood.

- Two inversion pulses are used. One is slice selective and the other inverts the whole sample.
- After the initial RF pulses, magnetization everywhere outside the slice is inverted, but the magnetization in the slice is untouched.
- During the ~500ms inversion time, blood in the slice (which is not inverted) flows out of the slice, and is replaced by blood that was inverted.
- At the end of the inversion time, the magnetization of the 'new' blood that has flowed into the slice has relaxed to the 'null' point of the inversion recovery sequence and, therefore, appears dark in the images. The static tissue (vessel wall) is always in the slice and, hence, was not inverted and appears bright (high signal). We are fortunate that the time from inversion to recovery to the 'null' point for blood means that when we can gate from the R-wave and acquire data in the late-diastolic period we obtain good suppression of the blood.

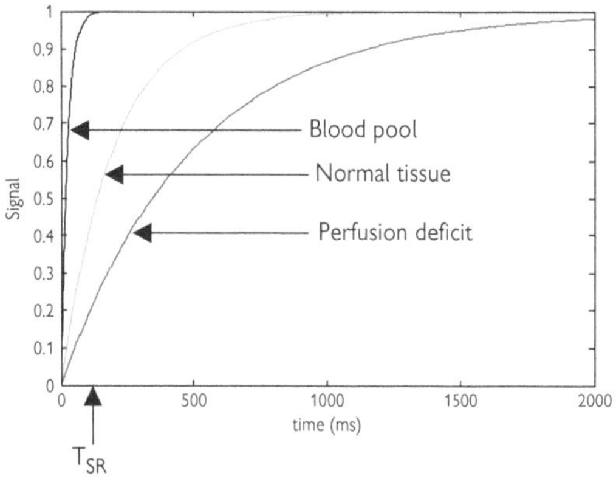

Fig. 1.18 Saturation recovery. Signal recovery curves after a saturation pulse are demonstrated. In a perfusion study, contrast agent concentrations are very high in blood (hence the rapid recovery of the signal). The contrast agent concentrations in the perfusion deficit will be lower than in the normal tissue resulting in longer T_1 and, hence, reduced signal intensity when we acquire images at the point T_{SR}.

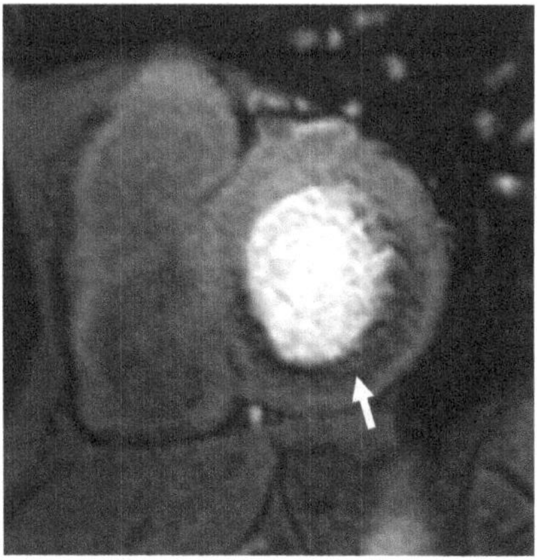

Fig. 1.19 Short axis image during first-pass perfusion of gadolinium through the myocardium, using a saturation recovery technique. The blood pool appears bright, with the normal myocardium mid-grey, and there is a large inferior perfusion defect, which appears dark due to the lower amounts of gadolinium in this ischaemic region (arrowed).

Cine imaging

- 'Cine' sequences involve imaging at different points through the cardiac cycle. These images are put together into a movie that shows the motion of the heart throughout the cycle. Valuable structural and functional information can be obtained in this way.
- Most sequences are acquired over several cardiac cycles and the data combined to form the movie.

Imaging sequences

The two different imaging sequences generally used for cine imaging are detailed below, with examples shown in Fig. 1.20.

Steady state free precession

The steady state free precession (SSFP) technique provides images with a very high signal to noise ratio (SNR), and a high level of contrast between the myocardium and the blood. The high SNR level is achieved by reusing the magnetization from one acquisition to the next. Consequently, it is a technically challenging sequence and can be prone to artefacts caused by field inhomogeneities (regions where the magnetic field is not constant). Table 1.2 details the manufacturers' brand names used for the SSFP sequence.

Fast low angle shot

This sequence uses a short repetition time (TR) to generate images quickly. The signal from the myocardium is low (dark) as the magnetization has no time to recover in between the pulses. The blood signal is high (bright) as the blood is constantly flowing into the imaging slice and is, therefore, unaffected by previous RF pulses. FLASH images suffer from poor contrast at the border between the myocardium and blood pool due to the slower motion of blood at the endocardial surface. It can also be affected by motion artefacts (turbulence) in blood, which appears dark from the dephasing of spins, although this can be advantageous in imaging valvular regurgitation or small shunts.

Speeding up the acquisition

The time needed to produce cine images can be reduced in a variety of ways, allowing shorter breath-hold times.

Shared phases

Some redundancy in the acquired data is utilized so that image data is shared between adjacent images in the cardiac cycle.

Parallel imaging

Spatial information from an array of receiver coils is acquired in parallel, reducing the amount of data from each coil and speeding up the acquisition. Complex algorithms are used to combine the data from the different coils allowing the images to be reconstructed. See Table 1.3 for the brand names.

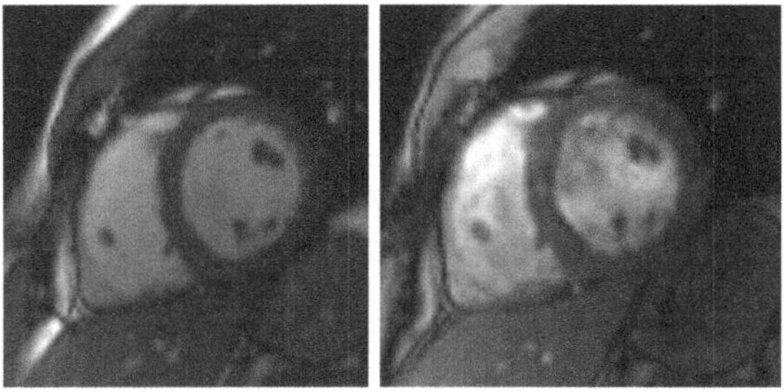

Fig. 1.20 Cine imaging. SSFP sequence (left); FLASH image (right).

Table 1.2 Manufacturer names for steady state free precession (SSFP)

Manufacturer	Acronym	Full name
Siemens	True-FISP	True fast imaging with steady state precession
General Electric (GE)	FIESTA	Fast imaging employing steady state acquisition
Philips	BFFE	Balanced fast field echo

Table 1.3 Parallel imaging techniques

Manufacturer	Acronym	Full Name
Generic	SENSE (image reconstruction)	Sensitivity encoding
	SMASH (k-space reconstruction)	Simultaneous acquisition of spatial harmonics
Siemens	iPAT (parallel imaging package)	Integrated parallel acquisition techniques
	mSENSE (image reconstruction)	Modified sensitivity encoding
	GRAPPA (k-space reconstruction)	Generalized autocalibrating partially parallel acquisition
General Electric (GE)	ASSET	Array spatial sensitivity encoding technique
Philips	SENSE	Sensitivity encoding

Artefacts

CMR artefacts are many and varied. The most common are listed below.

Susceptibility artefact

- Due to metallic objects (Fig. 1.21).
- All signal from a limited area is destroyed, due to interference with the magnetic field.
- The area affected is variable, and dependent on the size and type of metal object and the sequence used. Some sequences are more/less sensitive. Imaging of the object and the immediate area remains a significant limitation of MRI.

Signal-to-noise ratio artefact

- Significantly reduced SNR, usually due to imaging with the wrong coil (Figs 1.22 and 1.23).
- Can be caused by leaving the magnet room door open. In this case, additional noise can be seen in the image (sometimes yielding discrete streak artefacts).

Field of view artefact

Due to the field of view (FOV) being too small. This results in signal from peripheral parts of the body wrapping into the image. Either the FOV can be increased, or the slice rotated to include all the image (Fig. 1.24).

If it is important to retain the same imaging parameters, it may be possible to increase the FOV, but also to increase the parallel imaging acceleration factor (SENSE factor) to reduce the acquisition time enough for a single breath-hold.

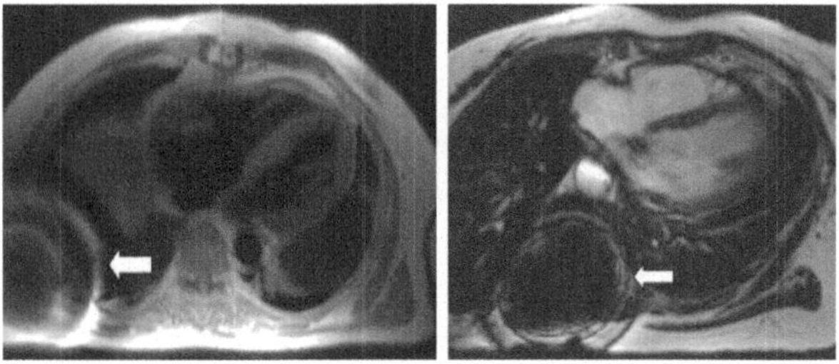

Fig. 1.21 Spin echo image (left) of a patient with a retained metal object in the subcutaneous tissue of the right lateral chest wall. SSFP image (right) of a patient with a metallic Harrington rod in the spine. Note the large artefact (arrowed) with destruction of image data from the inhomogenous field.

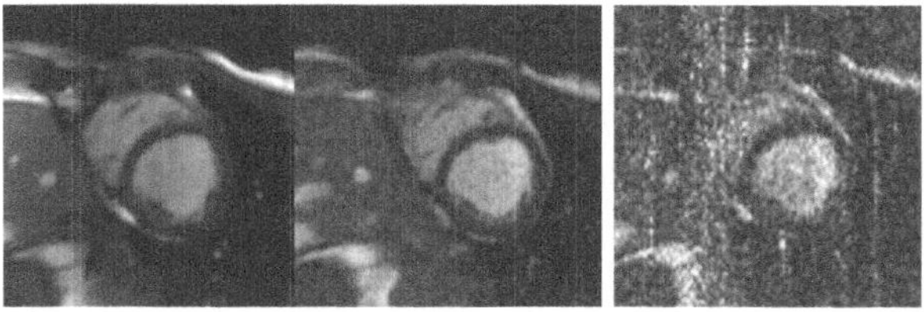

Fig. 1.22 SNR artefact: short axis SSFP images demonstrating optimal acquisition (left), and the poor image quality from lower SNR when only the integrated body coil is used (centre), or the door is left open (right, with streak artefact).

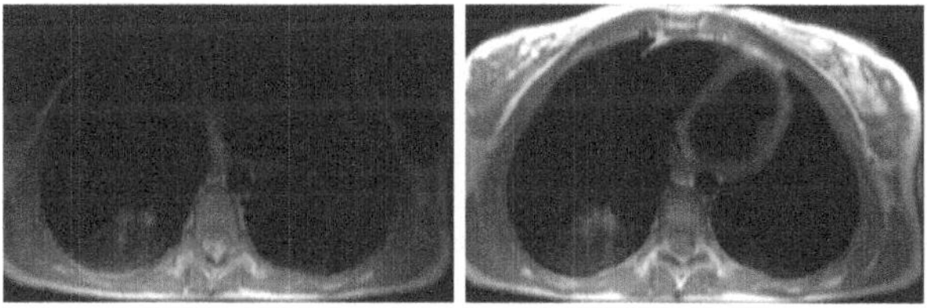

Fig. 1.23 The image on the left is acquired without the anterior coils switched on. The full image is shown on the right.

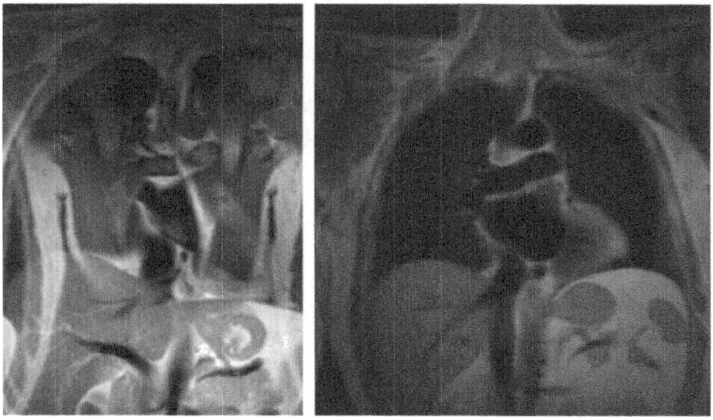

Fig. 1.24 Coronal image with 'wrap' (left) due to inappropriately small field of view in the phase direction. The same image (right) with correct field of view.

Motion artefact (breathing)

Breathing motion during image acquisition causes different sections of the image to fail to register correctly with each other.

Reacquire the data with a better breath-hold, or if that isn't possible, change to a real-time acquisition. Note the repeating pattern from the chest wall in Fig. 1.25

Parallel imaging artefact

Note the similarity of this artefact (Fig. 1.26) to the motion artefact. The difference is the spacing: in this case the distance between patterns will be the FOV divided by the acceleration factor. In the motion artefact, it will be the FOV divided by the number of heart-beats in the breath-hold.

To remove this, either decrease the acceleration factor or space the coils slightly away from the patient.

Gating artefact

Cardiac gating is essential for good quality CMR. Poor gating is often noticed during the acquisition (shown on monitoring equipment or non-uniform sounds from the gradient system; see Fig. 1.27).

Reacquiring the image with better gating is the only solution here (📖 p.46). Real-time non-gated acquisition methods can be used, but the image quality is inferior.

Steady state free precession artefact ('off-resonance' artefact)

SSFP has a characteristic artefact (Fig. 1.28), consisting of a dark line which can move during the cardiac cycle. It is a fundamental feature of this sequence, occurring when the magnetic field is not sufficiently uniform. It occurs more commonly at 3T, but has been shown at 1.5T, particularly in the right ventricle (RV) if there is a large amount of adjacent air in bowel loops. Solutions include:

- Shimming (to improve the magnetic uniformity in this region).
- Manually adjusting the frequency (to move this boundary to a region where it isn't detrimental).
- Using a different sequence (i.e. FLASH instead of SSFP).

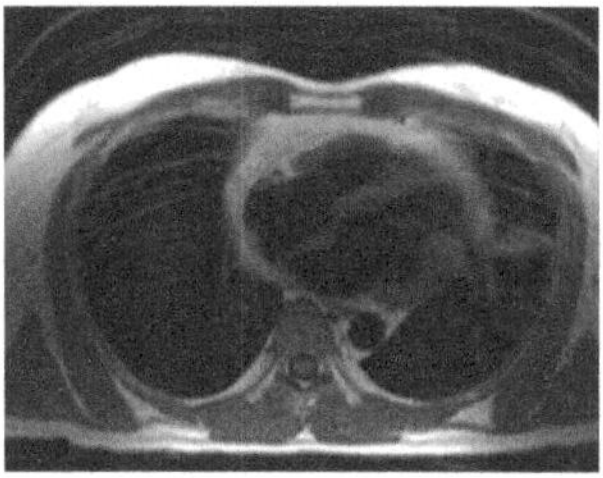

Fig. 1.25 Breathing artefact. Turbo spin-echo image showing the typical repeating chest wall pattern.

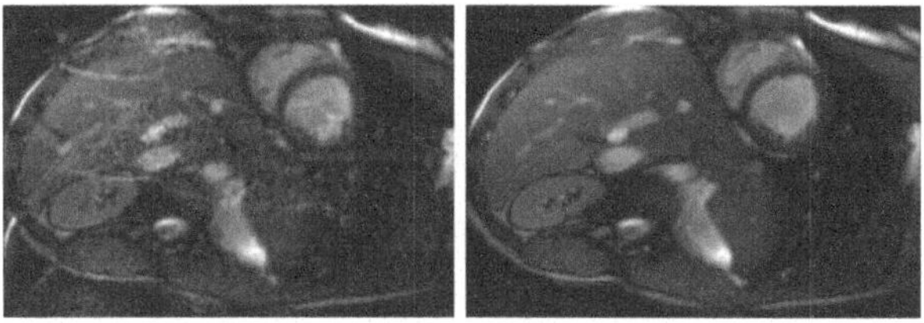

Fig. 1.26 Parallel imaging artefact. The image on the left has been acquired with an acceleration factor of 4, resulting in a repetitive artefact at a spacing of one-quarter of the FOV.

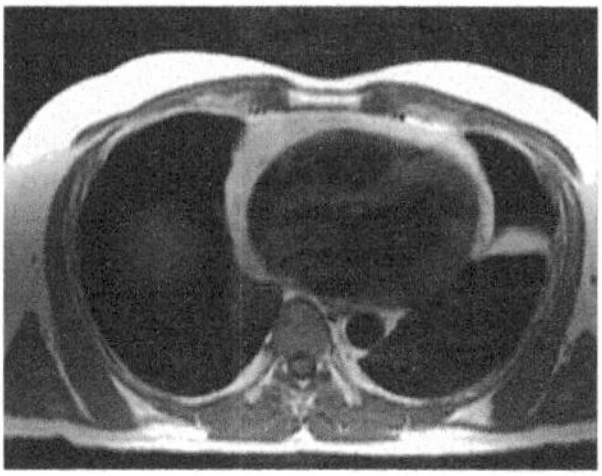

Fig. 1.27 Gating artefact. Note the blurred cardiac borders and cardiac 'ghosting' artefact in the phase-encode direction.

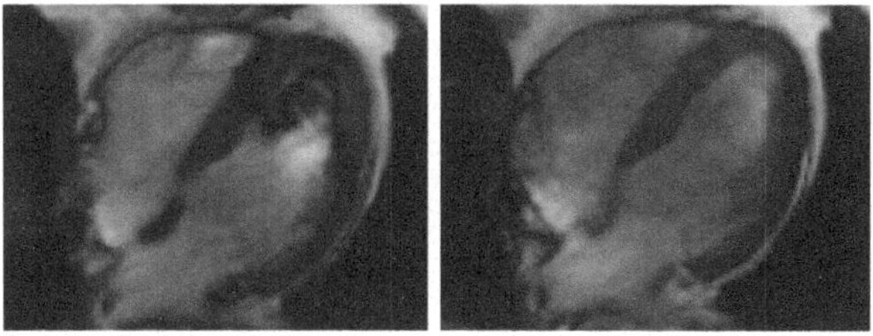

Fig. 1.28 SSFP image showing off-resonance artefact in the left ventricle at 3T (left) and resolution after adjustment of centre frequency (right).

Magnetic resonance contrast agents

The addition of even small amounts of certain molecules can cause large changes in relaxation times (T_1, T_2, and T_2*) within tissues, which results in significant changes in the MR image. These compounds are called MR contrast agents, and are based upon molecules or ions that are magnetically active (paramagnetic moieties). Iron (Fe), dysprosium (Dy), gadolinium (Gd), and oxygen (O_2) are used as these demonstrate the greatest effects. Contrast agent effects are regionally specific, i.e. affect the site of the contrast agent and by an amount that increases with concentration.

Types of contrast agent

T_1 contrast agents

Interact with the nuclear spins and shorten the T_1. Close contact between the agent and the protons is required.

T_2 and T_2 contrast agents*

These contrast agents shorten the T_2 and T_2* of the sample and do not need close interaction between the nuclei and the agent, as they occur over much larger distances.

Intravascular agents

Contrast agents are now available that remain within the vascular system, which would allow longer angiographic imaging, with potential improvements in image quality. Gadolinium is *not* an intravascular agent and angiography acquisition needs to occur when it is undergoing its first-pass through the vascular tree. Nonetheless, good quality images are usually obtained and it is used for most angiographic examinations.

Targeted contrast agents

By combining MR contrast agents with compounds that adhere to specific molecules (e.g. a monoclonal antibody), 'targeted' contrast agents can be created. This 'molecular imaging' is a promising future approach, but is currently in the experimental stage and none are licensed in humans yet.

Gadolinium

- The most commonly used agent. See Fig. 1.29.
- A small molecule which diffuses out of the vasculature.
- Generally chelated (e.g. with diethylene-triamine penta-acetate, DTPA) to render it non-toxic and safe for injection.
- Gadolinium (Gd) compounds act predominantly as T_1 contrast agents in the blood and myocardium, although where the contrast cannot freely mix with the observed water (i.e. in the brain because of the blood-brain barrier), their small T_2 and T_2* effects can also be observed.
- Gd-based contrast agents are approved for general clinical use, though licensing varies by country. These are not yet licensed for cardiac applications in the USA, although this will likely change in the future.

Iron-oxide particles

Predominantly affect the T_2 and T_2* of the tissue. In MR images the regions where these particles accumulate will decrease the signal in T_2-weighted images.

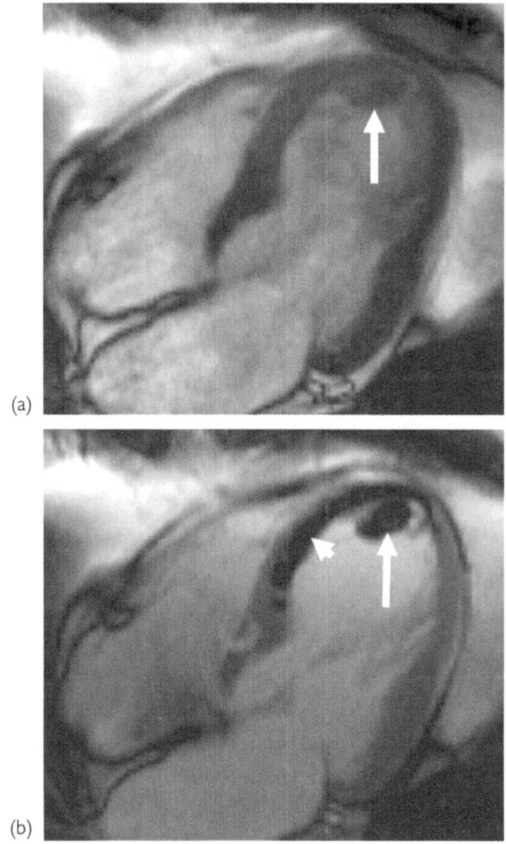

Fig. 1.29 Imaging pre and post-gadolinium injection. (a) 4-chamber view (SSFP sequence) showing a filling defect at the LV apex consistent with a thrombus (long arrow). (b) the same 4-chamber view imaged 1–2 minutes after gadolinium injection with a T1-weighted inversion recovery sequence. The filling defect seen above has no contrast uptake and appears dark (low signal, long arrow), in keeping with a thrombus. The contrast has now highlighted the adjacent myocardium (arrowhead), which also appears dark in comparison to the rest of the myocardium, indicating negligible perfusion in this region from a recent myocardial infarction.

Cardiac spectroscopy and non-proton imaging

The images produced by MR scanners are based on signals obtained from the hydrogen nuclei (protons) in water and fat molecules. However, many other molecules contain protons and there are many non-proton nuclei which produce an MR visible signal, e.g. phosphorus, sodium, and carbon. A vast amount of information can be gained from these different molecules and nuclei by utilizing various imaging and spectroscopy techniques. However, the application of cardiac spectroscopy is hampered by their low concentrations and/or poor sensitivity, and none of the following methods form part of routine clinical CMR scanning.

Proton spectroscopy

Proton spectroscopy can reveal important information about a range of important molecules in the heart, especially creatine and myocardial lipids. However, proton spectroscopy is hampered by the difficulties of shimming in the myocardium and the need to suppress the underlying signal from water in the blood.

Phosphorus spectroscopy

Phosphorus spectroscopy can provide a useful probe of the high-energy phosphates phosphocreatine (PCr) and adenosine triphosphate (ATP) within the heart (Fig. 1.30). The PCr/ATP ratio has been shown to be reduced in heart failure patients and is an independent predictor of mortality.

Cardiac phosphorus spectroscopy is challenging due to low concentrations of the element, low MR sensitivity, and contamination from the surrounding skeletal muscle and the liver.

Carbon spectroscopy

Carbon spectroscopy (Fig. 1.31) can yield information on a wide range of different molecules and provides a tool for the assessment of cardiac metabolism. However, the low natural abundance of the MR visible isotope of carbon (^{13}C) and a low MR sensitivity means that studies with carbon are very limited. New techniques of hyperpolarization are showing promise in the development of carbon spectroscopy by increasing the available signal for a short period of time.

Sodium imaging

Due to the short recovery time (T_1) and the relatively high concentration of sodium within the blood (~80mM), it is possible to generate sodium images of the heart (Fig. 1.32). Sodium levels are known to increase in regions of myocardial infarction (due initially to failure of the sodium-potassium pump), and later during the oedematous phase of ischaemia and, therefore, sodium images may provide a useful indicator of myocardial damage.

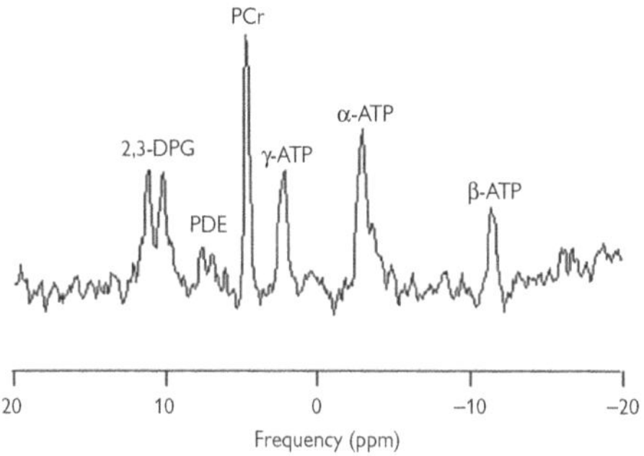

Fig. 1.30 A phosphorus spectrum of the heart collected over a 50ml volume of tissue. These peaks can be quantified to provide direct metabolic information.

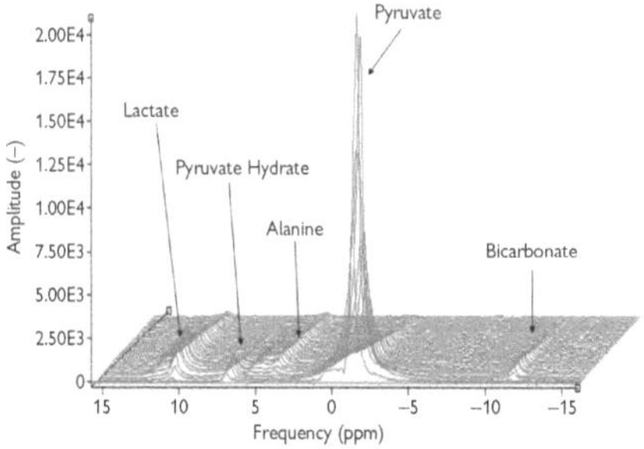

Fig. 1.31 Example of ^{13}C spectroscopy using hyper-polarization.

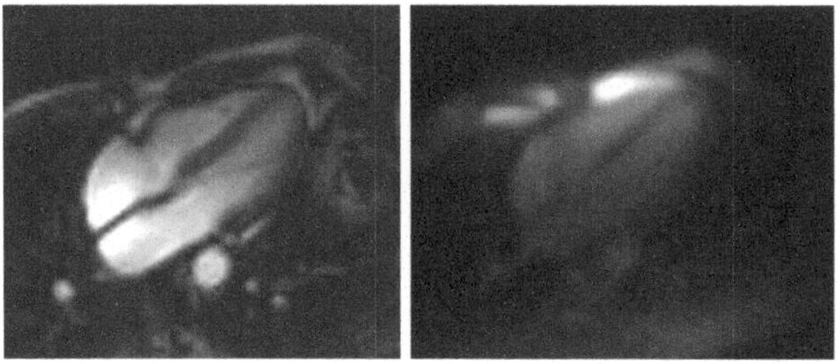

Fig. 1.32 Standard SSFP image (left) and sodium image (right).

Chapter 2

Scan set-up and optimization

Magnetic resonance safety

CMR presents many challenges for the safe imaging of patients with cardiovascular disease and it is vital that all staff involved are aware of the specific safety issues. Regular training and updates are essential.

General considerations

MRI is responsible for a large increase in exposure to strong magnetic fields, but there are currently no known harmful biological effects. The majority of cardiovascular MR is carried out at 1.5T, although increasing amounts are performed at 3T and the FDA (Food and Drug Administration) state that systems up to 8T are considered to be a 'non-significant risk' for adult patients. There are, however, a number of potential risks associated with the magnetic environment and these must be taken into consideration when performing CMR:

The static magnetic field

The main hazard associated with the magnetic field is that of ferromagnetic attraction and it should be remembered that the magnet is **ALWAYS** on. This is the main reason why all MR units have signs warning of the strong magnetic field (📖 p. 14). Staff and patients must be carefully screened prior to entering the magnet room to prevent any ferrous objects being taken in and inadvertently becoming dangerous projectiles. An example of a screening form is shown in Fig. 2.1. A more comprehensive form can be downloaded from www.mrisafety.com

Gradient switching

Noise damage

The gradient (or time-varying) magnetic field is only present during scan sequences and is responsible for the typical loud noises that patients associate with MRI. The noise level can reach up to 115dB at 1.5T during acquisition sequences, such as echo-planar (EPI), due to the extremely fast gradient switching and high gradient amplitude. Hearing protection is essential and headphones are advisable, sometimes combined with ear plugs for the noisiest sequences. The patient needs to hear and understand breath-hold commands, however, so a balance must be found. Most MR systems have an intercom system through the headphones.

Peripheral nerve stimulation

The gradient field has the potential to induce peripheral nerve stimulation (PNS) due to the induction of electrical fields. At sufficient exposure this is perceptible as tingling or tapping, and may be uncomfortable or even painful. The FDA consider MR procedures that use gradient switching sufficient to cause PNS to be a significant risk, and a high level of safety is therefore built into clinical systems. Prior to acquisition of a sequence likely to cause PNS, many systems display a warning message, allowing the operator to make a decision to acquire the data or adjust the acquisition parameters to minimize the effect. The site of PNS varies according to the gradient direction used and the patient may become aware of the sensation moving around the body.

CLINICAL MRI SAFETY SCREENING FORM

Please complete both sides

Patient name ____

Date of birth ________________ Weight ________ kg Height ________ m

Please carefully check the following. Some items can interfere with examinations, and may be hazardous to your safety. Your answers will be kept strictly confidential.

IF YOU HAVE ANY QUESTIONS THEN PLEASE ASK US BEFORE YOUR SCAN		
Do you have a heart pacemaker or pacing wires?	YES	NO
Have you had any heart surgery?	YES	NO
Have you had any surgery to your head (including eyes/ears/brain), neck or spine?	YES	NO
Do you have any implanted devices (e.g. programmable hydrocephalus shunt, nerve stimulator, cochlea implant, aneurysm clip)?	YES	NO
Have you had any operation involving metallic pins / plates / screws / wires?	YES	NO
Have you had any other surgical procedure of any kind? (Please write them here)	YES	NO
Have you ever sustained any injuries involving metal to the eyes or any other part of the body?	YES	NO
Have you ever had a serious accident (e.g. road traffic accident, explosion injury, shooting shrapnel injury?)	YES	NO
Have you ever had a fit or blackout, or do you suffer from epilepsy or diabetes?	YES	NO
Do you have any of the following (if yes please circle): Dentures with metal Hearing aid Artificial Limb or Prosthesis Body piercing/ jewellery Nitro patch Tattoos		
FOR WOMEN OF CHILDBEARING AGE: Could you be pregnant?	YES	NO
Have you removed your watch, bankcards, spectacles, hearing aids, keys, coins, jewellery, hairgrips and eye make-up?	YES	NO

IMPORTANT: NO METAL OBJECTS TO BE TAKEN INTO THE MAGNET ROOM

Patient signature ______________________________ Date of study ________________

Staff signature ___________________________________

Fig. 2.1 Example of a CMR screening form.

Radiofrequency energy

The RF energy used in MR imaging is also only transmitted during scanning. The majority of the RF power is transformed into heat within the patient's body, and the resultant thermoregulatory changes are dependent on the amount of energy absorbed. The dosimetric term to describe this energy absorption is the *specific absorption rate* (SAR) and is expressed in Watts per kg. The SAR at a normal operating level is 2W/kg and at 'first' level is 4W/kg. It is vital that the correct patient weight is entered into the system registration so that SAR levels are accurate.

SSFP sequences use large amounts of RF energy and the imaging parameters generally need to be altered to keep the energy delivery within a safe operating level. These changes (e.g. decreasing the flip angle, increasing the slice thickness or increasing the FOV) will result in a change in image contrast.

Patients with cardiovascular problems including hypertension, diabetes and obesity can be particularly challenged as their thermoregulatory system may be compromised. Drugs such as beta-blockers, calcium channel blockers and diuretics, used in the treatment of cardiovascular disease, can also affect the thermoregulatory system.

Implants and other devices

Many patients referred for CMR will have had some form of previous intervention. In practice, most patients can be scanned safely, but it is important to determine the nature of any surgical procedure, and the presence of any implant or other device, and the conditions under which the examination can be performed. The following need to be considered:

- What is it?
- Why is it there? Can it be removed, disabled, switched off?
- How long has it been there?
- What is it made of?
- Under what conditions can it be safely imaged?

For a precise risk assessment, the exact name, model, and manufacturer of the device is required, and the manufacturers information specific to the implant verified. Other information pertinent to the use and configuration of the device, and time since implantation, may also be necessary to determine the optimum conditions under which the patient can be examined. Device information can be obtained from various sources, e.g.:

- The implant/device card given to the patient after implantation.
- The patient's medical notes.
- The manufacturer's website.
- 'The reference manual for magnetic resonance safety, implants and devices' by Frank Shellock (Biomedical Research Publishing Group).
- www.mrisafety.com

Most prosthetic heart valves, coronary stents and joint replacements can be scanned safely. However, it is recommended that the individual device is verified against up-to-date information. A comprehensive list of devices is beyond the scope of this text.

Understanding the terminology

In 2005, the ASTM (American Society for Testing and Materials) developed a new set of terms and symbols for labelling implants, devices, and other equipment that may be used within the MR environment:

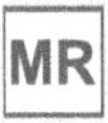

MR safe: this is an item that poses no known hazard in any MR environment. An example of an MR safe item is something made of a non-conducting, non-magnetic material, such as a plastic Petri dish. Items may be determined MR safe by scientific rationale or via stringent testing.

MR unsafe: this is an item known to pose hazards in all MR environments, e.g. a pair of ferromagnetic scissors or other surgical instrument.

MR conditional: this is an item that has been demonstrated to pose no known hazard in the MR environment under a set of pre-determined conditions, which include:

- The main (static) magnetic field strength.
- The gradient (time-varying) magnetic field.
- The RF pulse.
- Specific absorption rate (SAR).

Implants and devices classified as MR conditional have been sub-divided into Conditional 1–7 to further specify recommended scanning conditions. These sub categories are available from www.mrisafety.com

Previous terminology

Older terms were proposed in 1997 by the FDA, although these have been considered to be confusing and, in some cases, used interchangeably or used entirely incorrectly. They have now been superceded by the 2005 terms, but both sets of terminology are in use as items that were tested prior to 2005 have not been re-classified, and this may cause further confusion.

- **MR safe:** poses no additional risk to the patient or other person, but may affect the diagnostic quality of the scan. The conditions under which it was tested should be specified (e.g. field strength).
- **MR compatible**: shown to be safe as described above and does not significantly affect the diagnostic quality of the scan or, in the case of medical equipment, have its operational functions altered by being in the magnetic environment.

Optimizing the patient in the magnet

The best quality CMR images are acquired in a patient who is able to lie flat comfortably in the scanner, in regular sinus rhythm at a rate where repeated breath-hold sequences are possible. A typical volumetric study including localizers and long axis cine acquisitions includes ~20 breath-hold scans. The operator must be able to tailor the examination to the individual patient, scan quickly and effectively, and prioritize sequences according to the clinical question being asked.

Preparation of the patient

Having an MR scan can be a daunting prospect for many patients and it is vital that the patient is aware of what to expect, and their role in obtaining an optimum study, particularly with the additional complexities in CMR, e.g. ECG monitoring, intravenous access, BP monitoring, and pulse oximetry.

Clothing

The patient should preferably change out of their clothing into a gown. Many items of clothing contain small metallic fasteners/zips, and these can impair image quality and occasionally present a safety risk. A gown also removes the risk of ferromagnetic objects being carried into the magnet room in pockets. The gown should be fastened at the front, to allow easy access to the chest for placement of the ECG electrodes. For CMR, bras should normally be removed as these often contain metal adjusters or under-wiring, which significantly impair image quality. Other underwear can usually be worn under the gown.

IV access

IV access, if required, should be established prior to entering the magnet room. An extension line can be used so the patient remains in the magnet during contrast administration, and pre- and post-contrast images can be acquired in the same table position, allowing accurate comparison.

Coil placement and patient positioning See Fig. 2.2.

- Depends on the coil configuration used.
- A common configuration is to include a spine array coil embedded in the scan table and a flex array coil placed over the anterior chest wall.
- Ensure the upper limit of the anterior coil covers the sternal notch to ensure adequate imaging of the great vessels.
- When imaging the entire aorta in tall patients, additional extender coils may be used in combination with the anterior chest coil to ensure adequate anatomical coverage.
- Dedicated cardiac coils with a smaller FOV are available and these should be placed over the left hemi-thorax.
- A foam wedge or pillow should be placed under the patients' knees to decrease lumbar lordosis and ease patient comfort. Scan times can typically be 45–60min and comfort is important.
- An explanation of the breath-hold commands prior to the start of the examination is essential to ensure a reproducible diaphragm position. This is particularly important in volumetric analysis.

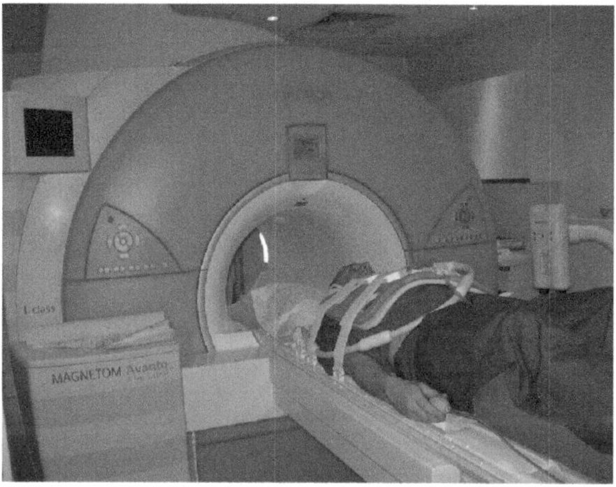

Fig. 2.2 A normal volunteer positioned on the imaging table ready for a typical CMR imaging examination. Note the theatre 'blues' (an alternative to a gown), anterior chest coil, the patient 'alert' button in the right hand, and the foam wedge under the knees. The spine coils are in the table 'bed'.

Patient anxiety and claustrophobia

Claustrophobia and anxiety remain two of the major problems associated with MRI, and can be exacerbated by the apparent complexity of CMR and the length of the examination. The patient lies with their head and upper body within the bore of the magnet, and with only their legs outside, which can increase their feeling of being confined. A rapidly increasing heart rate is often a good indicator of anxiety and the ECG display should be monitored continuously, especially at the start of the examination.

A number of measures can alleviate any anxiety/claustrophobia and allow the scan to be completed successfully:

- **BE PATIENT**. Take time to make the patient feel comfortable and, above all, not rushed into scanning. An anxious patient is much more likely to continue with the scan if they feel their concerns are responded to, rather than being pushed quickly into the scanner.
- Explain the procedure thoroughly, including breath-hold commands, noise levels during imaging, and any potential symptoms or side effects if pharmacological agents are used.
- Consider having a friend, relative, or partner within the magnet room during the procedure (appropriately screened, of course).
- Use prismatic glasses to enable the patient to see out of the scanner.
- Use of an eye mask or 'eye-pillow' containing lavender, linseed, or flax seeds to aid relaxation and detract from the surroundings.
- Aromatherapy.
- Music via a headphone system.
- Imaging the patient prone.
- Place the patient in the bore feet first. This is not always applicable for CMR, but some scanners facilitate this and some patients find this psychologically easier.
- Make use of sedatives or other anxiolytic medication. This can sometimes be helpful, although patients should not drive afterwards and need to be accompanied home, so prior preparation is required.
- Magnet technology is advancing and systems with a 70cm diameter are available. This helps alleviate the feeling of claustrophobia and also allows imaging of larger patients.

Obese patients

As obesity is associated with risk factors for cardiovascular diseases, many will present for CMR examinations. In addition, the prevalence is increasing, with the World Health Organization (WHO) predicting 2.3 billion 'overweight' adults by 2015, with 706 million 'obese' adults. It is important, therefore, to be able to adapt clinical protocols and imaging methods to deal with these patients.

Obesity is defined by the World Health Organization (WHO) using body mass index (BMI; see Table 2.1. However it is almost impossible to predict if a patient is able to fit into the magnet bore from the BMI measurement, weight or abdominal girth. Each patient needs to be assessed on an individual basis and performing a 'test run' beforehand may be very helpful.

Table 2.1 WHO body mass index

Body mass index (BMI) – kg/m^2 (= weight/height^2)	Definition
18.5–24.9	Normal weight
25–29.9	Overweight
30–39.9	Obese
40–49.9	Severely obese
≥50	Extremely obese

Fitting the patient in the magnet

- Take care of the elbows. These are the most likely to be difficult to fit in around a large girth and care should be taken when sliding the patient into the bore to ensure the elbows are not injured.
- The patient's arms should be covered so their skin is not in direct contact with the magnet bore to minimize the risk of RF burns.
- Scanning the patient prone with their arms above their head can help, and increases the size range of patients that can be imaged. In this case the flex array coil is placed over the upper back (Fig. 2.3).
- In very obese patients, imaging can be performed prone using only the integral body coil (Fig. 2.4). Disadvantages are a reduced SNR and image quality, and techniques that rely on coil technology, particularly parallel imaging techniques, e.g. SENSE or iPAT, either cannot be used, or breath-hold times will be significantly longer.
- Newer 70cm bore scanners facilitate imaging of larger patients.

Other problems

- Breathing while supine may be difficult due the weight of the abdomen.
- Breath-hold times may increase due to the need to perform phase over-sampling to avoid aliasing artefacts.
- Image contrast may be compromised due to the need to limit SAR (📖 p. 38), reducing the maximum flip angle that can be achieved. This can be a particular problem with SSFP cine sequences.
- Sweating during the examination may cause detachment of the ECG electrodes.

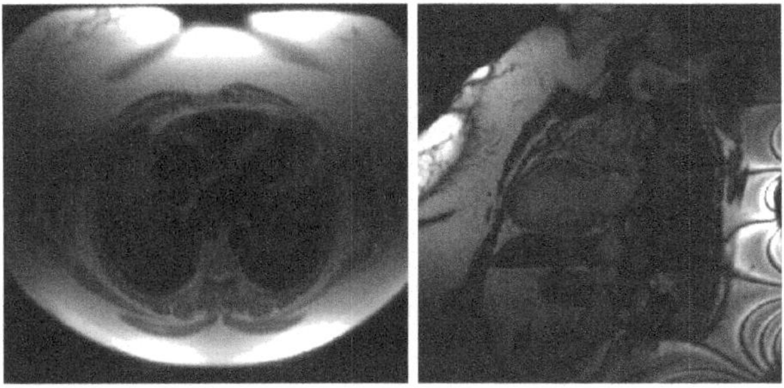

Fig. 2.3 A severely obese patient (BMI 54kg/m²) imaged prone using the spine array, with flex array coils placed over the back. Transverse HASTE image (left); short axis SSFP image (right) with typical moiré fringe (zebra stripe) artefacts often seen at the edge of the field of view, where the patient may be close to the transmit body coil.

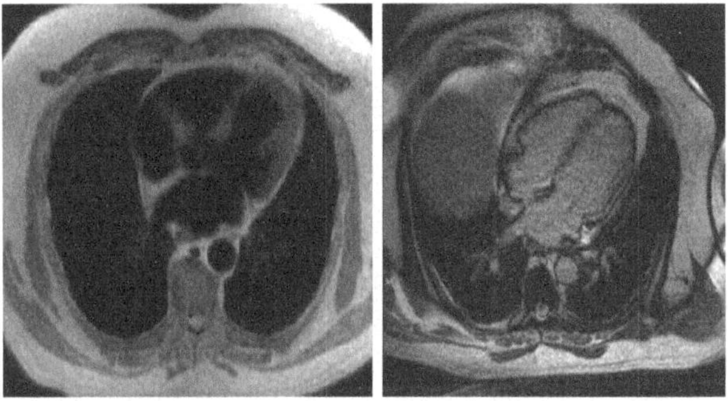

Fig. 2.4 A severely obese patient (BMI 46.9kg/m²) imaged prone with the integral body coil only. (Left) Transverse HASTE image. (Right) Diastolic frame from a SSFP cine, both showing a significant reduction in image quality.

Cardiac (ECG) gating

Timing the scan to the cardiac cycle is a vital part of CMR, in order to avoid motion artefact on static imaging and allow accurate, synchronized cine imaging. Time spent on ensuring a good signal pays dividends in the quality of images produced.

Choice of trigger

There are several physiological signals that can be used for gating, although the R wave of the ECG is the most robust indicator of the start of systole, being easy to identify and rapid in onset. Options include:

- ECG.
- Pulse signal, e.g. SpO_2 (pulse gating- sometimes referred to as PPG).
- Respiratory signal (e.g. from respiratory bellows).
- External signal: the signal from an ancillary monitoring unit is sent to the magnet via an external connecting cable.

These triggers do not occur at exactly the same time. However, Fig. 2.5 illustrates the time difference between ECG and SpO_2 signals, and explains why the pulse signal cannot be used for functional assessment using cines acquired with this method. It can, however, be used for the acquisition of static (single slice) anatomical images.

Preparation of the patient for the ECG

Preparation is the key to success. The ECG is crucial for good quality CMR images and the time spent getting it right saves much time later.

- Remove any excess hair.
- Remove any moisture/body lotion from the skin.
- Consider the use of specialist abrasive skin preparations. These can double the amplitude of the signal.
- Keep electrodes packed until you need them as this prevents contact gel drying out prior to use.
- Check electrode type. It must be MRI safe. RF burns have been associated with electrodes with metal connectors. Remove any other ECG electrodes left from previous ECG monitoring.
- Position electrodes and wait for the patient to lie still.
- Check that the scanner recognizes the ECG trigger correctly. Single shot techniques will not be adversely affected by a sub-optimal ECG, but cine imaging will be compromised making accurate volumetric analysis difficult. No trigger = No scan (as far as cine imaging is concerned).
- Move the position of the leads if necessary. Patient's body habitus, pathology, or previous surgery can affect the cardiac axis. A 12-lead ECG may help to determine this.
- **BE PATIENT**. Triggering may not be successful all the time due to background noise and gradient switching.

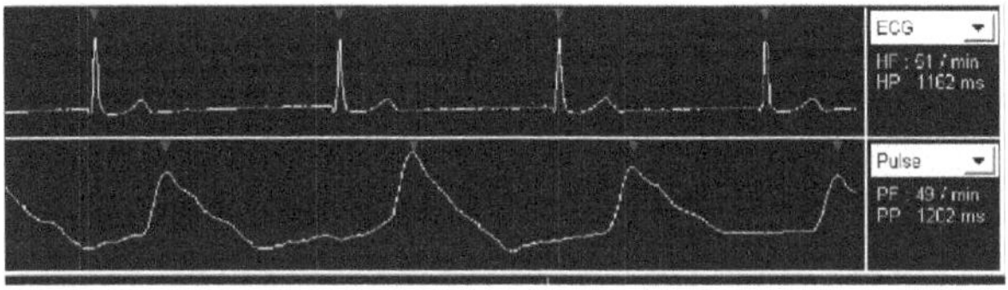

Fig. 2.5 Physiological signals – ECG (top) and pulse wave from pulse oximeter (bottom), acquired simultaneously. Note the time off-set of the two signals. Identification of each signal by the scanner is indicated by the triangle at the top of the trace.

ECG leads

There are various types of ECG cables available, depending on the system used, although most use a 3- or 4-electrode configuration. The cable may be connected to the MR system directly or via a wireless transmitter (the ECG is acquired at the patient and the signal transmitted to an integral receiver unit within the MR system).

The leads are usually coloured and labelled as follows. Where there are only three leads, the black lead is absent:

- **White:** RA (right arm).
- **Green:** RL (right leg).
- **Black:** LA (left arm).
- **Red:** LL (left leg).

Positioning the ECG cables

Figures 2.6 and 2.7 show suggested electrode positioning with a 4- or 3-lead configuration.

- The electrodes are generally placed close together and on the centre left-hand side of the chest. A better signal is obtained with the electrodes spaced more widely apart, but this results in more artefacts from gradient interference, so electrode placement is a compromise. Generally, the best signal is obtained with a good vector between the RA and LL leads using either 3- or 4-leads.
- The leads should not form loops as this could potentially cause an RF burn and some absorbent material should be placed under the cable so it is not in direct contact with the patient's skin.
- If a long cable is used this should be brought out of the magnet parallel to the magnet bore, which reduces potential electrical interference. This can also help prevent drift of the baseline ECG signal during respiration.

Electrocardiogram lead placement on the back

Although it is more usual to place the electrodes on the anterior chest wall, it is possible to place them on the patient's back, although the QRS complex detected is usually smaller in amplitude. It is useful if the patient is imaged in the prone position as the cable may be uncomfortable to lie on, but can also be very useful for:

- **Patients who have had radiotherapy to the anterior chest wall:** the skin may be reddened and fragile, and the patient may have applied aqueous cream to the region.
- **Patients with breast implants:** large implants may impede the electrical signal and prevent adequate ECG signal detection.
- **Obese patients.**

Both prospective and retrospective methods are used, and although these terms are often used synonymously, they differ in how the sequences are acquired and how much of the cardiac cycle is covered during cine acquisition. Anatomical images are usually acquired using a prospective triggering method and functional cine imaging or flow quantification can be acquired using either method.

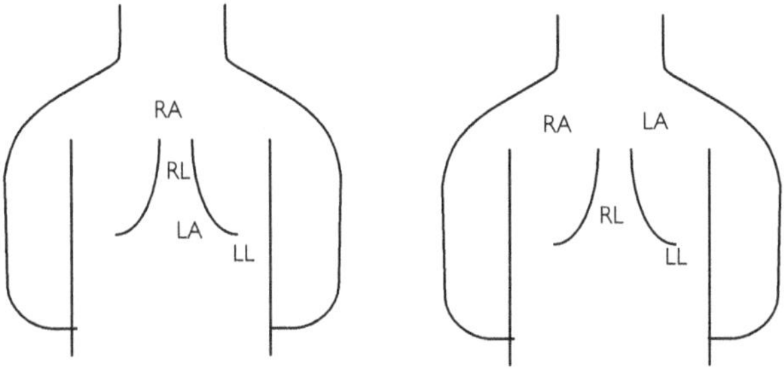

Fig. 2.6 ECG lead positioning options for a 4-lead system.

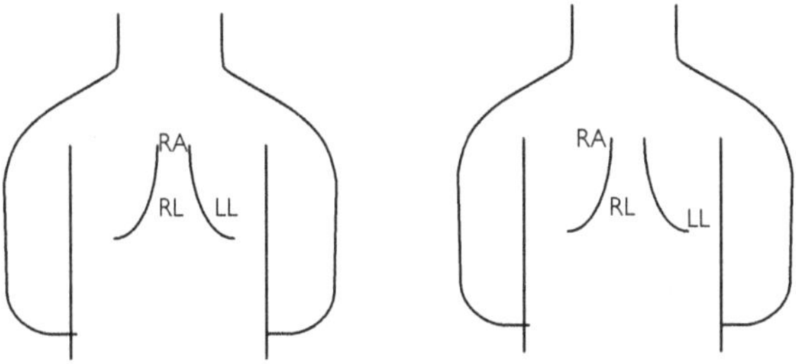

Fig. 2.7 ECG lead positioning options for a 3-lead system.

Problems with the ECG trace

The magneto-hydrodynamic effect

Moving blood induces a voltage when in the magnetic field of the scanner, which can interfere with the ECG trace. Flow perpendicular to the magnetic field (primarily from the ascending and descending aorta) causes ions in the blood to experience a force proportional to their charge (the Lorentz force), which creates an electrical field. This effect, known as the magneto-hydrodynamic effect, induces a voltage detected by the ECG leads. The signal is usually superimposed on the T wave, which can cause the T wave to be the largest waveform, creating problems with ECG triggering. It also means that interpretation of ECG changes (e.g. QRS morphology or ST segment shift), while in the scanner is problematic.

Factors affecting the magneto-hydrodynamic effect

- Field strength: the effects are greater with increasing field strength and can, therefore, be more problematic at 3T.
- Flow velocity within the vessel (effect is proportional to this).
- Vessel diameter: the effect is proportional to this.
- The angle of flow relative to the main magnetic field (B0).
- Orientation of the patient: whether positioned head first or feet first within the magnet.
- Respiration.
- Heart rate.
- Position of the ECG electrodes on the chest.

Value of the ECG within the magnet

Due to the magneto-hydrodynamic effect, interpretation of the ECG during the examination is limited. Evaluation of the P wave, ST segment and T wave is not feasible/diagnostic. Aspects that can be evaluated are:

- Heart rate (providing the QRS detection is good).
- Some rhythms, e.g. atrial fibrillation (AF).
- (Sometimes) the QRS pattern, e.g. left bundle branch block, especially if changes occur while the patient is within the scanner.

Problem ECGs

The ECG should always be observed during image acquisition as it may be distorted by patient movement and certain sequences. The type of ECG detection method used determines how sensitive it is to these forms of interference. The box opposite illustrates some examples of poor ECG traces.

Examples of ECG problems

A good ('normal') ECG within the magnet with a regular RR interval and good R wave detection with a positive QRS complex.

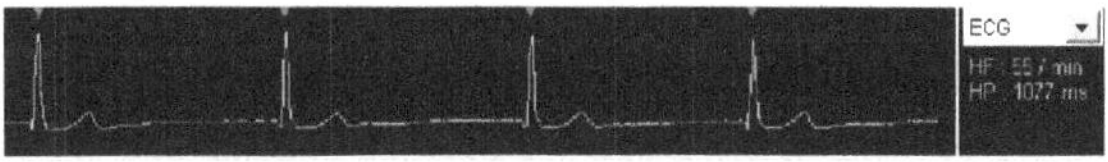

A similar ECG with an inverted R wave. Some systems will not recognize this as a trigger and the leads should be swapped so the R wave is positive.

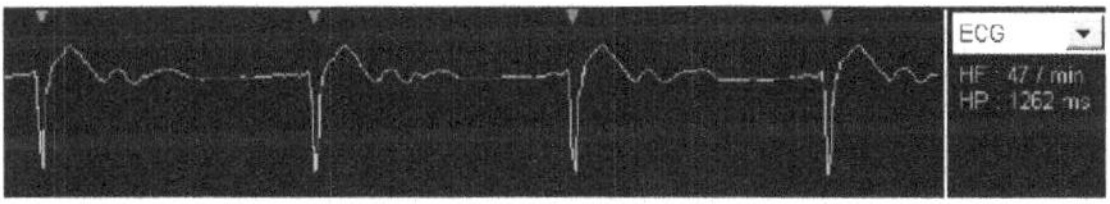

A poor ECG within the magnet. The R wave is small, there is baseline noise and the sequence is triggering erroneously.

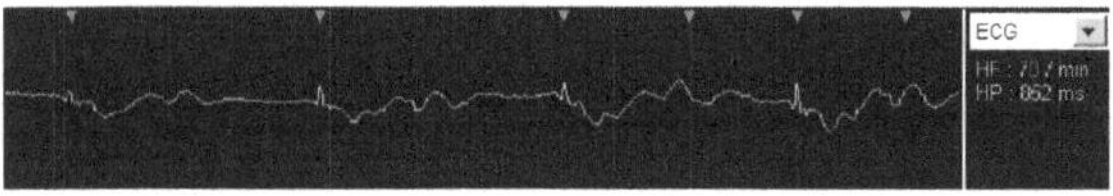

Distortion of the ECG due to gradient interference during the acquisition of SSFP localizer images.

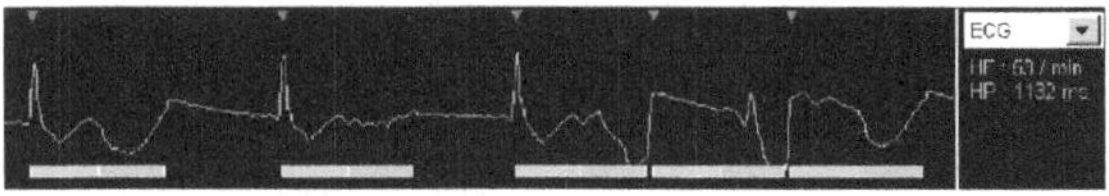

Erratic ECG detection due to an electrode becoming detached during acquisition. The patient may become warm during the scan and the operator should monitor the ECG display closely during the examination for changes in quality.

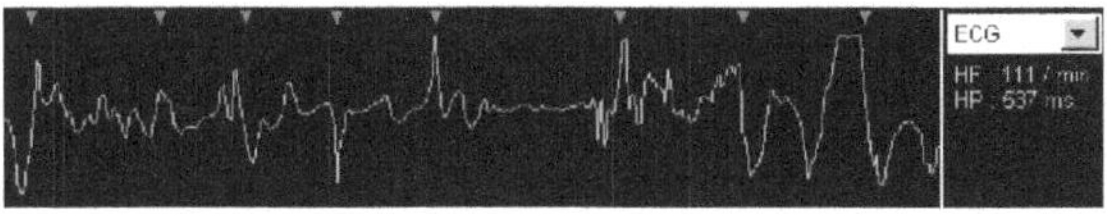

Types of triggering/gating

Prospective triggering

This method uses the R wave in the ECG (or other physiological signal) to trigger the acquisition (Fig. 2.8). For static images, these can be timed to a particular part of the cardiac cycle (often mid-diastole to minimize motion artefact). In prospectively triggered cine imaging, the acquisition starts immediately after the R wave and covers 80–90% of the cardiac cycle, missing end-diastole in order not to miss the subsequent R wave trigger (this would increase acquisition time and the length of the breath-hold). Consequently, there is a short pause in acquisition between one cardiac cycle and the next. Some systems can automatically 'capture' the cardiac cycle. This method usually allocates 90–95% of the cardiac cycle to imaging, but caution should be advised as the patient's heart rate can vary slightly during the study

Retrospective gating

With this method, no actual 'trigger' takes place and acquisition is continuous, independent of the pulse signal. The ECG and image data are acquired simultaneously and temporal assignment of the images to the corresponding cardiac phase is performed afterwards (retrospectively). The term 'gating' is not strictly correct, but is commonly used – a better description would be triggered retrospective imaging. Using this method, the whole of the cardiac cycle is acquired (Fig. 2.9). Retrospectively gated cines are helpful in the assessment of the diastolic portion of the cardiac cycle.

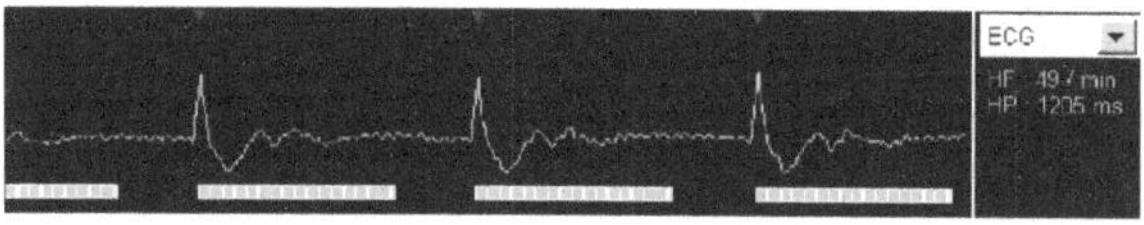

Fig. 2.8 Prospective ECG triggering during a cine sequence. The bar at the bottom of the screen represents the period of the cardiac cycle during which image acquisition will occur. There is a gap at the end prior to the subsequent R wave.

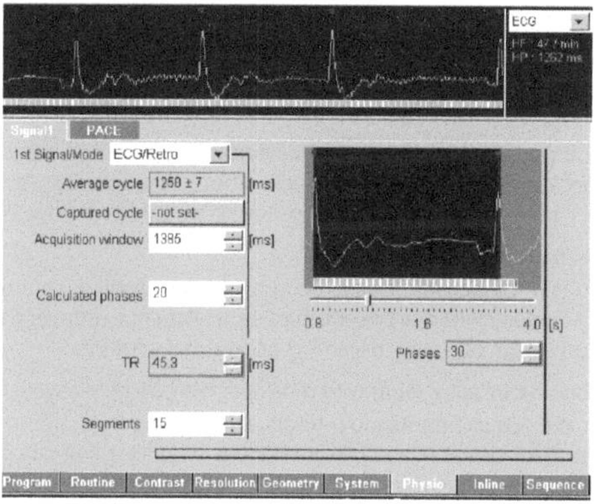

Fig. 2.9 Retrospective ECG gating. Data is acquired continuously, with retrospective construction of the cine sequence according to the position within the cardiac cycle. Usually, the sequence takes care of any parameters, but on some systems the operator must ensure the whole cycle is covered by setting the acquisition 'window' to ~20% more than the average RR interval either by manually entering the time in milliseconds in the acquisition window or by using the 'capture cycle' feature.

Cardiac arrhythmias

Sinus tachycardia

Cine imaging

The breath-hold time is reduced due to the faster heart rate and sinus tachycardia is not generally an issue with cine images, although the shorter R-R interval reduces the number of cardiac phases acquired.

Static imaging

Problems occur when using black-blood preparation techniques (e.g. HASTE, turbo spin-echo), in which adequate time is required for the tissues to recover from the previous excitation. It may be helpful to set the scan to acquire after every second or third R wave.

Irregular cardiac rhythms

Irregular cardiac rhythms present a particular problem for accurate cine imaging because mis-triggering reduces the image quality. Arrhythmia sequences can be used (as listed opposite) or treated as below.

Frequent ectopic beats

If a short run of ectopic beats occurs, the acquisition can often be repeated, hopefully without the ectopics again. Patients with very frequent ectopics or regular bigeminy/trigeminy pose a real problem.

Options for cine imaging *(both with a prospectively triggered sequence)*

- Shorten the acquisition window to allow triggering from the ectopic as well as the normal beats. This avoids mis-triggering and can produce acceptable image quality. If the ectopics produce significantly different LV contraction, the images can still be blurred however.
- Set the acquisition window to cover most of the cardiac cycle of a normal beat, but longer than the R-R interval for the ectopic beat. This will miss out the triggering from the ectopic beats, lengthening acquisition time and reducing late diastolic image quality, but acceptable images can often be achieved. It can still work if the first beat is an ectopic, as triggering from a normal beat usually occurs soon afterwards.

Atrial fibrillation (AF)

- If the rhythm is relatively slow or is regular, this should not present a problem. Carefully watch the R-R interval and choose an acquisition time ~10% shorter than the shortest R-R interval, with prospective ECG triggering. This misses out end-diastole for the longer R-R intervals, but this is usually acceptable and quantification of ventricular function is nearly always possible.
- Patients with a fast, irregular heart rate are problematic as the short R-R interval reduces the number of cine frames and the temporal resolution is often inadequate for the speed of contraction. The temporal resolution can be improved (increasing the number of cine frames acquired per cardiac cycle) by decreasing the number of K-space segments (lines per segment), but this increases the acquisition and breath-hold time. Ideally, patients in fast AF should have the rate or rhythm controlled prior to CMR scanning.

Arrhythmia sequences

Specific cine sequences exist for irregular cardiac rhythms. These are retrospectively gated and allow the operator to set an optimal R-R interval for the individual patient. A tolerance range is set and the system only accepts data when the R-R interval falls within these limits and 'ignores' those outside. Image quality is increased due to the lower heart rate variability. However, breath-hold times are increased and it is difficult to predict how long each acquisition will take, as the amount of 'ignored' cardiac cycles is unpredictable. Cine acquisitions of both cardiac function and blood flow can be acquired using this technique.

Reducing the acquisition time

As most sequences require several cardiac cycles to acquire the image data, the basic acquisition time is determined by the heart rate. However, patients with bradycardia or those who are short of breath may not be able to hold their breath for the required time, and it is important to know how to reduce breath-hold times, especially for cine imaging. This will improve image quality due to the reduction of motion or breathing artefacts and increase patient comfort and compliance.

The options for reducing image time are listed below.

- A view sharing technique, such as shared phases, which 'shares' similar data from adjacent image frames (📖 p. 24).
- A parallel acquisition technique, which acquires the data using several coil elements at the same time (in parallel). Examples include iPAT, SENSE, and ASSETT (📖 p. 24).

Both these techniques will reduce the acquisition time to roughly half that of a standard SSFP cine sequence. The trade-off with each is a reduction in overall image quality due to decreased contrast and increased noise within the image, although image quality usually remains acceptable. If very short scan times are required, these techniques can be used in combination, although image quality is reduced further.

The techniques can be used instead to reduce the overall scan time, e.g. two slices can be acquired in a single breath-hold, reducing the number of breath-holds required to complete the scan protocol.

Ultra-fast cine imaging

In patients who are very un-cooperative, unable to hold their breath or have a very variable heart rate, cine imaging using an ultra-fast technique can be helpful. Often termed 'real-time' imaging, these acquire many images a second and can provide a cine sequence in a single cardiac cycle, although are not truly 'real-time'. They can be useful in the visual assessment of ventricular function and are helpful in the diagnosis of pericardial constriction, when free-breathing imaging may be useful (📖 p. 294, 301), but currently the temporal resolution is too poor to quantify ventricular function accurately.

Breath-hold vs. non-breath-hold scans

Most CMR techniques rely on the patient being able to hold their breath for the duration of the sequence. However, this may not always be possible due to the patient's clinical condition or desirable due the lack of signal achieved in a short time, e.g. in coronary imaging. Other non-breath-hold techniques need to be used for these cases.

Anatomical (static) images

A stack of multiple contiguous images can be acquired using a single shot technique, such as HASTE or SSFP. There are several methods by which the breath-holding can be made easier:

Non breath-hold

Each slice will be acquired at the same point in the cardiac cycle, but are acquired at a different point in the respiratory cycle. The heart will be at a slightly different position within the thorax for each image. This provides reasonable images for general anatomy and position, but are not ideal for planning further breath-hold series due to the slightly variable position of the heart.

Multiple short breath-holds

The total number of slices can be divided into groups and each group acquired as a single breath-hold. Although the total time taken is longer, this provides good quality images, which can also be used for further image planning.

Navigator tracking

With this technique, the position of the diaphragm is monitored with a thin imaging 'column' and an accepted range of diaphragmatic positions is specified (i.e. at a specific point of the respiratory cycle, generally end-expiration); see Fig. 2.10. The data is only acquired when the diaphragm is within this range *and* at the required point in the cardiac cycle. The images are thus acquired at the same point in the respiratory cycle, improving image quality, but acquisition times are much longer due to the need to wait for the correct position of the diaphragm and the heart. Navigator sequences are commonly used for coronary imaging (📖 p. 404).

Single images

Single high-quality images (e.g. turbo-spin echo) are in general acquired in a single breath-hold and most scanners don't have sequences, which acquire the data over several breath-holds.

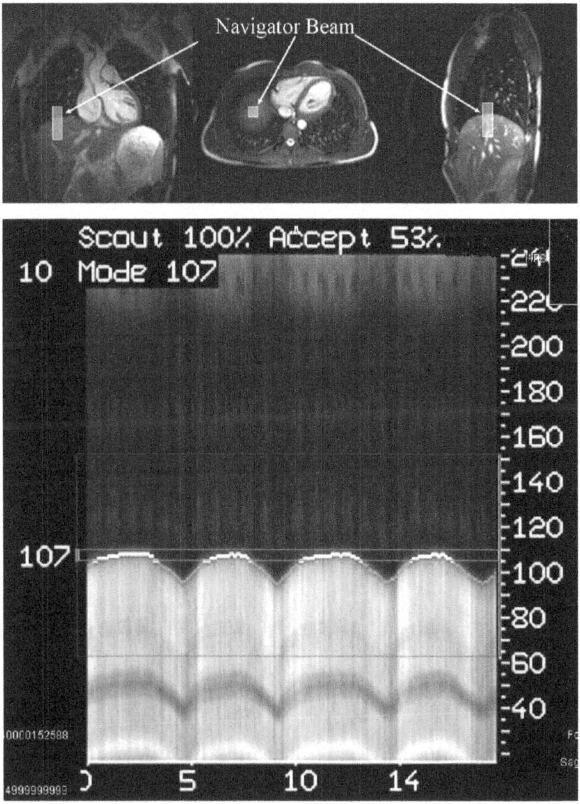

Fig. 2.10 Monitoring the diaphragm in a 'navigator' sequence. Top: position of the navigator column or 'beam'. Bottom: graph displaying the diaphragm position; the x-axis displays time (in seconds) and the y-axis the vertical position of the diaphragm. The acceptable range of positions (or 'window') is shown by the narrow parallel lines around the 107mm position, which is at end-expiration. Data is only acquired when the diaphragm position is between these lines.

Cine imaging

For functional analysis, the sequence of choice is a breath-hold SSFP, however this may not be possible in all patients. Ultra-fast sequences (📖 p. 56) can provide reasonable functional information, but the poorer temporal resolution does not allow accurate volumetric analysis.

An alternative method is to perform a gradient echo technique, such as FLASH, during free breathing and acquire the image over several respiratory cycles. Normally 3 or 4 copies of the same image are acquired to average out the artefact caused by chest wall motion. This significantly increases the total examination time and is rarely used nowadays, having been mostly superseded by the ultra-fast methods.

Flow

If breath-hold sequences are not feasible, longer free-breathing sequences have been developed which facilitate flow mapping. This is usually achieved by reducing the number of K-space lines acquired per RR interval (segments) and increasing the number of signal averages. The respiratory artefact is then averaged out over the duration of the scan, which is much longer (usually 2-4min depending on the heart rate and number of signal averages). This can also allow the number of phases per cardiac cycle to be increased (i.e. higher temporal resolution), which can be advantageous for certain parameters such as pulse wave velocity – this is not generally performed in clinical practice, but can be useful in some research protocols.

CMR in children

Older children

Many older children cope well with the MR environment and, above the age of 10 years, standard scanning methods are usually feasible. Extra care should be taken to ensure the child understands what is involved and why they are having a scan.

Younger children

Scanning without sedation or general anaesthesia can be achieved from the age of 6–7 years, although this is very dependent on the child and how well they respond to the environment. Take time to ensure the patient is happy, and see opposite for tips on achieving a successful scan. Very young children and those unable to tolerate the scanner may require general anaesthesia (📖 p. 64).

Technical aspects

The challenges of CMR are magnified when scanning small children, particularly the balance between image resolution, signal-to-noise ratio (SNR) and image acquisition time. The smaller size of structures, faster heart rates and reduced time for image acquisition (inability or difficulty with breath-holding) often compromise image quality.

Choice of coil

- Standard cardiac coils can often be used, though in neonates/very small children, a dedicated extremity coil (e.g. a knee coil) should be used.
- Specific paediatric cardiac coils have now been developed and may become increasingly used in the future.

Imaging small structures

Small anatomical structures require smaller fields-of-view and thinner slices. Although this leads to increased image resolution, there is a corresponding reduction in SNR. This can be compensated for by:

- Increasing the number of acquisitions, although this will ↑ scan time.
- Removing parallel imaging features – again with an ↑ in scan time.

If image quality remains poor despite these, a larger FOV may be necessary to increase image quality, albeit at the cost of reduced resolution.

Fast heart rates

See 📖 p. 54.

Motion artefacts

For children who have difficulty breath-holding, free breathing imaging can be performed with these possible compensation methods:

- Increase the number of acquisitions (NEX) from 1 to 3.
- Use respiratory compensation methods, e.g. navigator sequences (📖 p. 58), respiratory bellows or phase re-ordering algorithms.
- Use ultra-fast ('real time') imaging sequences (📖 p. 56).

Other

- Good manual shimming techniques are essential to minimize flow artefacts, particularly on balanced SSFP sequences.
- Gadolinium usually given at 0.2–0.4ml/kg for angiographic acquisitions.

Tips for scanning younger children

- Allow plenty of time for preparation of the patient. Be patient and flexible!
- Strong reassurance and good communication throughout.
- Minimize the scanning time – only image what is essential and scan the most important areas first, in case the child only manages a short time in the scanner.
- Involve the parents – many young children will appreciate having their parents present. The older the child, the less this is necessary and sometimes, parental anxiety can be counter-productive.
- Inspiratory breath-hold, rather than end-expiratory – this is easier for the young child to understand.
- Short sequences – a long breath-hold may not be feasible.
- Consider play therapy and/or pre-examination visits to the department – these can help the child overcome any anxiety.
- Consider installing a DVD/video system in the magnet room and allow the child to bring a favourite DVD/video with them. This is an excellent way to relax the child and achieve the best results. They are also more likely to remain in the scanner for longer.

General anaesthesia and CMR

General anaesthesia (GA) is usually only required for the youngest children (<8 years) who would be unable to tolerate the MR scanner while awake and in whom the scan provides important diagnostic information.

Performing general anaesthesia in the MR environment is challenging. The unit is often in a remote location and during the scan there is limited access to the patient and equipment. As well as the usual issues of anaesthesia in MRI, such as care with ferromagnetic equipment and the potential for RF interference with monitoring equipment, there are other factors to be taken into consideration when performing CMR in small children:

- Prolonged multiple breath-holds are required. In children, particularly with cyanotic heart disease, this can cause hypoxia. This may be minimized by limiting the number and duration of breath-holds and/or maintaining a positive end-expiratory pressure (PEEP) at a low level.
- The low ambient temperature in the scanning room produces a hypothermia risk, particularly to low birth weight newborn children.
- Extended breathing circuits impose additional dead space which can affect mechanical ventilation, so reliable respiratory gas monitoring and capnography are essential.
- An anaesthetist with cardiac experience is recommended. Ensure they are aware of the need to paralyse the patient for breath-holding, and of any other procedures that may be required under the same GA (e.g. central venous pressure measurement in patient undergoing MR to assess the bi-directional Glenn circulation).

Magnet room preparation

- MR conditional Boyles machine/ventilator situated inside the magnet room at a safe operating distance from the magnet bore.
- Extended breathing circuit from patient to anaesthetist in control room via wave guide, to facilitate breath-holding.
- MR conditional patient monitoring system inside the magnet room at a safe operating distance from the magnet bore. This should monitor patient ECG, O_2 saturations, BP, and end-tidal CO_2. A remote monitor should be placed in the control room for the anaesthetist to view during scanning. This is connected to the monitoring system either via the wave-guide, or a wireless connection designed for MR scanner use (Fig. 2.11).

Patient preparation

- Anaesthetic room (with MR safe trolley) situated in the MR unit with close proximity to the magnet room (does not need to contain MR conditional anaesthetic equipment).
- Patient metal check and safety questionnaire performed with parents *before* child anaesthetized. Remember to metal-check the parent if they are planning to sit in the MR scanner room during the procedure.
- Check patient's renal function if gadolinium use is planned.
- Wrap the patient to keep warm.
- Ensure patient trolley is free any of metallic items before transfer into scanning room (e.g. metallic O_2 saturation probe).

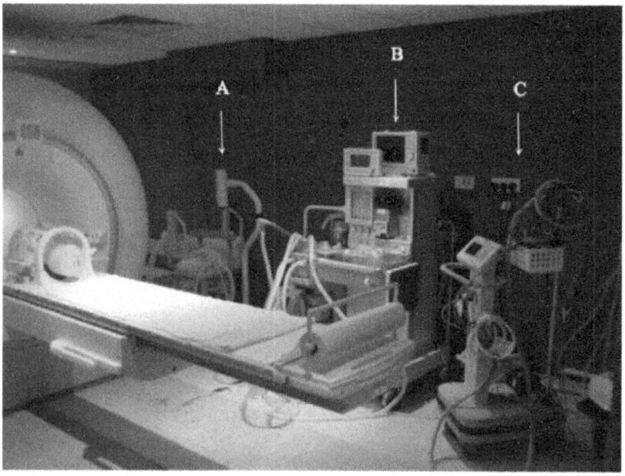

Fig. 2.11 MR scanner room set up for general anaesthesia. (A) Power injector. (B) Anaesthetic machine. (C) Patient monitoring system. Note the long length of airway tubing to enable the anaesthetist to perform breath-holding and monitoring from with the MR control room.

Safety issues with CMR under general anaesthesia

- MR safe/conditional equipment to be employed if used in the magnet room.
- Ensure that all anaesthetic staff are metal checked and aware of MR safety issues. MR safety training of all staff mandatory.
- Be aware of MR unsafe equipment brought into the department (e.g. ward trolleys, O_2 cylinders, syringe drivers/drip stands, etc.).
- Be careful when moving the scanning table to avoid possible extubation and trapping of long lines.
- RF filtered line extensions need to be correct length and snag free.
- Use ear defenders to protect against noise during image acquisition. Adhesive neonatal ear defenders employed for small patients.
- Ensure resuscitation drugs and equipment are readily available outside the scanning room.
- Make sure the team are aware of arrest procedure. Importantly, the child **MUST** be withdrawn from the MR room and metallic objects, such as resuscitation trolley **MUST NOT** be brought into the room.
- Ensure that there are clear signs within the MR unit that outline what to do in an arrest or if the child is seriously unwell.
- Ensure that local hospital resuscitation teaching highlights the importance of withdrawing the patient from the MR scan room, and not to enter the MR scan room with resuscitation equipment.

Pacemakers/ICDs and CMR

Permanent pacemakers and implantable cardioverter-defibrillators (ICDs) are generally considered an absolute contra-indication to MRI. When in a strong magnetic field, the reed switch in the generator box is held open and the device is unable to function normally. Even with a stable underlying rhythm, there are risks involved, mostly from the pacing wire:

- Generation of an electrical current in the lead, from the changing magnetic field (Faraday's law). During movement of the patient in/out of the scanner and gradient switching. The longer or more coiled the wire, the greater the risk. This may cause arrhythmias (~2% risk, mostly ventricular ectopic beats, lower risk of ventricular tachycardia), or may inappropriately inhibit the pacemaker.
- Increased pacing thresholds post-scan, likely due to inflammation and/or fibrosis from lead tip heating. May require a change in pacing settings (up to 10% risk).

The most likely risks are therefore cessation of pacemaker function while in the magnet (nearly all), a deterioration in pacing parameters, and a small, but important, risk of a potentially life-threatening arrhythmia (VT/VF).

When CMR may be considered

In exceptional circumstances, there may be overwhelming reasons for performing a CMR study in a patient with a pacemaker, when the information provided by the scan is vital for the management of the patient, cannot be provided by other means, and the risks of not having the information outweigh the risks of the scan. This balance of risks **MUST** be assessed on an individual basis by a senior clinician in the MR unit, preferably the clinical director, in discussion with the patient's clinical team. Importantly, the risks must be discussed with the patient and informed consent obtained. The scan should be performed in a unit with the appropriate CMR and electrophysiological expertise following appropriate clinical governance procedures. It is essential to ensure good documentation of the discussion of risks/benefits. There are several steps that should be taken to minimize the risk (see box p. 67).

Temporary pacing systems

These are particularly risky, with long, bulky leads and external pacing generators increasing the risk. MR scanning should not be performed.

Retained epicardial pacing wires

Following previous cardiac surgery where temporary epicardial pacing was required. In some cases, the wires are unable to be removed completely and these are cut close to the skin, leaving the tips behind, with the skin healing over the top. They are more common following childhood cardiac operations. In general, the sections of wire are short and pose a minimal risk for MR scanning, even with standard cardiac sequences. Close ECG monitoring of the patient is a sensible precaution however during the scan. Screening with lateral chest X-rays in uncertain cases is no longer routinely required (see www.MRIsafety.com)

Steps to minimize the risk of adverse events

▶ The patient must not be pacing dependent – an acceptable underlying rhythm is essential.

- The pacemaker should be checked beforehand by an experienced cardiac technician/electrophysiologist, and either switched off or into a non-sensing mode (e.g. VOO).
- Sufficient clinical staff should be present to aid in case of an emergency.
- Adequate resuscitation facilities should be available within the MR unit, including a 'crash cart'.
- Continuous ECG monitoring of the patient should occur while in the magnet room, in addition to BP and oxygen saturation monitoring, and continuous verbal contact with the patient.
- The scan should be as short as possible, with only essential images acquired.
- Every attempt should be made to minimize the delivery of RF energy to the patient, with careful selection of sequences to achieve this. Expert advice sought if necessary and some MR systems have specific modes to facilitate this. A compromise in image quality may be required, but diagnostic images can still be obtained. SSFP sequences should be avoided due to the higher RF power deposition.
- After the scan, the pacemaker should be checked again and any changes in parameters noted. These should be communicated to the patient's clinical team to determine if any action is required. The pacemaker should be returned to its usual functional mode.

MR-conditional permanent pacemakers

The first MR-conditional pacing system is now available (Medtronic SureScan™), which has several modifications to improve the resilience of the pacemaker to the magnetic field. Pacing during the scan may even be achieved. However, this has currently only been tested for non-thoracic MR imaging and no data exist for cardiac imaging, for which the device does not have a license. Cardiac imaging involves a greater risk, due to the proximity of the pacing system to the magnet isocentre, and the fast acquisition sequences required, with strong gradient switching and high RF energy deposition (both increase the risk of inducible currents and lead tip heating).

Further reading

🖱 www.MRIsafety.com

Levine GN, Gomes AS, Arai AE *et al.* AHA statement. *Circulation* 2007; **116**: 2878–91.

Faris OP, Shein M. FDA perspective. *Circulation* 2006; **114**: 1232–3.

Nazarian S, Roguin A, Zviman HH *et al.* Clinical utility and safety of a protocol for non-cardiac and cardiac magnetic resonance imaging of patients with permanent pacemakers and implantable cardioverter defibrillators at 1.5 Tesla. *Circulation* 2006; **114**: 1277–84.

Cardiovascular magnetic resonance at 3.0 Tesla

Currently, the majority of clinical CMR is performed on a 1.5T system but cardiovascular imaging at 3T is becoming more widely available and accepted into clinical practice. Despite the 100% increase in signal to noise ratio (SNR) at 3T, there are other technical challenges including increased artefacts, which pose problems for CMR at 3T, and these need to be considered.

The main issues are:

- Increased susceptibility artefact.
- Increased chemical shift artefact.
- Off resonance artefacts due to RF inhomogeneity.
- Increased magneto-hydrodynamic effect on the ECG (📖 p. 50).
- Increased RF deposition, limiting TR and decreasing image contrast. This may also decrease the maximum number of slices allowed in one acquisition, and a time delay before subsequent sequence acquisition is required.
- Longer T_1 times and, therefore, longer inversion times for late gadolinium imaging for the same contrast dose and time delay.
- Shorter T_2 and T_2* times.

All these effects need to be taken into account during protocol optimization and adjustment of the scan parameters needs to be made on an individual basis.

Benefits

Despite the technical challenges, there are some aspects of cardiac imaging which are better at 3T due to the superior SNR, including:

- Single shot techniques.
- Parallel imaging techniques.
- Perfusion imaging.
- BOLD (blood oxygen level dependant) imaging (📖 p. 462).
- Spectroscopy.

SSFP cine imaging

Functional cine imaging in CMR is mostly acquired using SSFP sequences, which are particularly vulnerable to artefacts due to off-resonance effects. At 3T these appear as dark bands within the image and can be problematic, depending on their location within the image. Optimization of each sequence and sometimes for the same sequence in each different orientation, is required to avoid the artefacts. As a consequence, cine imaging at 3T can be time-consuming.

- To minimize the effects, a pre-scan 'scout' image can be acquired to determine the optimum excitation frequency, and the relevant adjustments made to subsequent acquisitions (Figs 2.12 and 2.13). This may need to be repeated as the slice orientation changes during the study.
- The implementation of high order shimming over a selected volume within the image may also help in reducing any susceptibility artefacts in the area of interest.

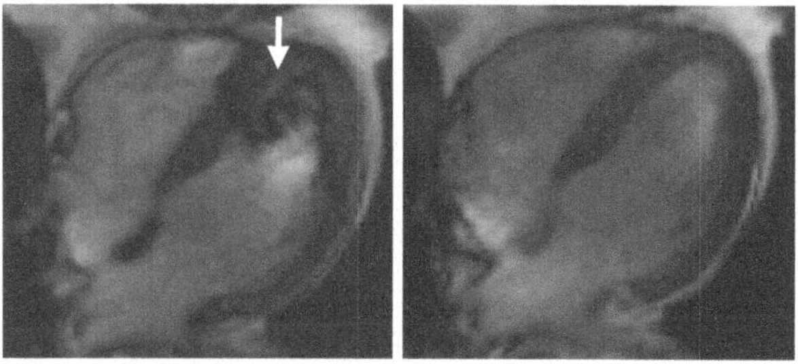

Fig. 2.12 SSFP cine sequence at 3T before (left) and after (right) adjustment of the centre frequency. Note the artefact at the LV apex on the left hand image (arrow).

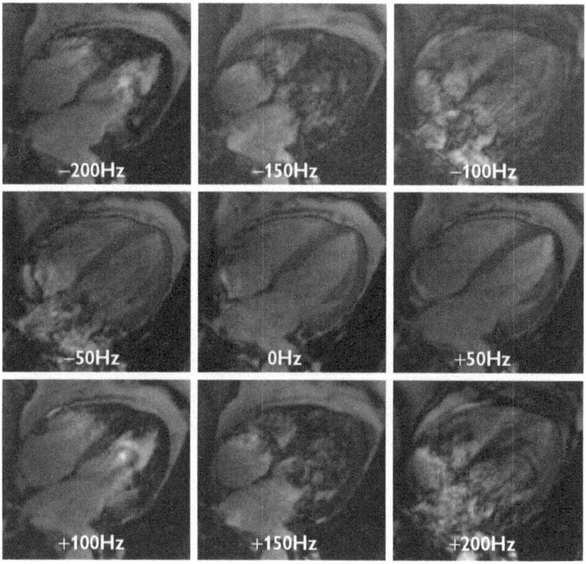

Fig. 2.13 Frequency scout series demonstrating the off resonance artefact for each centre frequency off-set. In this case, no off-set is required as zero (0Hz) off-set provides the optimal image.

Chapter 3

Image acquisition and standard views

Introduction

CMR requires a more complex set-up and imaging protocols than other areas of MRI, due mostly to the variable orientation of the heart within the thorax and its constant motion. Acquiring cardiac images requires unique imaging planes, and an understanding of the wide range of normal cardiac orientation and anatomy. It also requires moving (or cine) image sequences and sometimes velocity mapping.

The importance of operator interaction during the scan

It is important for the operator(s) to view the acquired images, and modify subsequent image acquisitions as appropriate. This may mean repeating images if quality is poor, refining image positions if the plane is incorrect (sometimes several times), and choosing unplanned image planes or sequences (e.g. flow, tissue characterization). This requires a high level of interaction *during* scanning from the operator and/or the reporting physician, and pre-set scanning protocols – of the 'fire and forget' type (running without further interaction) – are almost never suitable for CMR.

A 'standard' CMR dataset

The wide variety of CMR techniques and the unlimited image planes preclude a 'standard' image dataset, from which most diagnoses are made (as exists for a full echocardiographic study). A tailored approach is required, depending on the indication and CMR findings. It is possible, however, to suggest a basic dataset, applicable to many CMR studies, to which other sequences can be added as appropriate. There may be some CMR studies that do not require all of these:

- Transverse ± coronal multi-slice static imaging (e.g. HASTE) of the thorax, timed to mid-diastole to reduce cardiac motion.
- Cine imaging (usually a SSFP sequence) in the three standard long-axis planes of the left ventricle (LV) – horizontal long-axis (HLA) or 4-chamber view (📖 p. 82), vertical long axis (VLA) or 2-chamber view (📖 p. 84) and left ventricular outflow tract (LVOT) views (📖 p. 86).
- ± Short axis cine image stack (SSFP usually) if LV/RV volume/mass analysis is required (📖 p. 88).
- ± Late gadolinium enhancement images in the 3 standard LV long axes and short axis stack, if assessment of viability, inflammation or infiltration is required (📖 p. 112).

It is also possible to define standard imaging protocols applicable to specific applications/indications, and these are described in the relevant sections of the book.

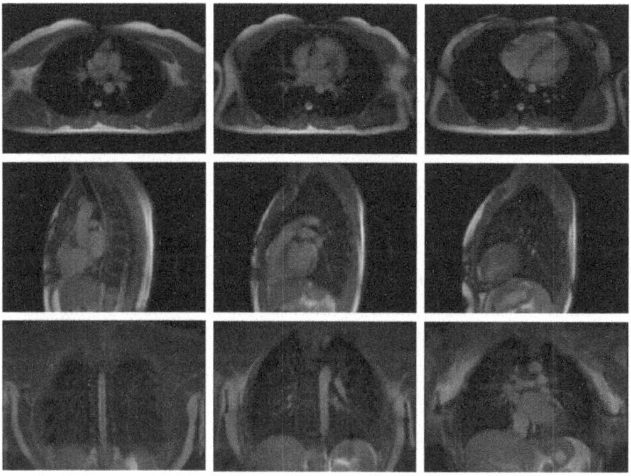

Fig. 3.1 A typical series of localizer images in transverse (top), sagittal (middle), and coronal (bottom) planes.

Choice of image sequence

Several image sequences are more commonly used for cardiac imaging. A detailed description of the sequences is included in Chapter 1, and specific applications are included in the relevant sections. Table 3.1 lists the manufacturers' names for the sequences.

Static images

Ultra-fast gradient echo 'localizers'

A whole image acquired in a single heart beat, but with low spatial resolution. Good for initial localizer images.

Single-shot turbo spin echo (e.g. HASTE)

Reasonable spatial resolution and tissue discrimination. Good for general multi-slice anatomical imaging.

Turbo spin echo

High spatial resolution, acquired over several cardiac cycles. Good for tissue discrimination and T_1 or T_2 tissue characteristics (📖 p. 18) can be examined. Fat saturation pulses (📖 p. 22) can also be applied.

Inversion recovery

High spatial resolution and good for tissue discrimination. The sequence used for late gadolinium enhancement (📖 p. 20); it can also be used to highlight T_2 characteristics, especially with triple inversion recovery sequences.

Gradient echo multi-slice

Relatively high spatial resolution and good for highlighting blood vessels, due to its inherent 'white blood' aspects.

SSFP multi-slice

Can be used for blood vessel imaging, though gradient echo is more commonly used. It is most useful for high resolution '3D' imaging (📖 p. 405).

Moving (cine) images

SSFP multi-frame

Standard CMR cine sequence. High spatial and temporal resolution, with high contrast between blood and myocardium make it ideal for cardiac imaging. More susceptible to artefacts and inhomogenous magnetic fields.

Spoiled gradient echo

Good spatial and temporal resolution. Contrast between blood and myocardium is not as high as for SSFP, but less susceptible to artefacts.

Ultra-fast 'real-time' imaging

Rapid acquisition not requiring breath-holding, but with low spatial and temporal resolution.

Flow/velocity cine sequences

All flow/velocity imaging uses gradient echo sequences, termed phase velocity mapping. Velocity can be measured in blood moving through the image plane, or within the image plane, along the major axes. (See, 📖 p. 100 for a more detailed description.)

Table 3.1 Sequence branding of the major CMR manufacturers

Sequence type	Siemens	GE	Philips
Spin echo	Spin echo, SE	Spin echo, SE	Spin echo, SE
RARE (rapid acquisition relaxation enhancement)	Turbo spin echo, TSE	Fast spin echo	Turbo spin echo, TSE
Half-Fourier single shot turbo (fast) spin echo	HASTE	SSFSE	Single shot TSE
Spin echo black blood (cardiac)	Dark-blood prepared TSE, HASTE	Double IR FSE, FSE-XL with blood suppression	Double inversion BB T_1 or T_2
Spin echo black blood null fat (cardiac)	TRIM	Triple IR FSE, FSE-XL IR with blood suppression	Black blood pre pulse plus SPIR
Gradient echo	Gradient echo, GRE	GRE, GRASS	Fast field echo, FFE
Spoiled gradient echo	FLASH	SPGR	T_1 FFE
Steady state free precession	True FISP	FIESTA	Balanced-FFE
Ultra-fast gradient echo	Turbo flash	Fast GRE, fast SPGR	Turbo field echo, TFE
3D ultra-fast	MP rage	3DFGRE, 3D fast SPGR	3D TFE
Gradient and spin echo	Turbo GSE, TGSE	GRASE	GRASE
Inversion recovery	IR, Turbo IR, TIR	IR, MPIR	IR-TFE (or TSE)
Short tau IR	STIR	STIR	STIR

With thanks to Cindy Comeau, Carnegie Hill Advanced Cardiovascular Imaging, New York.

Standard orthogonal image planes

Localizers

A set of multi-slice, multi-planar images is acquired first to determine the patient's position within the magnet. These usually comprise three transverse, three coronal, and three sagittal images acquired using an SSFP or gradient echo sequence acquired in a single breath-hold (Fig. 3.1). If the patient position is incorrect, repeat images can be required after altering the table position slightly.

Transverse plane

Transverse multi-slice images are planned from the localizers, and are used for most CMR scans. The slice group should extend from above the arch of the aorta superiorly to the lower border of the right ventricle inferiorly (Fig. 3.2). Ensure the anterior array coil is positioned high enough on the patient's chest to ensure adequate signal at the origin of the head and neck vessels. The field of view (FOV) may be adjusted in the (phase-encoding) antero-posterior (AP) direction to minimize acquisition time

Imaging sequences that may be used include:

HASTE

Single shot technique (i.e. one heart beat per slice), which can be acquired either breath-hold or non breath-hold. It is predominantly T_2-weighted and is a black-blood technique (Fig. 3.3 and p. 20).

Turbo spin echo

Higher resolution than HASTE, but requires multiple heart beats per slice and breath-holding, so multiple breath-holds are usually required. Can be either T_1- or T_2-weighted for tissue characterization (Fig. 3.3 and p. 20).

SSFP

Although commonly used for cine imaging, this can be useful as a single shot technique for anatomical imaging. It is a white blood technique, and can be useful in differentiating blood vessels and airways (Fig. 3.3 and p. 24).

Advantages of the transverse plane

- General anatomical survey.
- Most structures are easy to identify.
- Demonstrates the relationship of the cardiac chambers and great vessels (Fig. 3.4).
- Pericardial visualization is possible.
- Assessment of any potential thoracic pathology.

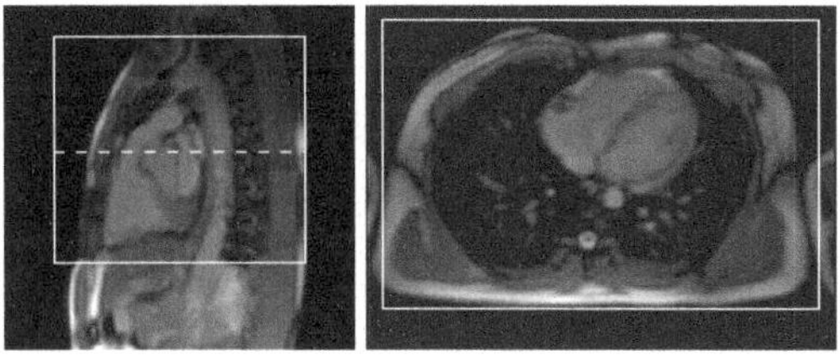

Fig. 3.2 Position of the transverse slice group, ensuring coverage from the head and neck vessels to the inferior border of the RV. (Left) The slice group positioned on a sagittal localizer. (Right) a representative slice position on a transaxial localizer.

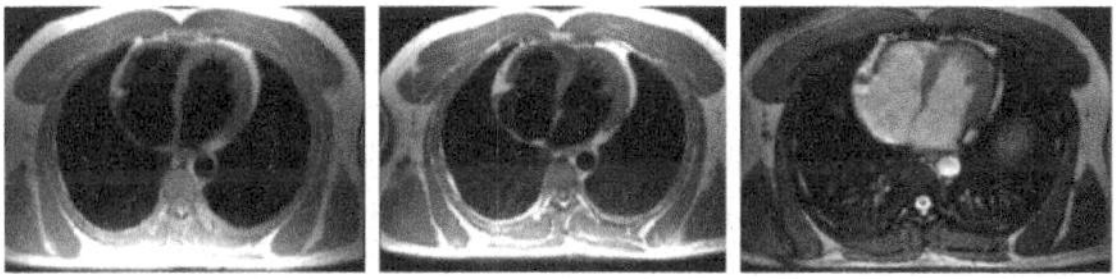

Fig. 3.3 Examples of a transaxial plane through the mid-thorax. (Left) HASTE image. (Middle) Turbo spin echo (TSE). (Right) SSFP multi-slice.

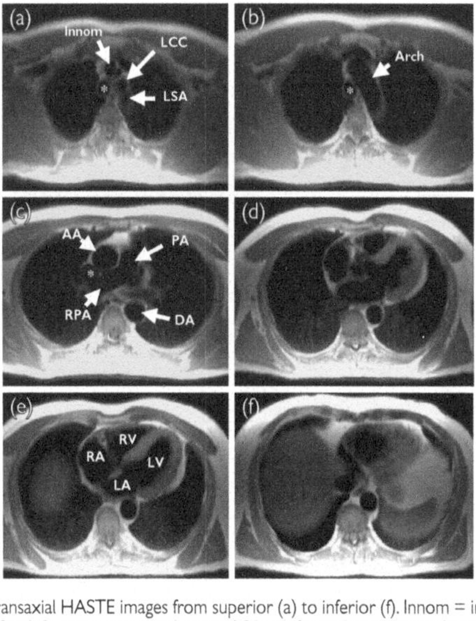

Fig. 3.4 Transaxial HASTE images from superior (a) to inferior (f). Innom = innominate artery; LCC = left common carotid artery; LSA = left subclavian artery; * = SVC; AA = ascending aorta; DA = descending aorta; PA = pulmonary artery; RPA = right pulmonary artery. RA = right atrium; RV = right ventricle; LA = left atrium; LV = left ventricle.

Coronal plane

A coronal multi-slice image stack is often used in addition to transverse imaging. It is planned from the transverse image stack and positioned from the posterior border of the descending aorta to the anterior border of the right ventricle (Fig. 3.5). It may be necessary to increase the FOV ± over-sample in the phase-encode direction to avoid any aliasing (wrap-around) artefact (📖 p. 26)

Structures usually well visualized in the coronal plane

See Fig. 3.5.

- Aortic valve.
- Left ventricular outflow tract and proximal ascending aorta.
- Descending aorta.
- Upper pulmonary veins.

Sagittal plane

Planned from the transverse multi-slice sequence. The slice group should cover the entire heart from medial to lateral borders (Fig. 3.6).

Structures usually well visualized in the sagittal plane

See Fig. 3.7.

- Superior vena cava.
- Inferior vena cava.
- Right ventricle and pulmonary outflow.
- Descending aorta.

Oblique sagittal plane

This oblique plane is helpful in the assessment of the thoracic aorta, and can provide the classical 'hockey stick' or 'candy cane' view. It is planned from the transverse multi-slice group and runs parallel to the ascending and descending limbs of the aorta (Fig. 3.6).

It is often helpful to plan an odd number of slices, typically 7–11 (depending on the dimensions of the aorta), with the middle slice positioned through the centre of both ascending and descending limbs (Fig. 3.6). The aorta may not lie perfectly within this plane, and further imaging may be required, potentially using a 3-point planning tool (📖 p. 96).

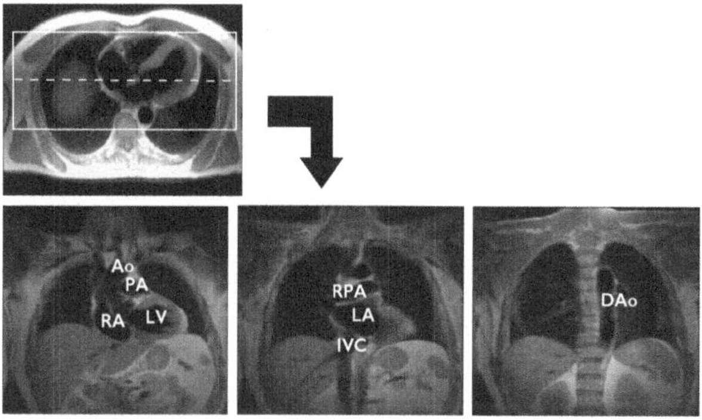

Fig. 3.5 Position of the coronal image group (top left), from the RV free wall anteriorly to the descending aorta posteriorly, viewed on a transaxial image. The read-out (phase-encode) direction is normally head-foot, with the phase direction left to right (**NB.** The FOV should extend beyond the lateral chest wall to avoid wrap-around artefact). (Bottom) Resulting coronal HASTE images from anterior (left) to posterior (right). Ao = aorta; PA = pulmonary artery; RA = right atrium; LA = left atrium; LV = left ventricle; RPA = right pulmonary artery; IVC = inferior vena cava; DAo = descending aorta.

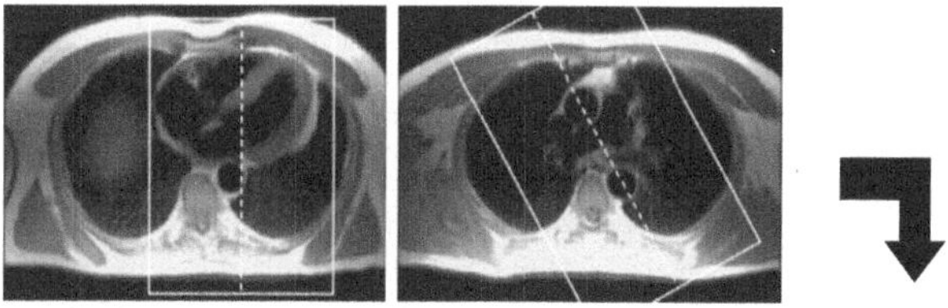

Fig. 3.6 Position of the sagittal (left) and oblique sagittal (right) slice groups.

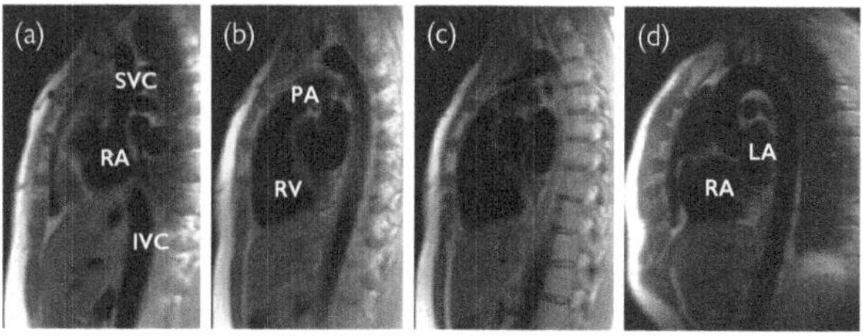

Fig. 3.7 Resulting HASTE images – sagittal group (a–c) and central slice from the oblique sagittal group (d).

Left ventricular function

The standard orthogonal planes described above refer to the planes of the body and not the cardiac axes. To assess cardiac function accurately, imaging planes along the cardiac axes must be specifically planned for each patient. The LV can be thought of as a cone, with an outlet (aorta) adjacent to the inlet (mitral valve).

- SSFP cine sequences are the sequence of choice for functional imaging.
- See chapter 5 for details on assessing function.

Standard views for the left ventricle

Horizontal long axis (HLA)

Equivalent to the echocardiographic apical 4-chamber view.

Vertical long axis (VLA)

Equivalent to the echocardiographic apical 2-chamber view.

Short axis stack

Left ventricular outflow tract (LVOT)

Equivalent to the echocardiographic 3-chamber view.

Pilot (scout) images

- These allow accurate positioning of the long axis cine images.
- Pilot images should be acquired using a rapid single-shot sequence, similar to the localizers, taking one cardiac cycle per image to acquire the data, and timed to diastole.
- Alternatively, a low temporal resolution cine may be used to assess the amount of descent of the atrioventricular ring during the cardiac cycle, and determine systole and diastole.
- Some systems have a real-time inter-active planning mode, which allows the operator to continuously acquire data, whilst manipulating the imaging plane, reducing the need for pilot images. Once the specific view or anatomy has been identified, the plane can be stored and used for further planning. This method relies on good anatomical knowledge and spatial orientation, but can be time saving with experience, and can be useful in congenital heart disease to identify abnormal connections/ conduits.

VLA pilot

Using the (breath-hold) transaxial localizer images, position the slice along the long axis of the left ventricle, running through the mid-point of the mitral valve and the apex (Fig. 3.8).

HLA pilot

Using the VLA pilot, position this slice along the long axis of the left ventricle using the same anatomical landmarks (mitral valve and apex, Fig. 3.9).

Short axis (SA) pilots

Using the VLA and HLA pilot images, acquire 3–5 short axis slices with the most basal slice parallel to the atrio-ventricular groove in both planes (Fig. 3.10). In a patient with distorted left ventricular geometry, it may be necessary to acquire up to 7–9 SA slices.

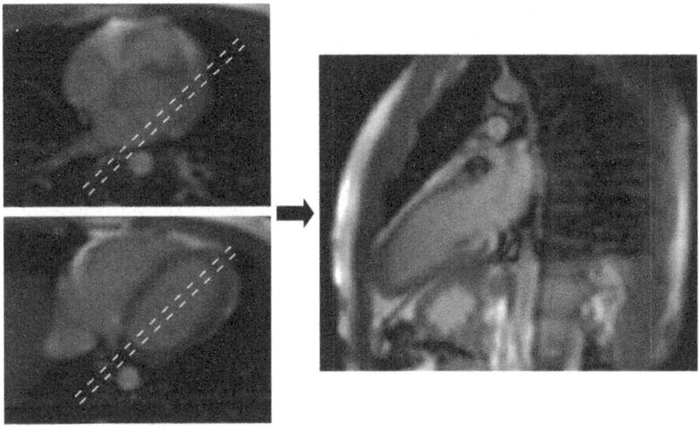

Fig. 3.8 Planning the vertical long axis (VLA) localizer image (right) from the transaxial localizer images (left).

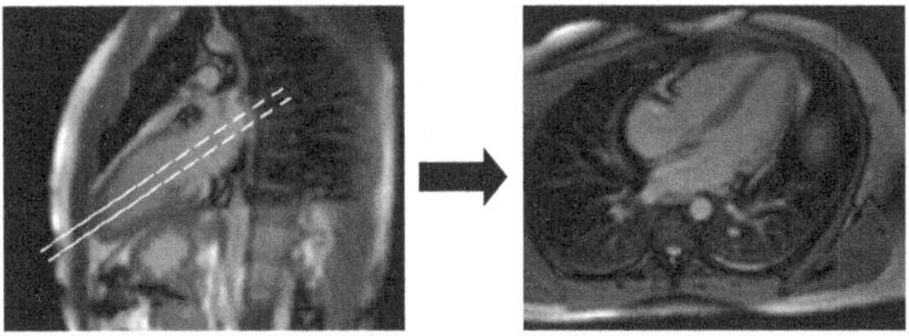

Fig. 3.9 Planning the HLA localizer (right) from the VLA localizer (left).

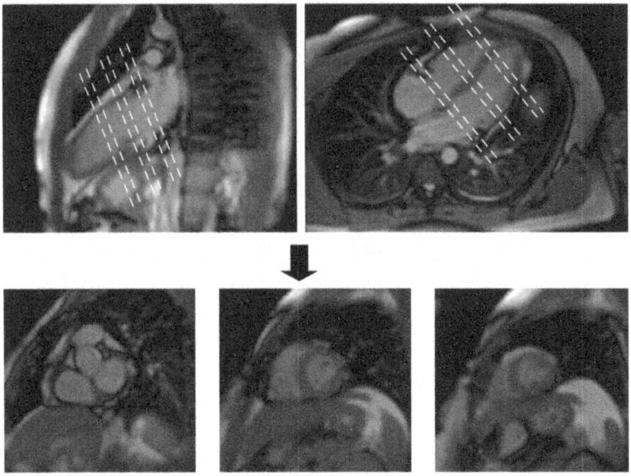

Fig. 3.10 Using the VLA (top left) and HLA (top right) localizers to plan the short axis localizer images (below). These should be positioned at the base along the atrioventricular (AV) groove, at the mid ventricular level and towards the apex.

Horizontal long axis view

- Using the SA pilots, choose a mid-ventricular image and position the slice through the maximum lateral dimensions of both ventricles, avoiding the left ventricular outflow tract (seen on the basal SA image).
- The image should pass through the middle of the mitral valve and the LV apex. If necessary, the VLA pilot image can be used to angle the slice towards the apex.
- Remember to concentrate on the LV long axis (the central axis of the LV) and resist attempting to include all of the atria.

Provides an assessment of:

- Overall atrial and ventricular size and function.
- Mitral and tricuspid valves.
- Regional wall motion – septum, lateral wall, and apex of the LV and free wall of the RV.

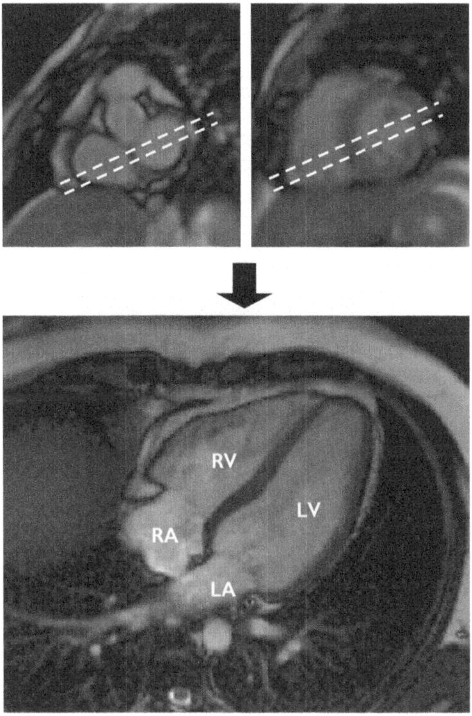

Fig. 3.11 Planning the HLA cine from the short axis localizer images. The VLA localizer can also be used to align the plane through the apex. RV, right ventricle; RA, right atrium; LV, left ventricle; LA, left atrium.

Vertical long axis view

- Using the SA pilots, position the slice through the maximum dimensions of the left ventricle, roughly parallel to the insertion points of the RV and aligned through the LV apex (Figs 3.12 and 3.13).
- Positioning can be checked using the HLA cine (end-diastolic frame).
- The plane is approximately 60–90° from the HLA.

Provides an assessment of:
- Left ventricle: anterior and inferior walls, and apex.
- Mitral valve.
- Left atrium.

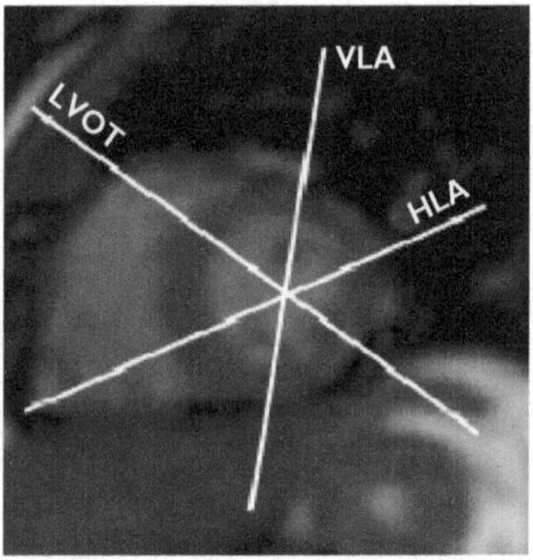

Fig. 3.12 Relative orientation of the three long axis, at ~60° to each other. LVOT, left ventricular outflow tract; VLA, vertical long axis; HLA, horizontal long axis.

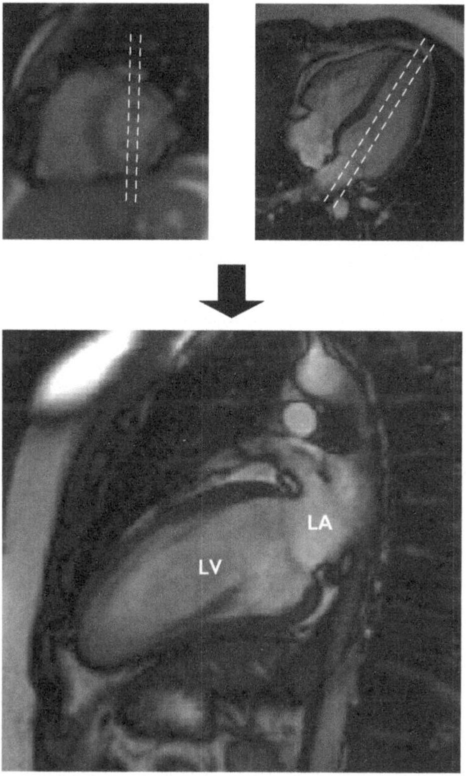

Fig. 3.13 Planning the VLA cine from the short axis localizer images. The HLA cine can be used to align the plane through the apex. LV, left ventricle; LA, left atrium.

Left ventricular outflow tract view

- Using the basal SA pilot, position the slice through the aortic valve and perpendicular to the lateral atrial/ventricular wall.
- This can be refined on a coronal image passing through the aortic root (if available). Angle the slice to pass through the proximal aorta.
- See Fig. 3.14.

Provides an assessment of:
- Left ventricle: septum, LVOT, posterior wall.
- Mitral valve.
- Aortic valve.
- Aortic root.

'Coronal' LVOT view

- An additional view orthogonal to the initial LVOT view can be useful in the assessment of patients with aortic valve or proximal aortic disease.
- The slice is positioned perpendicular to the LVOT cine, through the aortic valve and into the proximal ascending aorta.
- See Fig. 3.15.

Provides an assessment of:
- Aortic valve.
- Ascending aorta.

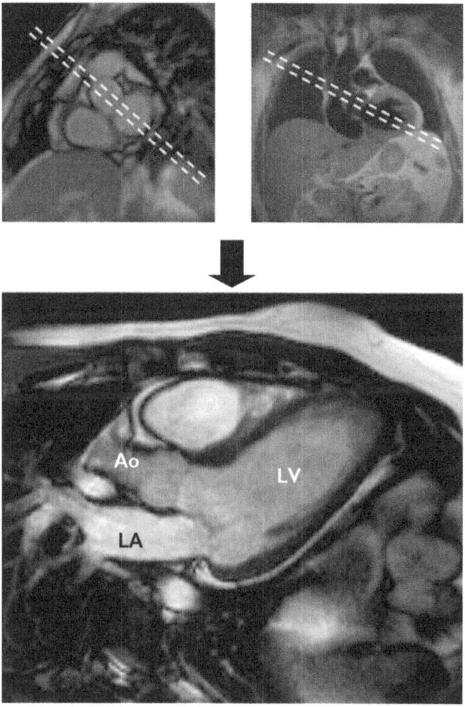

Fig. 3.14 Planning the LVOT cine from the basal short axis localizer image (top left), using a coronal HASTE image (top right) to refine orientation. LV, left ventricle; LA, left atrium; Ao, aorta.

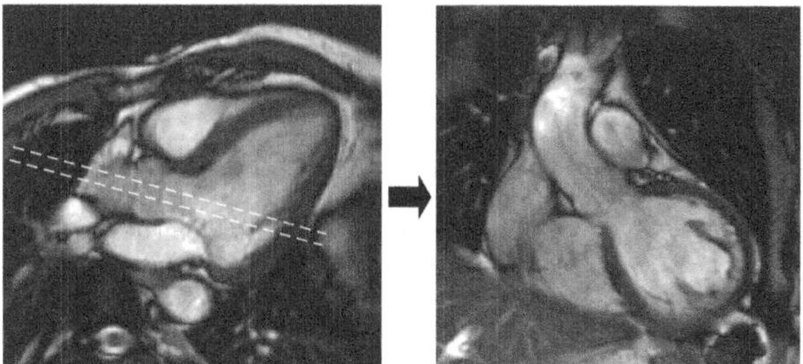

Fig. 3.15 Planning the coronal LVOT from the standard LVOT view (left), with the resulting image (right).

Short axis cine stack

- Using the diastolic frame from both the HLA and VLA cines, plan the first slice through the AV groove on both views, to lie at the base of the LV (Fig. 3.16).
- On the HLA view, the basal SA slice should pass from the left AV groove to the right AV groove, ignoring the septum/LVOT. The right coronary and circumflex arteries can often be seen in cross section.
- Parallel cines are then acquired until the whole ventricle has been covered, usually with the leading edges at 1cm intervals, e.g. a slice thickness of 7mm with a 3mm interslice gap, or 8mm slice thickness with a 2mm interslice gap (Fig. 3.16).

Basal slice positioning

This is crucial for accurate LV function measurements, and care must be taken in planning. Ideally, the first slice lies just within both ventricles in diastole (and in the atria in systole due to long axis contraction of the heart). This is the first slice to be included in LV analysis and should ideally have the entire circumference surrounded by ventricular myocardium in diastole (as a minimum, 50% of the circumference should be surrounded by ventricular myocardium).

If helpful, an additional slice just within the atria can be acquired, for comparison with the ventricular slices, and to help identify any partial volume effects (📖 p. 128).

What the stack provides

- Forms the basis for LV and RV volumetric, mass, and quantitative functional analysis that is a major component of CMR.
- Regional assessment of the entire circumference of the LV and RV in each slice (septum, anterior, lateral, and inferior walls of the LV) and free wall of the RV.

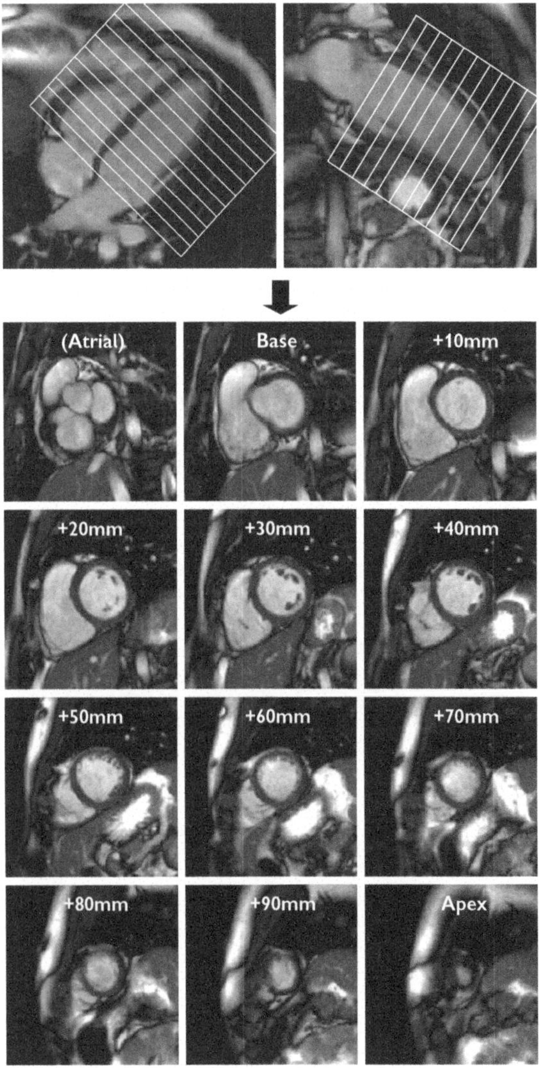

Fig. 3.16 Planning the short axis image stack from the HLA (top left) and VLA (top right) diastolic cine image frames. **NB.** The short axis image slices should extend to the edge of the thorax – they are shortened here for ease of visualization.

Right ventricular function

The RV is a complex shape, but is perhaps best thought of as a half cone lying parallel to the LV, with a long tubular outflow tract (infundibulum) lying anterior to the inlet (tricuspid valve). The complex shape requires specific views and quantitative function is virtually impossible to calculate without the full volumetric analysis possible with a CMR image stack.

Right ventricular views

- Horizontal long axis (as for LV function, 📖 p. 82).
- Right ventricular outflow tract (📖 p. 92).
- 'Horizontal' RVOT (📖 p. 92).
- RV 2-chamber view (📖 p. 94).
- RV 3-chamber view (📖 p. 94).
- Short axis stack.
- Transaxial cines.

Short axis cine stack

The same stack acquired for the LV can be used to quantify RV volumes.

Transaxial cines

The RV free wall is best visualized on standard transaxial cine images, as it lies roughly parallel to the anterior chest wall, and both long axis contraction and fine detail of regional function can be assessed.

The slice positions can be copied from the transverse anatomical images. Usually an image stack is imaged from the RVOT to the inferior wall of the RV at 1cm intervals (similarly to the short axis stack).

Right ventricular outflow tract view

- The slice is positioned perpendicular to the transverse multislice anatomical series (often a HASTE sequence). Align the slice through the main pulmonary artery, the narrowest point of the RVOT and into the RV (Fig. 3.17). This is usually an oblique sagittal view.
- The RVOT should be visible within the plane throughout the cardiac cycle. If it moves out of plane in systole, the image slice should be repositioned, usually by angulating the slice towards the apex, to allow for the significant long axis shortening of the RV. If this fails, the 'horizontal' RVOT cine can be used to fine-tune the position.

Provides an assessment of:

- Right ventricle: anterior free wall and outflow tract (infundibulum).
- Pulmonary valve.
- Proximal pulmonary artery.

'Horizontal' RVOT view

A second view, perpendicular to the standard RVOT can be helpful in further evaluating the pulmonary outflow tract (Fig. 3.18). This is helpful for visualizing most aspects of the outflow tract and for planning through-plane flow sequences perpendicular to the outflow tract (Pulmonary valve 📖 p. 268).

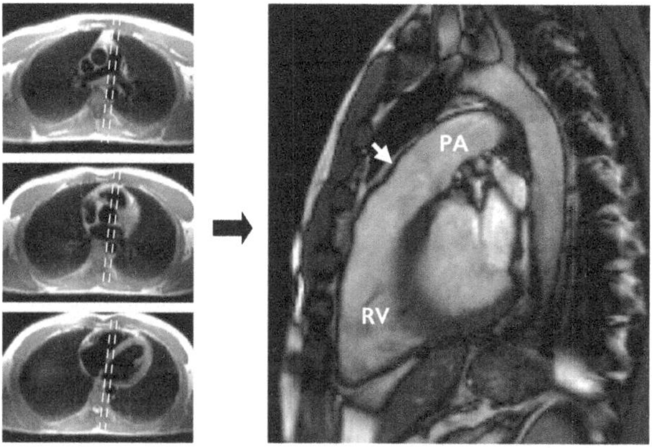

Fig. 3.17 Planning the RVOT view (right) from multiple transaxial HASTE images (left). The right ventricle (RV) and pulmonary artery (PA) can be visualized well, though the pulmonary valve is often difficult to see in still frames (the base of the annulus is arrowed).

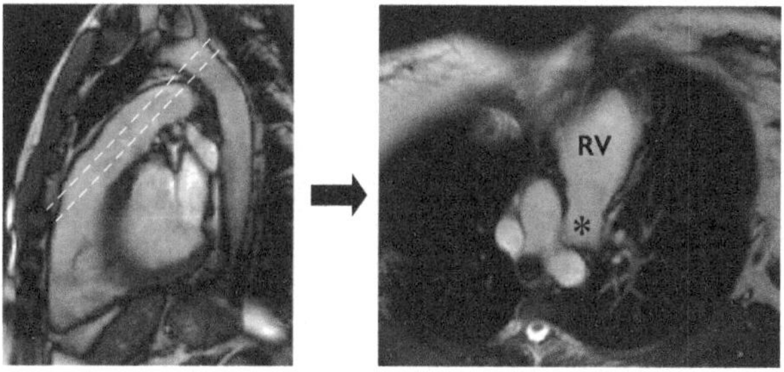

Fig. 3.18 Planning the 'horizontal' RVOT image (right) from the standard RVOT image (left). The right ventricle (RV) infundibulum can be seen, and the proximal pulmonary trunk (*).

Right ventricular 2-chamber view

This is planned from the HLA cine and positioned through the right atrium, tricuspid valve and right ventricle, almost parallel to the septum (Fig. 3.19). It may be useful to include a systolic frame in planning, due to septal motion in the cardiac cycle.

Provides an assessment of:

- Right atrium.
- Right ventricle (anterior and inferior walls).
- Tricuspid valve.

Right ventricular 3-chamber view ('inflow-outflow' view)

This can visualize both inflow and outflow tracts and is useful in suspected RV pathology (e.g. Arrhythmogenic right ventricular cardiomyopathy, 📖 p. 184) and congenital heart disease (Chapter 12, 📖 p. 309). It can be planned from the transverse anatomical images using the tricuspid valve, right atrium and ventricle and SVC (Fig. 3.20).

Provides an assessment of:

- Right atrium (and SVC sometimes).
- Tricuspid valve.
- Right ventricle – body and infundibulum.
- Pulmonary valve.

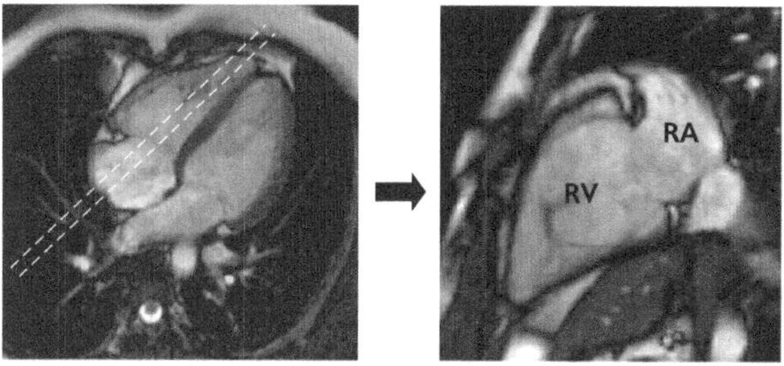

Fig. 3.19 Planning the RV 2-chamber view (right) from the HLA cine (left).

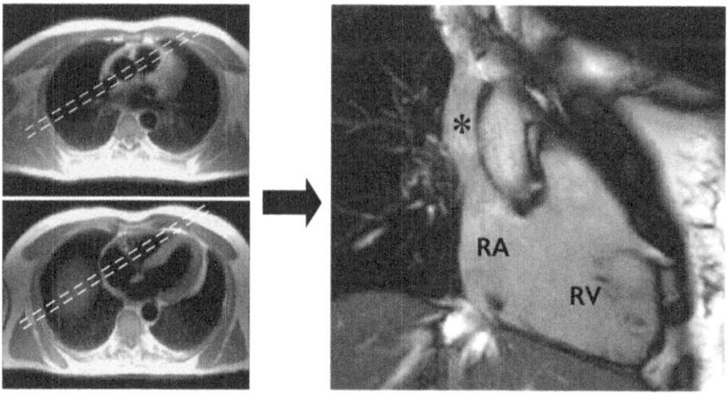

Fig. 3.20 Planning the RV 3-chamber view (right) form the transverse HASTE images (left). The plane through the SVC in addition to the right atrium (RA) and ventricle (RV).

Planning an unusual image plane

A unique advantage of CMR is the ability to acquire images in infinite orientations. Standard image planes are described earlier in this chapter, and specific advice is given in later chapters where relevant, but unusual image planes are sometimes required to visualize specific structures. They are especially useful for unusual anatomy, tortuous vessels, anomalous connections, or surgical conduits (e.g. in congenital heart disease).

Options for image positioning

Use an existing image plane

An existing plane can be used to plan a subsequent perpendicular image, positioned through the area of interest (the standard approach to image positioning). This can be repeated multiple times if necessary, using the new image plane each time, to plan the next image.

Three point planning tool

This is available on many systems and involves defining a unique plane by placing three points on existing images. The points can be placed on any image and can be a powerful tool for unusual slice positioning. A common use of this technique is to place the 3 points on multiple images along the path of a conduit or outflow tract (Fig. 3.21). Experience is required for optimal use of the technique.

Real-time inter-active planning

This technique, available on some systems, allows the operator to continuously acquire data, while manipulating the imaging plane, which can also be stored and used for further planning. It requires good anatomical knowledge, but can be time saving.

3D imaging

A 3D image can be acquired covering the volume of interest. On some systems, multi-planar reconstruction can be performed, generating the slice of interest in the desired orientation, which can be used for planning of subsequent slices.

Avoiding partial volume effects

When imaging thin structures (e.g. the atrial septum or an aortic dissection flap), the image plane should be planned perpendicular to the structure. This maximizes the in-plane resolution to produce crisper images with greater image contrast between the structure and surrounding anatomy, and minimizes partial volume effects (Fig. 3.22).

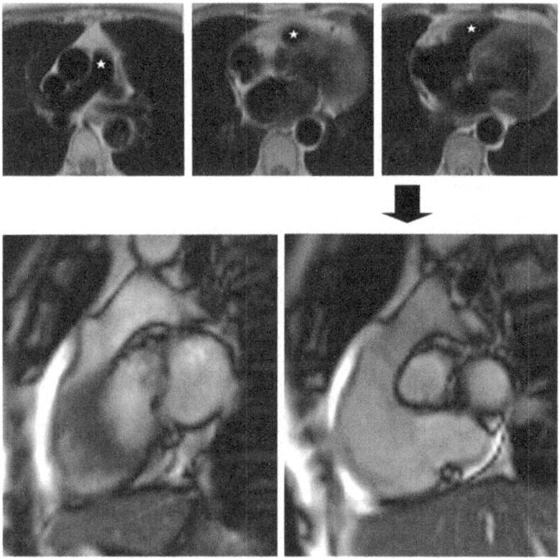

Fig. 3.21 3-point planning. The oblique sagittal RVOT (bottom left) had poor views of the infundibulum, so 3-point image plane positioning was used: the three transaxial HASTE images at the top show the position of the 3 points (stars) used to define the image plane, in the proximal pulmonary artery (left), the infundibulum (middle) and the mid-RV (right). The resulting RVOT view is shown bottom right.

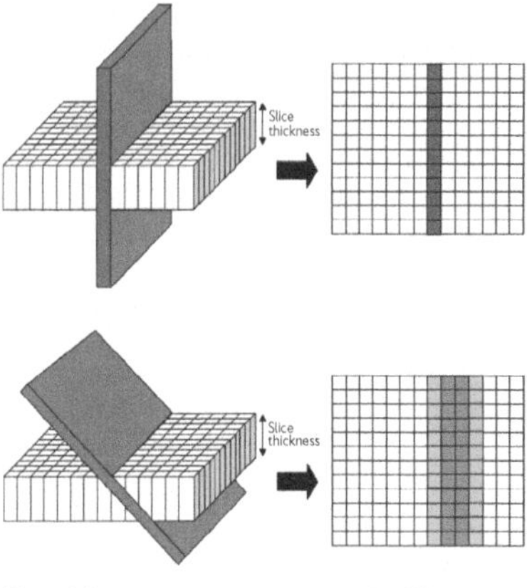

Fig. 3.22 The effect of slice orientation on image quality. The representative image slice at the top is perpendicular to the thin grey wall (left), so that the rectangular voxels are parallel to the wall and maximize the effect of in-plane resolution, with a resulting crisp image (right). The image slice at the bottom is at an oblique angle to the thin wall (left), with the signal from the wall spread over several voxels, producing a partial volume effect and resulting in a blurred, lower intensity image (right).

Tissue characterization sequences

One of the advantages of CMR is the ability to exploit different MR characteristics of different tissues to visualize the different tissue types (see 📖 p. 18 for more information on the different sequences). Examples include:

- High-resolution T_1 and T_2-weighted turbo spin echo (TSE).
- Fat suppression pulses (usually used with TSE sequences).
- Inversion recovery.

Optimizing turbo spin echo sequences

ECG gating

T_1-weighted images are acquired every cardiac cycle ('trigger 1') and T_2-weighted images, every other cardiac cycle ('trigger 2') to obtain the longer TR necessary for adequate T_2-weighting.

Echo time (TE)

The echo time of the T_2-weighted sequence needs to be longer (around 70–110ms) compared to the T_1-weighted sequence.

Repetition time (TR)

Obtaining good T_1 and T_2 images is heavily dependent on the R-R interval, determined by the patient's heart rate. Ideally, the TR should finish in mid–late diastole when cardiac motion is least and the heart has returned to its baseline position. If the TR is too short, the myocardium has not returned to the same position as when the black-blood pulses were applied at the R wave, and there is little signal from the myocardium. With an optimal TR, the myocardium is mid-grey and the blood pool black, with good definition at the endocardial border. If the TR is too long, the blood pool appears grey and the myocardial/blood pool border may be indistinct. It may be necessary to acquire several images with different TR's to determine the best contrast between myocardium and blood pool (see Fig. 3.23 for examples).

Fat saturation

The high signal from fat on T_1- and T_2-weighted TSE sequences can be effectively 'removed' by a saturation pulse prior to data acquisition (📖 p. 22). This technique is specific for fat (which has a slightly different resonant frequency to water) and can be extremely useful in determining the nature of tissue (Fig. 3.24).

Gadolinium contrast

T_1-weighted images before and after the administration of gadolinium contrast may be helpful in determining the vascularity of any mass lesion. This is considered in more detail in Imaging with gadolinium contrast, 📖 p. 106.

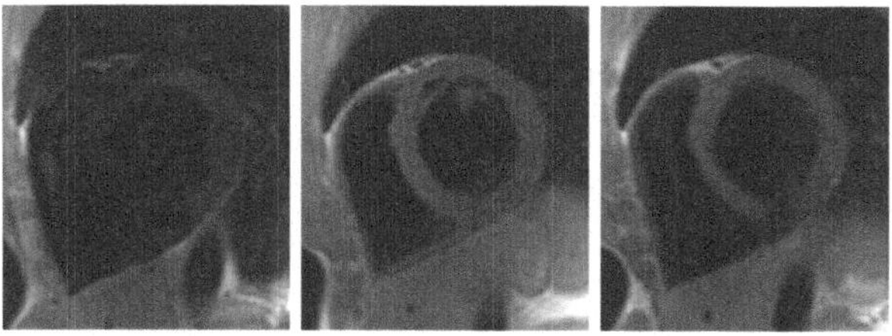

Fig. 3.23 A series of T_1-weighted TSE images demonstrating the optimum TR. Left: TR too short (note the absence of myocardial signal). Middle: Optimal TR. Right: TR too long (note the blurred myocardial borders due to movement).

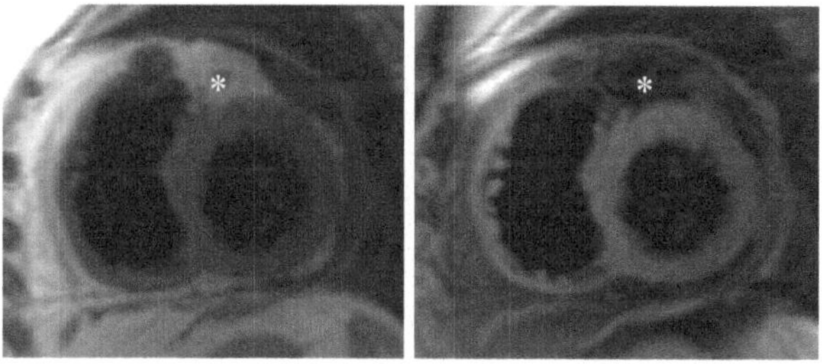

Fig. 3.24 T_1-weighted short axis TSE (left) showing high signal from significant pericardial fat, especially in the interventricular groove (*). Right: The same image with fat saturation, demonstrating the 'removal' of adipose tissue.

Flow imaging

CMR is able to measure tissue velocities, both through an image slice and within the slice in a single orientation. It is mostly applied to the flow of moving blood, and can be used to assess the severity of a stenotic valve or vessel, or by combining spatial information with through-plane velocity measurements, CMR has the unique ability to measure flow through a selected slice.

The physics of flow imaging: phase velocity mapping

The technique utilizes the properties of resonating protons as they move through a magnetic field gradient. Their phase changes relative to their position along the gradient, so faster moving protons will be in a phase further away from baseline than slower moving ones. When an equal and opposite (reverse) gradient is applied, static protons revert to their baseline 0° phase, but moving protons acquire a new phase proportional to their position along the gradient, which is determined by their velocity. The phase can be determined with phase-sensitive data collection, and the velocity can be determined from this using the gradient strength and the time interval between switching gradients.

Both velocity (*phase-encoded*) and anatomical (*magnitude-encoded*) information is acquired simultaneously, and displayed in separate images for each frame of the cine (Figs 3.25 and 3.28). The spatial resolution of the anatomical image is reduced, but still acceptable. The signal intensity on the phase image reflects the velocity.

In-plane velocity mapping

- Velocities can be measured along a single direction within an image plane, allowing visualization of a flow jet and the different velocities along its course (see 🕮 p. 140 for analysis).
- Choose the correct direction for velocity measurement within the plane (the options will be along either the x- or y-axis of the image plane) and rotate the image plane so the measured velocity direction is parallel to the desired jet/vessel.
- Can also be useful for positioning a through-plane flow slice at the peak velocity of a stenotic jet.

Partial volume effects

If a flow jet is narrow, the image slice (5–7mm thick) may contain voxels with both high velocity flow and surrounding lower velocity flow, resulting in an underestimate of the true velocity (Fig. 3.26). Through-plane flow mapping is better in this situation, as the in-plane image resolution (~1mm) is superior (Fig. 3.27). The in-plane flow could be used to position the through-plane slice at the point of highest velocity.

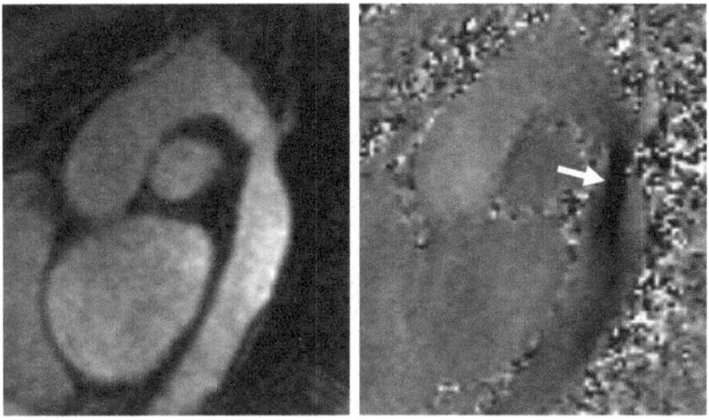

Fig. 3.25 In-plane flow mapping in a patient with coarctation, with the velocity direction aligned with the direction of flow. Magnitude image (left); flow image (right) showing the higher velocity jet arising from the coarctation (arrowed).

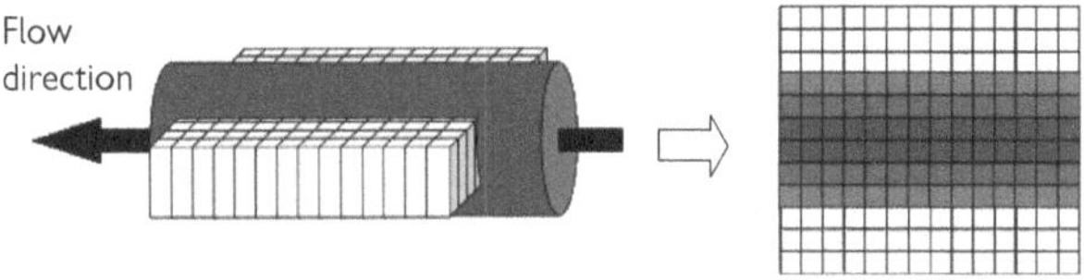

Fig. 3.26 Representation of in-plane velocity mapping. The long axis of the rectangular voxels is across the direction of flow, which can result in partial volume errors in small jets. The image obtained allows visualization of velocity along the whole path of the flow jet, although it does not allow flow quantification as the whole cross-sectional area is not covered.

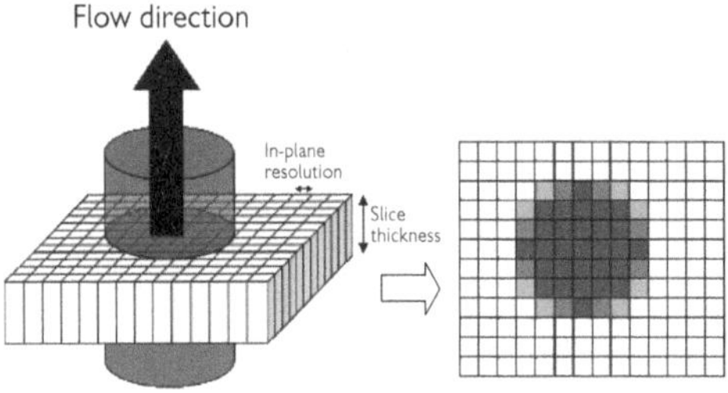

Fig. 3.27 Representation of through-plane velocity mapping. The long axis of the rectangular voxels is in the direction of flow, resulting in a higher spatial resolution across the flow jet and is also better for narrow jets. The full coverage of flow in the region of interest and good spatial resolution allows for flow quantification.

Through-plane velocity mapping

- Measures velocities through (perpendicular to) the slice of interest.
- High in-plane resolution is good for narrow jets.
- Doesn't visualize flow along the length of a jet, so careful positioning of the image slice is important, especially if peak velocity is required. If necessary, an in-plane flow sequence can show the location of the peak velocity for subsequent through-plane velocity mapping.
- It is important to be perpendicular to the flow jet for accurate measurement of velocity. If the jet is angulated relative to the direction of flow measurement, only the component of velocity in the flow direction is measured (i.e. the cosine of the true velocity), and errors can also occur due to partial volume effects.
- The imaging sequence can be either breath-hold or a longer sequence with free-breathing. The latter has superior temporal resolution, but the images are slightly more blurred. If breath-holding is likely to affect flow (e.g. if there are differences throughout the respiratory cycle), free-breathing sequences may be a better option.

Flow quantification

Flow through a slice can be measured by summing the velocities from all the pixels in a given region of interest, incorporating the cross sectional area (measured from the image), and integrating over the whole cardiac cycle. This provides the total flow volume per cardiac cycle (see 🕮 p. 136 for analysis techniques). Both forward and reverse flow can be measured, and the technique is typically applied to vessels (e.g. measurement of aortic and pulmonary flow in suspected cardiac shunts), and the quantification of valve regurgitation (🕮 p. 242, 260, 270).

Important limitations

Temporal resolution

The temporal resolution of velocity mapping is reasonable (typically 25–45ms), but may not be enough to capture the short time at the peak velocity of stenotic jets, so a slight underestimation is possible. By comparison, continuous wave Doppler echocardiography has a 10-fold higher temporal resolution and may be more accurate for measuring peak values in high velocity jets (e.g. aortic stenosis) *if* the correct beam alignment can be obtained. The advantage of CMR is the ability to align velocity measurement precisely with the direction of flow.

Phase shift errors

Flow quantification relies on a homogenous magnetic field and laminar (non-complex) flow. Several factors can affect these and cause phase shifts, introducing errors in velocity measurement:

- Field inhomogeneities and Eddy currents.
- High velocity jets (generally above 3.5–4m/s).
- Turbulent flow.

These are minimized by avoiding the measurement of highly turbulent flow, and ensuring the imaging plane is at the isocentre of the magnet (where field homogeneity is best and Eddy currents are minimized) – some scanners position the patient automatically.

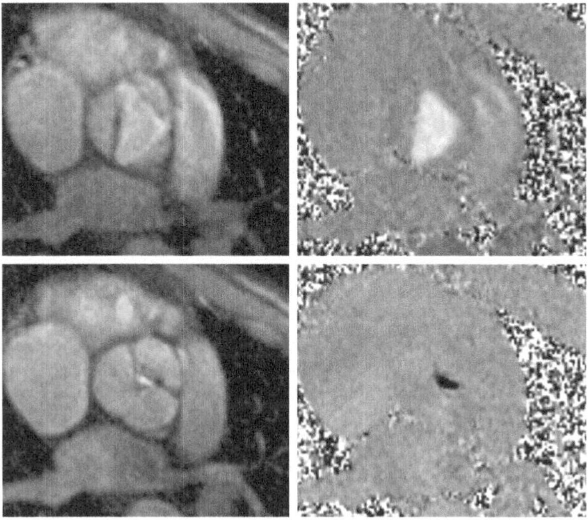

Fig. 3.28 Example of through-plane flow sequence in a patient with aortic regurgitation. (Top) Systole, with the open valve visible on the magnitude image (left), and forward flow visible in white on the flow image (right). (Bottom) Diastole, demonstrating the closed valve with failure of co-aption centrally on the magnitude image (left), and reverse flow in black on the flow image (right). On the flow images, note the mid-grey signal intensity from the static tissues, and intense 'noise' (multiple black and white specks) from the lung fields, due to the paucity of signal.

Arrhythmias

Very irregular rhythms (e.g. uncontrolled AF) reduce the accuracy of flow measurement. The sequences are acquired over several cardiac cycles (typically 10–12), and data is acquired in a complex manner and reconstructed based on the assumption of a regular rhythm. In subjects with an irregular rhythm, the complexity of the data acquisition means that, although acquired over several cardiac cycles, the flow is not averaged over these, as might be expected, and large variations in flow can occur.

Where beat-to-beat variability is low (e.g. AF with a controlled rate), these errors are usually not clinically significant. Very irregular rhythms (uncontrolled AF, multiple ventricular ectopics) can present a challenge, however. Intelligent timing of data acquisition to the ECG (📖 p. 54) can offset some of the problems, but this does not work for all patients and caution should be exercised in interpreting the flow data.

Specific arrhythmia sequences now exist (📖 p. 55), which ignore data from cardiac cycles with R-R intervals outside a specified range and can improve flow accuracy. Acquisition time is increased however due to the disregarding of some data.

Imaging with gadolinium contrast

Gadolinium-based contrast agents are used in 40–50% of all patients undergoing MRI, and up to 65% with CMR due to the high utility of gadolinium contrast in many areas, including perfusion imaging, visualization of intra-ventricular thrombus, determining myocardial viability, contrast-enhanced angiography, the assessment of cardiomyopathies, and characterization of tumours and masses.

There are a number of pharmacological preparations available (see Table 3.2). It should be noted, however, that not all products are licensed for cardiac use worldwide, e.g. gadolinium contrast is not currently licensed for cardiac imaging in the USA.

Safety

In general, gadolinium contrast agents are extremely safe, with a low incidence of adverse effects. The safety profile of the different preparations is similar, and the most common reactions are (~1% each):

- Nausea and vomiting.
- Headaches.
- Urticaria.

A myriad of other non-specific effects have been reported, although none are common and many are unproven. Cardiovascular symptoms have been reported, including:

- Hypo and hypertension.
- Vasodilatation.
- Tachycardia.
- ECG changes.

These may be difficult to determine, but the patient should be monitored closely for any signs of change in their clinical status.

Anaphylaxis

As with many intravenous medications, there is a very rare risk of a severe anaphylactic reaction (~1 in 100,000–500,000). Such reactions are commonly associated with a previous history of asthma or other respiratory problems and allergic drug reactions. It is, therefore, essential that emergency policies and procedures are in place, and that appropriate drugs and other resuscitation equipment are available.

Pregnancy and lactation

There are no reports of any harmful effects to either mother or foetus during pregnancy, though data is limited and a sensible precaution would be to avoid gadolinium contrast in pregnant women unless it is particularly important for diagnosis.

Gadolinium can be excreted in breast milk, but the amount is ~100-fold lower than concentrations routinely given during neonatal MR scanning. Manufacturers recommend abstaining from lactation for 24 hours after gadolinium administration, though some may regard this as not essential given the very low amounts excreted. A pragmatic approach may be to discuss it with the patient and explain that no harm has been reported, but she may wish to avoid breast feeding for up to 24 h.

Table 3.2 Gadolinium compounds

Brand name	Generic name	Charge	Concentration	Elimination	Protein binding (= remains intravascular)
Omniscan (GE Healthcare)	Gadodiamide	Non-ionic	0.5mmol/ml	Kidney	Nil
OptiMARK (Mallinkrodt)	Gadoversetamide	Non-ionic	0.5mmol/ml	Kidney	Nil
Magnevist (Bayer Schering)	Gadopentetic acid	Ionic	0.5mmol/ml	Kidney	Nil
Multihance (Bracco)	Gadobenic acid	Ionic	0.5mmol/ml	97% Kidney; 3% liver	<5%
Vasovist (Bayer Schering)	Gadofosveset	Ionic	0.25mmol/ml	91% Kidney; 9% liver	>85%
ProHance (Bracco)	Gadoteridol	Non-ionic	0.5mmol/ml	Kidney	Nil
Gadovist (Bayer Schering)	Gadobutrol	Non-ionic	1.0mmol/ml	Kidney	Nil
Dotarem (Guerbet)	Gadoteric acid	Ionic	0.5mmol/ml	Kidney	Nil

Nephrogenic systemic fibrosis

Nephrogenic systemic fibrosis (NSF) was described as an independent disease in 2000, having been first termed nephrogenic systemic dermopathy in 1997. It is a systemic disease involving fibrosis, and contracture of the skin and internal organs (although not the kidneys!), sometimes with severe consequences.

In 2006, a link was established between the development of NSF and prior administration of gadolinium contrast in a small number of patients with severely reduced renal function [glomerular filtration rate (GFR) <30ml/min]. The contrast was given up to many years prior to the development of the condition. The proportion of patients who develop NSF is unknown, but to date a few hundred cases worldwide have been reported, which represents a very small proportion of the total receiving gadolinium contrast (~100 million). The best estimate in the highest risk group (those with end-stage renal failure) is a 1–2% lifetime risk of NSF (based on a single study), although the risk is unknown for patients with less severe degrees of renal dysfunction. No reports of NSF have occurred in patients with a GFR >30ml/min.

The condition has led to caution in the use of gadolinium contrast in patients with significantly reduced renal function, although practice is not uniform. Patients referred for CMR may have an increased risk of renal disease (age >65 years, hypertension, diabetes) and operators should be aware of the issues. Local policies and procedures should be devised and followed.

A suggested practical guide

All patients who require gadolinium contrast should be screened for renal dysfunction, especially if >65 years. This usually involves obtaining a serum creatinine measurement and calculating the estimated glomerular filtration rate (eGFR) using either the Cockroft and Gault, or modification of diet in renal disease (MDRD) formula. On-line calculators are available, e.g. http:/nephron.com/cgi-bin/CGSI.cg ☞.

- **GFR >60:** no limitation to gadolinium contrast.
- **GFR 30–60:** gadolinium contrast can be given if the clinical indication outweighs the theoretical risk (no cases of NSF have been reported in this group) – gadolinium is usually appropriate, although it is wise to inform the patient of the potential risks and obtain their consent.
- **GFR <30:** a strict individual risk/benefit analysis needs to be made, assessing the diagnostic information the gadolinium may provide against the small risk of NSF. Patients should be made aware of the risks, and consent obtained. Contrast should only be given if benefit >> risk.

Available guidelines on nephrogenic systemic fibrosis

The Royal College of Radiologists (UK). Available at: ☞ www.rcr.ac.uk/docs/radiology/pdf/bfcr0714_gadolinium_nsf_guidancenov07.pdf

Medicines and Healthcare products Regulatory Authority (MHRA) – UK. Available at: ☞ www.mhra.gov.uk

Food and Drug Administration (FDA) – USA. Available at: ☞ www.fda.gov

European Agency for the Evaluation of Medicinal Products (EMEA). Available at: ☞ www.emea.europa.eu

Tissue characterization post-contrast

Post-contrast imaging adds significantly to myocardial tissue characterization, a major strength of CMR.

Gadolinium shortens the T_1 of tissues, and T_1-weighted TSE sequences can be used pre- and early post-gadolinium to characterize contrast uptake of the tissues (see 📖 p. 194 for use in myocardial inflammation and 📖 p. 218 for use in tumours/masses.

The most useful technique for characterizing the myocardium is late gadolinium enhancement. This involves imaging 10-20 minutes post gadolinium administration, when the contrast has washed out of the normal myocardium, but persists in any expanded interstitial space, which can occur in several disease processes, e.g. infarction, fibrosis, inflammation. A full account of the technical aspects of the method can be found in Chapter 1, 📖 p. 20 and details of the pattern in different diseases is found in the relevant chapters (though see Fig. 3.29 for a general guide). This section will focus on techniques for optimizing image acquisition.

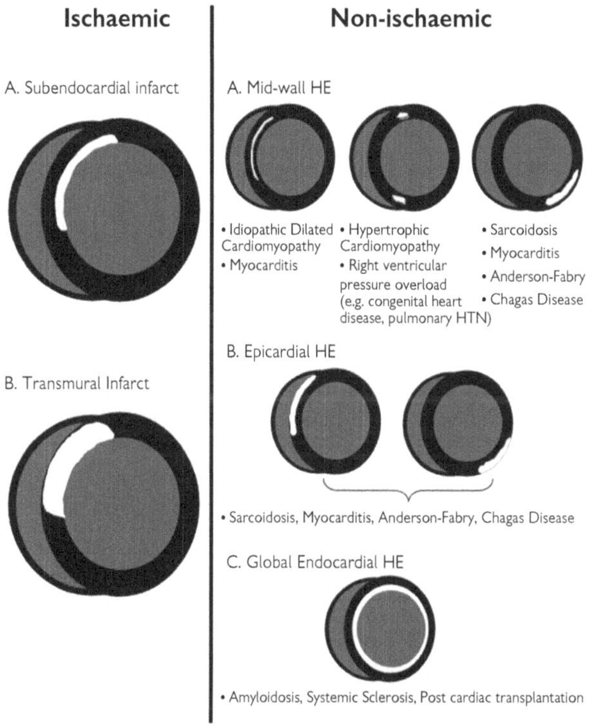

Fig. 3.29 Examples of delayed hyperenhancement patterns. Ischaemic damage (infarction, left side) always involves endocardial enhancement while mid-wall or epicardial enhancement suggests a non-ischaemic aetiology (right side). Reproduced from Shah *et al.* in: Edelman RR *et al.* (2005) *Clinical Magnetic Resonance Imaging*, 3rd edition, New York: Elsevier Press, copyright 2005, with permission of Elsevier.

Late gadolinium enhancement

General scanning technique

- Administer IV bolus of 0.1-0.2mmol/kg gadolinium.
- Consider early gadolinium enhancement imaging under 2min, if thrombus detection is required.
- Allow ~10min from gadolinium administration before delayed imaging to allow the contrast to wash out of the normal myocardium and distribute into the interstitial space. The time can be used for flow imaging, or LV function imaging if maximal time efficiency is required.
- Perform late gadolinium enhancement (LGE) imaging using an inversion recovery sequence, with the same LV slice positions as the cine images. Normal myocardium should be 'nulled' or black, and areas of persistent gadolinium should be bright or 'enhanced'.

Early gadolinium enhancement

To identify LV thrombus, image as soon as possible (max. 2min) after gadolinium administration, using the same inversion recovery technique, but with a long inversion time (450–500ms). Both blood pool and myocardium will be moderately bright, but thrombus has no contrast uptake and thus appears dark, allowing easy identification (Fig. 3.30). The LV long axis views are usually imaged, to ensure coverage of the apex.

Determining the optimal inversion time

Optimizing the inversion time is essential to obtain the best image contrast between normal myocardium, blood pool, and any areas of enhancement, and is the main technical challenge. If the TI is too short, the myocardial signal is not suitably 'nulled' and a 'white streak' effect occurs. If the TI is too long the myocardium appears grey (Fig. 3.31). In both cases, the amount of true enhancement may be unclear, leading to both over and under-estimation. A number of aspects affect the TI.

Contrast dose

A standard dose is 0.1mmol/kg; higher doses shorten the T_1 to a greater extent and require a shorter TI.

Time from injection

As gadolinium gradually washes out (and T_1 shortening is diminished), the inversion time needs to be increased to maintain optimal image quality. A general guide is to estimate the likely TI required and adjust accordingly to ensure good nulling of the normal myocardium. Once the optimal TI is determined, the rate of increase in TI is ~10–15ms/min.

- A typical inversion time would be ~300ms at 8–10min post-contrast dose of 0.1mmol/kg, using a turbo-FLASH sequence. Earlier imaging requires a shorter TI; later imaging requires a longer TI.
- Phase-sensitive sequences are much less inversion-time dependent.

Helpful sequences

Some sequences help determine the correct TI (e.g. TI scout or Look locker). A series of images are acquired with a range of TI's and the optimum time can then be applied (Fig. 3.32).

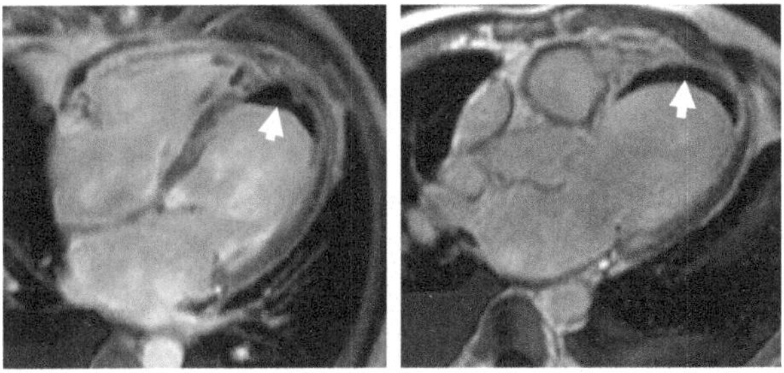

Fig. 3.30 Early gadolinium imaging – inversion recovery sequence in the HLA (left) and LVOT (right) views at 1min, with an inversion time of 450ms. There is a large thrombus at the apex and extending onto the septal wall (arrows), easily identified by its very low signal in contrast to the adjacent myocardium and blood pool, both with intermediate-high signal.

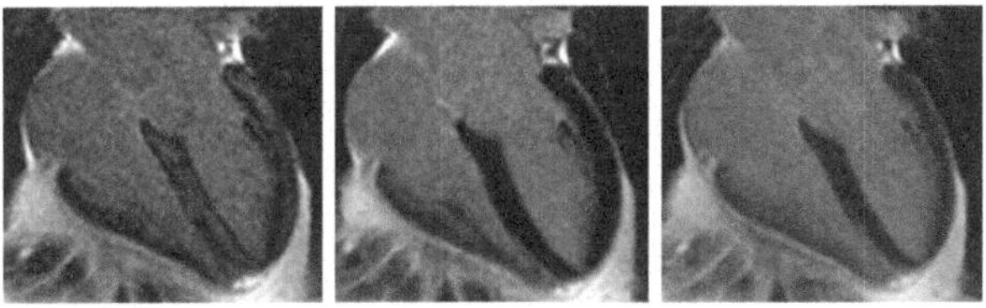

Fig. 3.31 A series of late gadolinium enhancement images in the HLA view with different inversion times. (A) The TI is too short; note the 'white streak effect' within the myocardium. (B) Correct TI. (C) The TI is too long and the myocardium appears grey, due to increasing signal as the myocardium is past its null point.

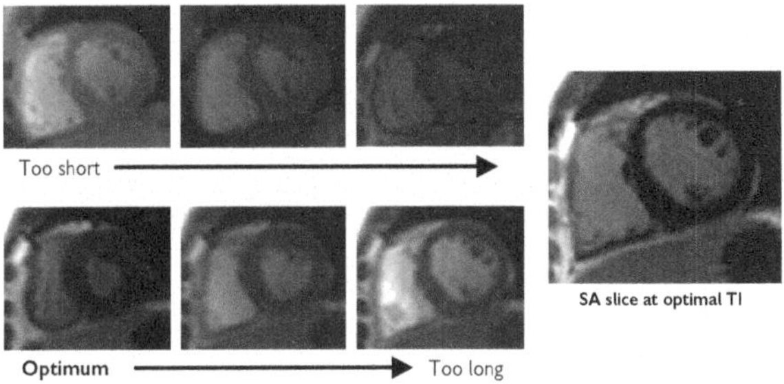

Fig. 3.32 A series of TI scout images to determine the optimum inversion time for late gadolinium imaging. Each frame is at a different inversion time (and also a different time in the cardiac cycle, hence the apparent change in myocardial thickness). On the right is a short axis image acquired at the optimum TI. The myocardium is nulled (black) with the blood pool grey; no areas of enhancement are seen.

Choice of sequence

There are several different sequence for LGE.

Segmented inversion recovery fast gradient-echo

The most commonly used and provides good quality images. Tends to be more sensitive to an incorrect TI.

Turbo-FLASH phase sensitive inversion recovery (PSIR)

Less dependent on a precise TI and can be valuable for easy imaging (Fig. 3.33). It may not be necessary to increase the TI during imaging.

Single-shot SSFP or Turbo-FLASH sequence

A rapid sequence that can be used with free-breathing, so good for patients with difficulty breath-holding (Fig. 3.34). An alternative is to use parallel imaging techniques to speed up imaging.

Avoiding artefacts

Artefacts are common with LGE and care should be taken with any small areas of enhancement to differentiate between artefact and true pathology. Consider:

- Repeating the same slice position with the phase encode direction swapped (e.g. from AP to head foot). Artefacts often occur in the phase-encode direction, so if the area of enhancement is still present with a different phase-encode direction, it is likely to represent true enhancement (Fig. 3.35).
- Repeating the same slice with a different LGE sequence. If real, the enhancement should be persistent.
- Planning a second plane perpendicular to the current one, cutting through the area of enhancement. This can also help define the extent of the enhancement in a different plane (Fig. 3.36).

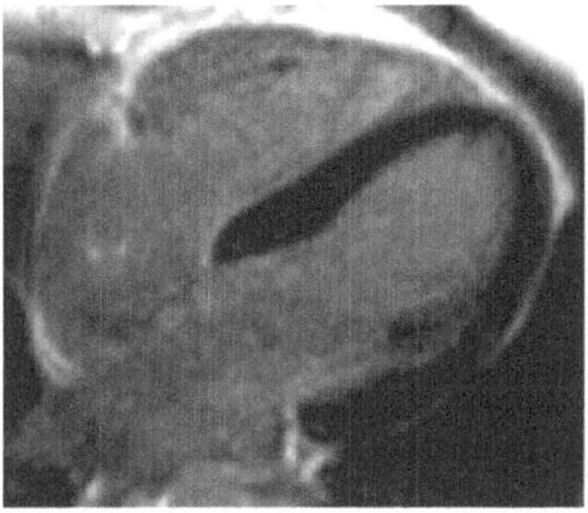

Fig. 3.33 Late gadolinium imaging in the HLA view, with a phase sensitive (turbo flash inversion recovery) sequence, 10min post-injection of 0.1mmol/kg gadolinium with an inversion time of 300ms.

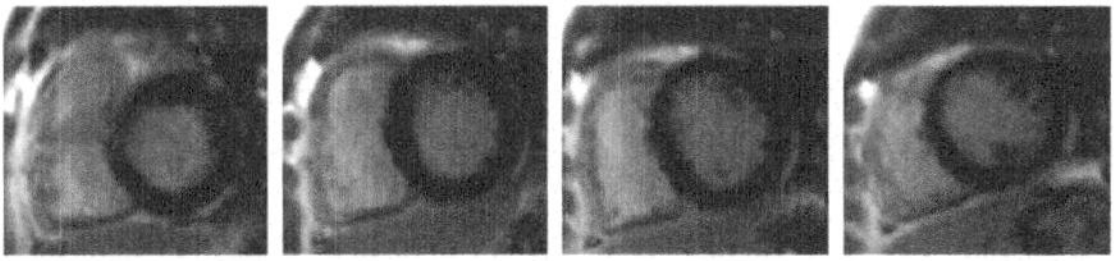

Fig. 3.34 A series of shorts axis images from a single shot SSFP sequence. 10min post-0.1mmol/kg gadolinium with an inversion time of 360ms; non-breath hold.

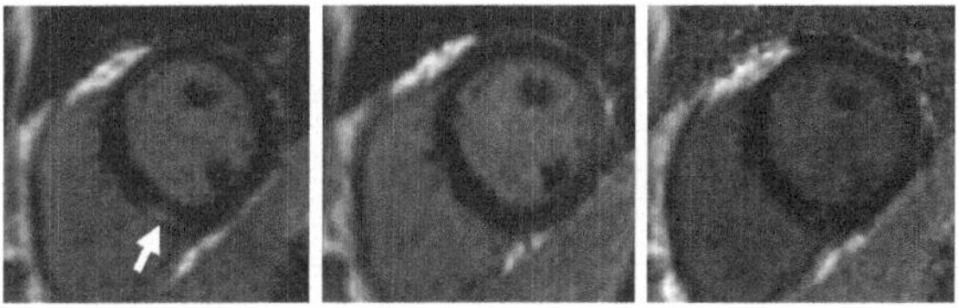

Fig. 3.35 Short axis turbo-FLASH LGE image with a small area of enhancement at the inferior LV/RV junction (left, arrowed). The same slice is shown with the phase-encode direction swapped (middle) and with a phase-sensitive sequence (right); the area of enhancement has disappeared in both additional images, indicating artefact.

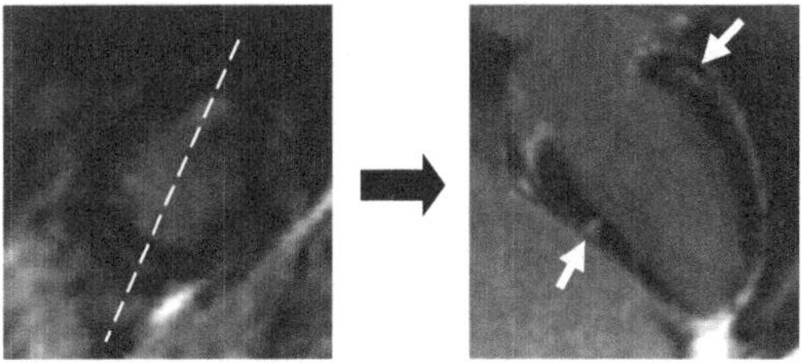

Fig. 3.36 Small areas of enhancement on a SA view (left) are confirmed with a modified VLA view passing through the relevant areas (right, arrows). The patient had sarcoidosis, and the scan confirmed cardiac involvement.

Contrast-enhanced magnetic resonance angiography

Contrast-enhanced MR angiography (CE-MRA) is invaluable for the assessment of many vessels, including aortic coarctation, pulmonary vein anatomy and congenital heart disease.

The principle is straightforward – a fast bolus of contrast (often 20ml) is administered, followed by a saline bolus (~20ml), and a large image volume containing the area of interest is acquired as the contrast passes through. The main challenge is determining the optimum time between contrast injection and data acquisition. Acquire too early and the contrast has not arrived in the vessel of interest (Fig. 3.38); too late and the contrast has already passed through the region and re-circulation of the contrast dose may already have occurred. Both result in a poor contrast-to-noise ratio and reduced image quality.

The other major factor in obtaining good CE-MRA is the site of venous access and the size of cannula used. Ideally, a 19g cannula sited in the ante-cubital fossa should be used. This ensures that the contrast can be delivered at 5–6ml/s and the bolus is not unduly spread out with slower administration through a smaller peripheral vessel.

Orientation of the image plane is dependent on the vessel concerned – see relevant sections for more information. Processing of the data to generate 3D angiograms is covered on 📖 p. 142.

Methods to optimize timing

Automatic bolus detection

Acquisition is triggered when the contrast reaches the region of interest (detected by the increase in signal intensity). This may be difficult to combine with breath-hold techniques.

Fluoroscopic triggering

This method can be used in peripheral angiography where the transit time is a little longer, the injection rate slower (~2ml/s) and breath-hold is not required. The contrast injection is given and a dynamic series started simultaneously. When the contrast reaches the target vessel (e.g. aorta at the level of the renal arteries if the aorto-femoral, iliac, and tibial arteries are to be imaged) the angiogram sequence is manually started and a moving table technique may be used. See also Peripheral arteries, 📖 p. 394.

Test bolus (timing run)

A small amount of contrast (~2ml) is injected and a series of images is acquired at short intervals (e.g. every second) to determine the transit time to the vessel of interest. The time to maximum signal intensity in this vessel is noted, either on visual inspection or a time-intensity curve can be generated (see Fig. 3.37). The transit time is then used to calculate timing of the contrast injection and data acquisition. This is further complicated by needing to factor in the time for the operator to issue breath-hold instructions. Careful practice and good teamwork and communication are essential – see box Calculation of the timing for contrast angiography, 📖 p. 118.

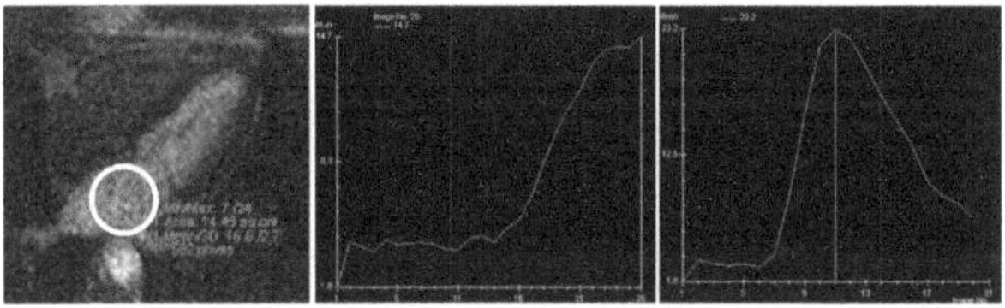

Fig. 3.37 (Left) dynamic timing run for a pulmonary venous angiogram with the region of interest drawn within the left atrium. (Middle) resulting time/signal intensity curve following injection in the dorsum of the hand. The upslope of the curve is shallow and the time to peak is difficult to determine. Maximum intensity had not been reached after 26s and the scan was stopped early. (Right) The cannula has been re-sited in the antecubital fossa, producing a brisk upstroke and clear peak intensity; the transit time shown is 11s. TR of the sequence is 1000ms (i.e. one image/s).

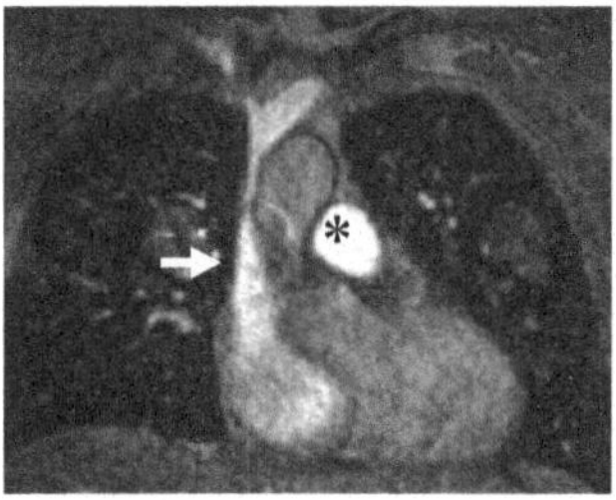

Fig. 3.38 Coronal slice from a pulmonary venous angiogram where the acquisition was too early. Contrast is still in the main pulmonary artery (*) and the SVC (arrow).

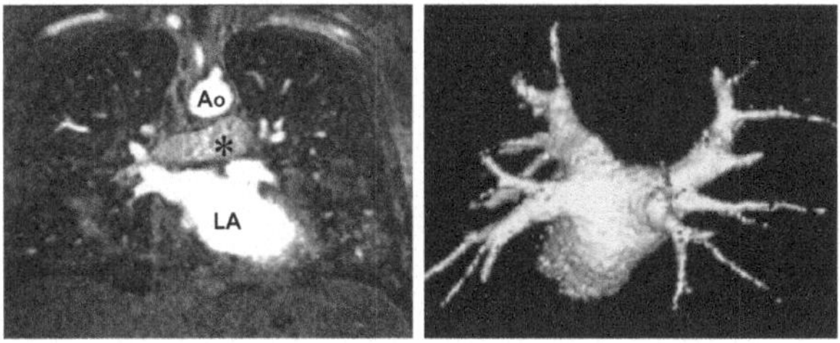

Fig. 3.39 Correct timing for a pulmonary venous angiogram – coronal view (left) with contrast in the left atrium (LA) and significantly reduced signal from the pulmonary artery (*); Ao = aortic arch. (Right) The resulting 3D reconstruction of the pulmonary veins.

Calculation of the timing for contrast angiography

Scan delay time (delay between injection and acquisition) =
transit time – time to central k-space + ½ contrast injection time

Example

- Transit time = 11s (determined as above).
- Time to central k-space = 7 seconds (defined by the sequence).
- 20ml contrast given at 5ml/s: time for injection = 4 s (4/2 = 2s).

Scan delay time is therefore (11 – 7) + 2 = 6s

In this case, the injection is given first and the acquisition started 6s later. If the transit time is very fast, e.g. in a patient with tachycardia, then the time may be a negative number and, therefore, the acquisition starts first and the injection given at the identified time afterwards.

Factoring in the breath-hold instruction time

The time it takes for the operator to give the breath-hold instruction can be determined during acquisition of the localizers, mask images, or timing run, but it is important to be consistent.

Example

If the operator takes 10s to instruct the patient, in the example shown above, the injection is started 4s after the start of the instructions and image acquisition started after a further 6s.

Some systems have the facility to enter a countdown time in the display, but the acquisition usually needs to be started manually.

Perfusion imaging

Myocardial perfusion can be assessed with CMR as a bolus of contrast passes through the myocardium ('first-pass perfusion'). This differs from nuclear cardiology methods (e.g. gated SPECT), which use the accumulation of radio-labelled tracer over a slightly longer time, with imaging performed a short while (several minutes) after the injection. With CMR, the myocardium is imaged both at rest and after pharmacological stimulation ('stress'). Physical exercise would be impractical in the MR environment. Several studies have shown excellent sensitivity (80–90%) and very good specificity (70–80%) for detecting myocardial ischaemia.

Mechanism of pharmacological stress

In CMR perfusion, the vasodilator adenosine is the most commonly used agent, due to its ultra-short half-life (<10s) and transient nature of the side effects. It produces near-maximal vasodilatation in normal coronary arteries, causing an increase in coronary blood flow 4–5 times above normal. In diseased arteries, resistance at the arteriolar level is already reduced in the resting state in order to maintain regional myocardial blood flow (i.e. coronary vasodilator reserve has been utilized), and minimal further increases in blood flow can occur. This results in relative hypoperfusion distal to a coronary stenosis.

Safety during perfusion imaging

The intravenous administration of vasoactive drugs requires extra care during scanning, particularly given the difficulties of the MR environment. It is recommended that at least 2 experienced operators are present, one of whom should be a physician. In addition, the following should be in place:

- Adequate monitoring equipment during scanning (BP, ECG, intercom).
- Emergency evacuation procedure for rapid removal of the patient from the magnet, with regular practice sessions.
- Emergency resuscitation policy and available equipment (incl. defibrillator and emergency drugs).
- Contraindications to the vasoactive drug should be known and checked beforehand (see box Agents used for pharmacological stress, 📖 p. 121).

Additional aspects during the scan

- Reassure the patient – maintain good communication via the intercom and ask about symptoms.
- Watch carefully for hypotension and bradycardia.

Agents used for pharmacological stress

Adenosine

- The most widely used for CMR perfusion.
- An endogenous nucleotide, with powerful vasodilator properties to most vascular beds, except for hepatic and renal arterioles.
- The effective half-life of <10s provides a high degree of control, as effects disappear rapidly after discontinuation.
- Products containing caffeine or other methylxanthines (coffee, tea, chocolate, theophylline) should be withheld for 24h before the scan.
- **Dose:** 140μg/kg/min for 3–6min.
- **Contraindications:**
  - High-grade (2nd or 3rd degree) AV block
  - Asthma or bronchoconstrictive disease
  - Sinus bradycardia
  - Systemic hypotension (BP <90mmHg).
- Side effects:
  - Transient heart block
  - Transient hypotension
  - Transient tachycardia
  - Bronchospasm.
- In the rare situation of persistent adenosine-related side effects, aminophylline reversal may be needed and should be available.

Dipyridamole

- An indirect vasodilator. It blocks cellular uptake of adenosine, increasing the endogenous levels of adenosine and causing vasodilatation.
- Its prolonged duration of action (~30min), makes it less controllable and, therefore, not ideal for perfusion CMR.
- Dose: 0.56mg/kg IV over 4 min.
- Similar to adenosine, patients need to avoid methylxanthine-containing products for 24h before the scan.
- Side effects can be countered with 50–100mg of aminophylline injected slowly over a period of 1min. Aminophylline injection may be repeated up to a total dose of 250mg.

Dobutamine (*p. 164*)

- Powerful positive inotropic agent, which mimics the effects of exercise. It increases heart rate and myocardial contractility.
- Its use is limited primarily for stress wall motion analysis (i.e. detection of inducible ischaemic wall motion defects) and viability studies, because the increased heart rate associated with dobutamine is problematic for perfusion CMR.

Patient preparation

Consent, contraindications and explanation of the procedure

- Avoid any products that interfere with adenosine for 24h prior to the scan:
  - Caffeine (e.g. coffee, tea, chocolate)
  - Drugs (e.g. xanthines, theophylline).
- Consent the patient and explain the procedure in detail, with particular emphasis on adenosine-related side-effects (e.g. flushing, chest pain, dyspnoea).
- Ensure the patient has no high-grade atrioventricular (AV) block (perform or request an ECG) or asthma, as these are the main contraindications to adenosine.

Set-up

- Connect two IV lines, ideally placed in both arms (antecubital veins). The first is for contrast (16–18G cannula) and the second for adenosine (18–20G cannula). This avoids injecting a bolus of adenosine when the contrast agent is delivered, which can lead to high-grade AV block.
- Place the blood pressure cuff on the arm with the contrast agent, to avoid interference with the administration of adenosine.
- Prepare an adenosine infusion pump outside the scanner room and connect to the patient by a long line (6–8m; volume of adenosine within the line itself is ~4.5–6ml). Set the rate to 140μg/kg/min.
- Prepare the contrast injector: contrast dose 0.05–0.1mmol/kg gadolinium (see box Dose of contrast, 📖 p. 123), rate 3–6ml/s, with a normal saline flush of 15–30ml.
- Place the O_2 saturation probe on the arm with the adenosine infusion.
- Ensure a good quality ECG tracing – this is essential for successful CMR perfusion and the signal is often degraded by the perfusion sequence.

Scanning protocol

Image preparation

- Choose the perfusion sequence (see box Perfusion sequences, 📖 p. 125).
- Identify suitable short-axis (SA) slice positions: aim for good coverage of the LV without being too close to the LVOT (check on the end-*systolic* long-axis views). Plan the basal slice ≥1cm below the LVOT to allow for the additional long axis motion during stress.
- Adjust the timing and number of images so that all SA slices are imaged every cardiac cycle during stress (i.e. allow for an increase in heart rate). Usually 3–4 SA slices can be imaged, but if this is not possible (e.g. tachycardia), you may need to reduce the number of slices.
- Run a test perfusion scan (with no contrast or adenosine) with 10–20 measurements to check ECG triggering and slice position. Wrap (fold-over) artefacts into the LV should be avoided.
- Measure baseline blood pressure.

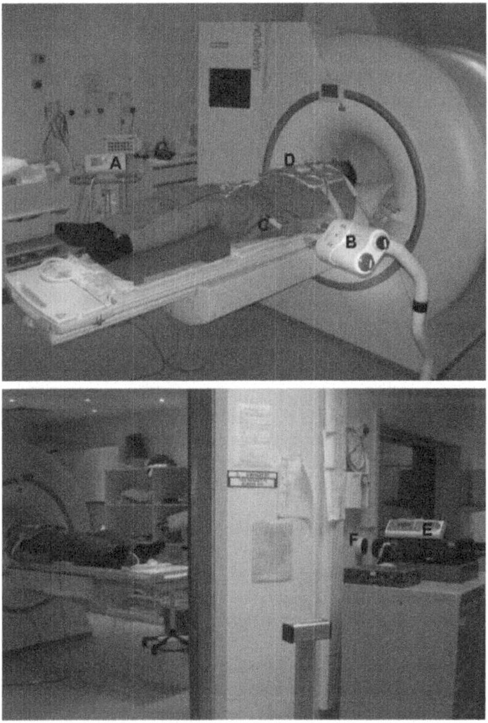

Fig. 3.40 Scanner set-up for stress perfusion CMR. Note (A) the blood pressure monitor unit, (B) the power injector for contrast administration, (C) the oxygen saturation probe, (D) the anterior coil, and (E) the syringe-pump for adenosine, which is situated outside the scanner room. A 6m line connects the driving syringe with the subject through the wave-guide (F) in the wall.

Dose of contrast

Qualitative (visual) assessment (📖 p.170)

The standard technique for clinical scans. A standard dose of 0.1mmol/kg gadolinium is used.

Quantitative assessment (📖 *p. 172*)

This relies on a linear relationship between contrast concentration and signal intensity, and requires a low contrast dose (<0.05mmol/kg). This is more difficult to achieve and is currently reserved for research studies.

Stress perfusion

- Copy the test perfusion sequence (to maintain any adjustments made), ensuring you have selected 40–60 measurements (40–60 heart beats).
- Inform the patient before starting the adenosine infusion, remind him/her of the potential adverse effects and provide reassurance.
- Start the adenosine infusion at a rate of 140μg/kg/min.
- After about 1min, most patients show a rise in heart rate of ~10–20bpm and feel the first adenosine-related symptoms. Maintain communication and provide reassurance.
- Check BP every minute during the infusion, and for at least 2min afterwards. A slight reduction (<15mmHg) is usual.
- Continue the infusion for 3–6min to ensure maximal vasodilatation.
- Discontinue the infusion earlier if:
    - Patient request (intolerant of side effects)
    - Persistent or symptomatic 3rd degree AV block
    - Severe hypotension (systolic BP <90mmHg)
    - Bronchospasm.
- When you are ready to scan, ensure the last BP reading has been successful and the BP cuff is not inflating when you inject the contrast.
- Instruct the patient to hold their breath for as long as they can and then to breathe shallowly until the end of the acquisition. Breath-holding can be at either inspiration or expiration, although ECG-triggering is often worse at end-inspiration.
- Start the scan and inject the contrast after 3 cardiac cycles, followed by the saline flush.
- Stop the adenosine infusion when the first pass of the contrast agent is completed (usually 20–25 beats after injection). Select an inline display to show the image as each is reconstructed.
- When the perfusion sequence is complete, reassure the patient that the symptoms will subside within 1–2min.
- Allow at least 10min for contrast wash-out before rest perfusion imaging. Other imaging can be acquired during this time – see 🕮 p. 175 for an efficient scan protocol.

Rest perfusion

- Rest perfusion is performed using the same sequence parameters and dose of contrast agent as for stress perfusion.
- Although it is a slightly longer scan (because of the lower heart rate at rest), patients find it easier to hold their breath as they do not experience the effects of adenosine.
- Following rest perfusion, late gadolinium enhancement imaging can be performed (🕮 p. 112). A top-up dose of gadolinium may be needed, depending on the total contrast dose and the time between stress and rest perfusion aim for 0.1–0.2mmol/kg).

Perfusion sequences

CMR perfusion sequences involve a series of T_1-weighted images that follow the dynamic passage of the contrast bolus through the heart. T_1-weighting is usually obtained using saturation recovery preparation pulses (📖 p. 22). The sequences need high temporal resolution to allow acquisition of at least 3 slices every heartbeat (for sufficient anatomic coverage), and need high spatial resolution to identify sub-endocardial defects (<3mm in-plane resolution).

Main perfusion sequences

Turbo-FLASH (gradient echo)

- The most commonly used sequence.
- Reduced image artefacts compared with the other two sequences.
- Can also be used for absolute quantification as it has been validated in animal experiments against blood flow measurements with labelled microspheres.
- Lower signal-to-noise ratio compared with SSFP.
- Benefits substantially from the higher signal-to-noise ratio at 3T. This improves the confidence of the reader and results in improved diagnostic accuracy at 3T compared with 1.5T.

SSFP

- Higher signal-to-noise ratio (improved contrast enhancement).
- More susceptible to artefacts, particularly at 3T.

Hybrid echo-planar (gradient echo-EPI or hybrid EPI).

- Potential for high temporal resolution, as echo-planar sequences involve the acquisition of several K-space lines following a single RF excitation.
- Fewer artefacts compared with SSFP.
- However, lower contrast to noise ratio.

Further reading

Kellman P, Arai AE. Imaging sequences for first pass perfusion – a review. *J Cardiovasc Magn Reson* 2007; **9:** 539–47.

Chapter 4

Image processing

Ventricular volumes and function

A major strength of CMR is the accurate and reproducible measurement of ventricular volumes, mass and function, and it is widely regarded as the 'gold standard' for these measurements. Analysis is based on a stack of 2D contiguous short axis cine datasets, encompassing both ventricles from base to apex (📖 p. 88 for acquisition). Volumes are calculated using Simpson's or the rectangle rule (see Fig. 4.1), with mass determined from the end-diastolic images by multiplying myocardial volume by its specific density (1.05g/cm^3).

Image analysis is usually performed off-line using a variety of commercial software. For an experienced operator, post-processing time is ~15min, depending on image quality and the software used.

► The basal slice is crucially important for accurate analysis – inclusion/exclusion of a slice makes a large difference to the volume and is the main source of error. Good slice positioning during image acquisition is important and avoids problems (Fig. 4.2), making processing easier.

General steps in manual processing

- Define end-diastole (this is usually the first phase) and end-systole (phase with the smallest cavity).
- Define the basal ventricular slice for both end-diastole and end-systole (see below). The latest processing software significantly aids this by allowing identification of the mitral and tricuspid valve positions on long axis images to automatically separate atrial from ventricular slices.
- Draw the endocardial and epicardial borders on the short axis slices at end-diastole, and the endocardial borders at end-systole (see Fig. 4.3).
- The software usually calculates the volumes ± mass automatically by summing the areas from each slice.

LV volume/mass analysis: the basal slice

- A general 'rule of thumb' is that all ventricular slices are surrounded by a rim of thicker ventricular myocardium (see Fig. 4.2A). Slices in which <50% of the circumference is surrounded by ventricular myocardium are likely to be predominantly atrial and can be excluded.
- Compare the first (end-diastolic) image with subsequent systolic frames. The ventricle initially decreases in size and longitudinal contraction pulls the atrium into the imaging plane. A change in shape, decreasing wall thickness and/or increasing chamber size may be seen (Fig. 4.4). The atrium enlarges during ventricular systole (*atrial* diastole).
- Compare the basal slice in question with the slices above and below. Is there a change in wall thickness or chamber size? Is there contiguous endocardium?
- The basal slice at end-systole is usually 1–2 slices more apical than at end-diastole, due to the longitudinal movement of the base towards the apex (assuming normal LV function). The degree of movement diminishes with decreasing LV function.
- The epicardial border can be difficult in the anterior and lateral walls, adjacent to the lung. Optimizing the image contrast and viewing the cine loop is helpful.

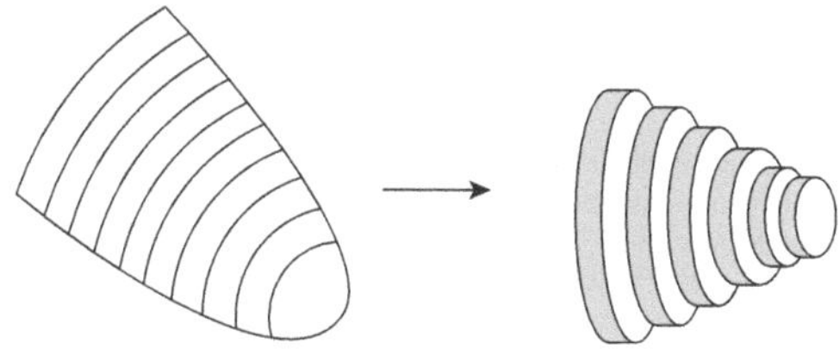

Fig. 4.1 Left ventricular volume calculation by Simpson's rule, summing the endocardial area measured from each slice, multiplied by the inter-slice distance.

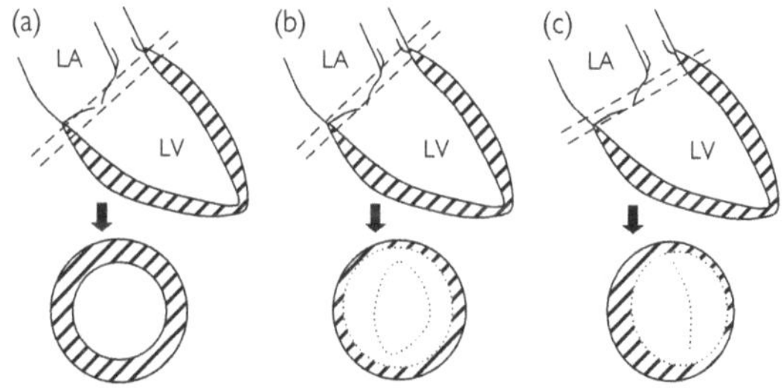

Fig. 4.2 Basal slice positioning in the LV. (A) correct position of the basal image slice (dashed parallel lines) with subsequent circular ventricular image with clear border definition. (B) Basal slice mid-way between the ventricle and atrium, with the resulting image showing partial volume effects from the thick image slice. Note the less distinct endocardial border, larger cavity, and wall thicknesses mid-way between atrium and ventricle. The mitral leaflets can sometimes be seen in faint outline. (C) Skewed basal slice with one half of the image in ventricle (thicker wall) and the other half in the atrium (thinner wall). The anterior mitral leaflet is often seen between the two.

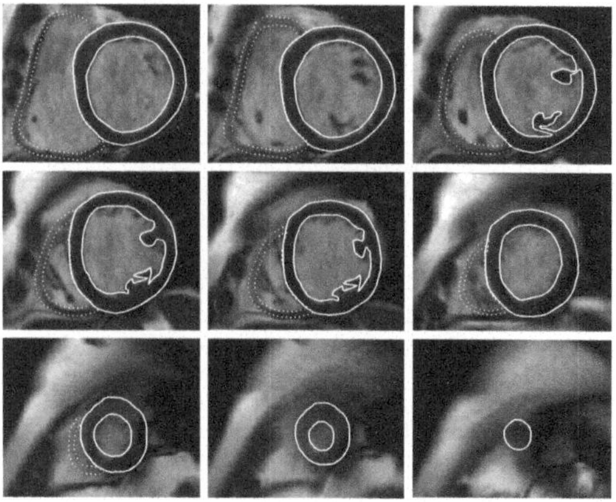

Fig. 4.3 Examples of contours on diastolic frames of an SSFP short-axis image stack. LV (solid lines) and RV (dotted lines).

Papillary muscles

The papillary muscles should be included with the LV mass (and excluded from LV volume) for greatest accuracy. They can either be outlined separately or included in the endocardial contour with a thin 'stalk' connecting them to the endocardium. On some software packages, including the papillary muscles is difficult and, in this case, it is feasible to exclude them from LV mass (including them within LV volume), which introduces a small, but usually reasonably acceptable error. It is important, however, to be consistent with the method used, and their inclusion or exclusion should be the same as that used in the normal reference ranges.

RV volume/mass analysis

Basal slice selection

- Basal slice selection is even more difficult in the RV because of its complex shape, and experience is important.
- Similar rules to the LV apply – comparing the diastolic image with subsequent images in the cardiac cycle, and to the diastolic images above and below can be helpful. Look for sudden changes in wall thickness and endocardial contours.
- Through-plane motion of the RV during systole is considerable at the base, and it may move 2–3 slices towards the apex, pulling the RA into the image plane. Therefore, expect the end-systolic RV basal slice to be 2–3 slices more apical (assuming normal RV function). Look for a change in the shape/size of the chamber or wall thickness, or the tricuspid leaflets coming through the plane, or chamber expansion during ventricular systole – all indicate an atrium moving into plane.
- Remember the tricuspid valve is more apical than the mitral valve, so if the LV is no longer in plane, it is unlikely that the RV is either.
- Look out for the tricuspid valve – it is not uncommon to have a small area of the RV outflow tract in the image slice *and* a portion of the RA more posteriorly, particularly in systole. Either discount the slice entirely, or include only the RVOT portion.

Trabeculations

- The RV is more heavily trabeculated than the LV and generally speaking, these trabeculations are included within RV chamber volumes, particularly as partial volume effects can increase their apparent size.
- Towards the apex, partial volume effects can make endocardial definition challenging, but the errors here are usually small.

RV mass measurement

- This may not always be necessary, but can be performed for selected cases, or if software facilitates easy measurement.
- The septum is generally considered part of the LV, so only the RV free wall mass is measured.
- The normal RV is thin-walled (<4mm), which can make epicardial border definition difficult and there is greater variability in RV mass measurements compared with the LV.

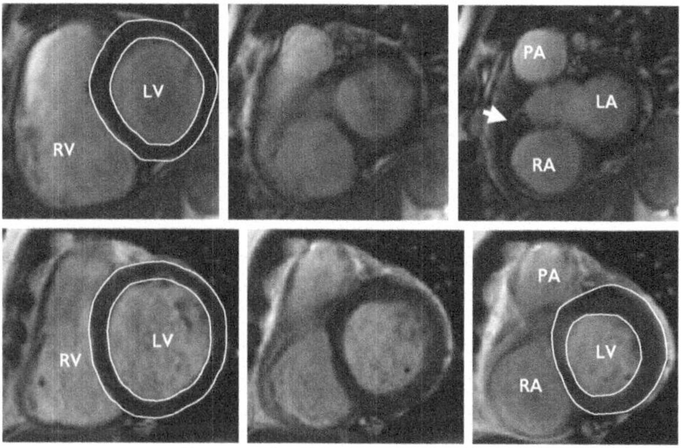

Fig. 4.4 Basal short axis image slice in two different patients (top and bottom rows) showing the progressive, but variable movement of the atria into the image planes due to the longitudinal contraction of the heart. (Top row) End-diastole (left), with both RV and LV in the image plane and LV contours shown. Mid-systole (middle) with partial volume effects due to both atria and ventricle being in plane. End-systole (right) with both atria in the plane and LV contours would be inappropriate. The right coronary artery can also be seen in the atrioventricular groove (arrow). (Bottom row) RV long axis contraction is significantly greater than the LV and only the right atrium comes into plane in systole. (Left) End-diastole with both RV and LV in the image plane and LV contours shown. (Middle) Mid-systole with partial volume effects due to both right ventricle and right atrium being in the image plane. (Right) End-systole containing the right atrium and the LV (with appropriate contours). LA = left atrium; RA = right atrium; PA = pulmonary artery.

Commercial software packages

Several commercial software packages are available for CMR volumetric analysis. Most of them follow the principle of manual definition of epicardial and endocardial borders; however, some offer additional advantages:

- Semi-automatic endocardial and epicardial contour detection (enables rapid processing).
- Identification of mitral and tricuspid valve positions on long axis slices to automatically include/exclude basal slices (using the 3D positioning data available in DICOM-based imaging).
- Fully automated contour detection is also available, but manual checking ± correction is usually needed.
- See Figs 4.5–4.7 for examples.

Future developments

Automatic boundary detection methods are expected to improve substantially in the future, and post-processing analysis for LV and RV function should become easier and quicker, leading to more efficient workflow and helping to increase the utilization of CMR in clinical practice.

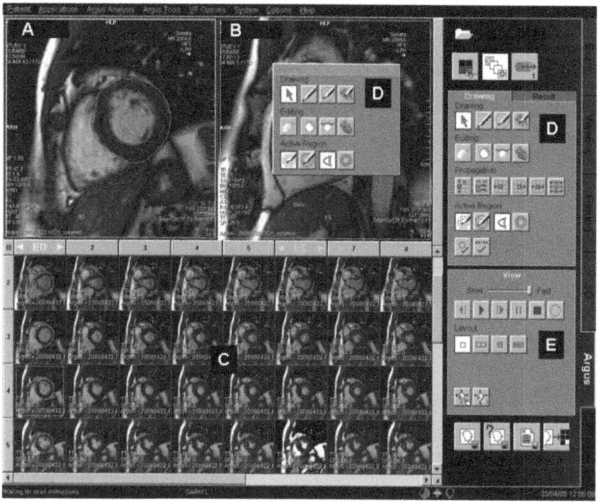

Fig. 4.5 Left and right ventricular analysis using Argus software® (Siemens Healthcare, Erlangen, Germany). (A, B) Two large screen segments for main image viewing or simultaneous display of end-diastole and end-systole. (C) A multi-phase/multi-slice screen display. (D) Drawing and editing tools. (E) Video and layout controls. The epicardial contours are drawn only on the end-diastolic frames.

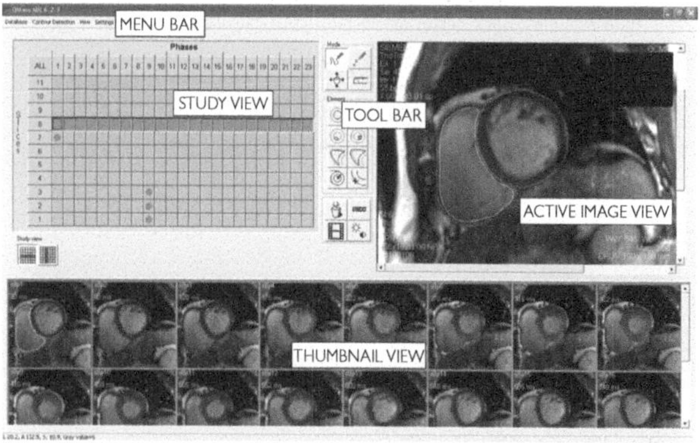

Fig. 4.6 Left and right ventricular analysis using QMass MR® (Medis Medical Imaging Systems B.V. Leiden, Netherlands). The menu bar contains most of the required commands. The study view shows a representation of the images in the currently loaded study. The thumbnail view shows the images in the slice selected from the study view. The active image view shows the image selected from the study or thumbnail views, and can also display some of the image properties.

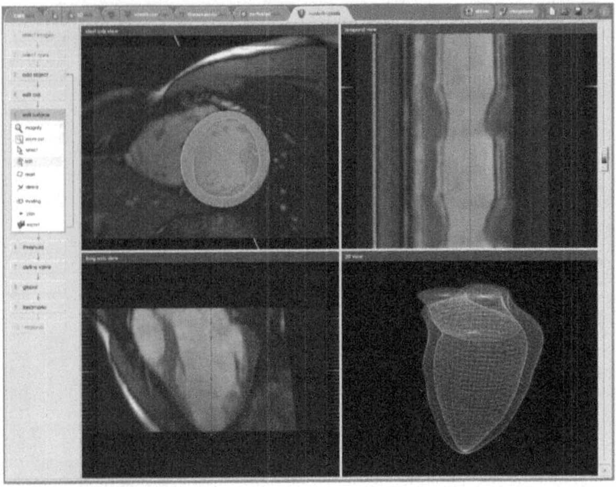

Fig. 4.7 Semi-automated analysis of ventricular mass and volumes using LVtools®, part of CMRtools® (Cardiovascular Imaging Solutions, London, UK; www.cmrtools.com). Four main views are shown: short axis (top left), reconstructed long axis (bottom left), temporal (top right), and 3D wireframe (bottom right). This model calculates the contours for all slices from user-defined guide-points and is fully adjustable. The long axis image enables checking of consistency through planes and time. A threshold technique is used for the blood pool, which automatically accounts for papillary muscles and trabeculations. Lastly, the mitral and tricuspid valve planes are defined on the long-axis cines in diastole and systole to automatically include/exclude basal slices from the ventricular calculations.

Further reading

Maceira AM, Prasad SK, Khan M, Pennell DJ. Normalized left ventricular systolic and diastolic function by steady state free precession cardiovascular magnetic resonance. *J Cardiovasc Magn Reson* 2006; **8:** 417–26.

Moon JC, Lorenz CH, Francis JH *et al.* Breath-hold FLASH and FISP cardiovascular MR imaging: left ventricular volume differences and reproducibility. *Radiology* 2002; **223:** 789–97.

Myerson SG, Bellenger NG, Pennell DJ. Assessment of left ventricular mass by cardiovascular magnetic resonance. *Hypertension* 2002; **39:** 750–5.

Flow analysis

The quantification of flow is a unique strength of CMR and can be achieved by processing through-plane phase velocity mapping sequences. 'Magnitude' images (anatomical data) and flow images (velocity data) are acquired simultaneously, as a series through the cardiac cycle, typically with a temporal resolution of 25–45ms.

Steps in through-plane flow quantification

- Flow is measured through a specific area in the image (e.g. the aorta) by outlining the 'region of interest' in each image in the series. A contour is usually defined on the magnitude image, which is automatically transferred to the corresponding flow image (Fig. 4.8). Many software programs allow copying of the contour from one image to all the frames to speed up the process. The copied contours often require modification, however, to correct for cardiac and vessel motion during the cardiac cycle. Some software offers an adaptive copying tool, which attempts to follow the structure outlined in the initial image, although this process is rarely perfect and manual checking is still advised.
- The velocities from each voxel are integrated with the area of the region of interest to obtain the instantaneous flow at that time point.
- All the frames from the sequence are then integrated over time (the cardiac cycle) to obtain the flow/cardiac cycle.
- The results are typically displayed in a flow-time graph (Fig. 4.9) as well as numerical values for both forward and reverse flow.
- Peak velocity is also usually displayed, although this tends to be slightly underestimated (see important limitations, 📖 p. 102).

Tips for accurate flow measurement

Ensure the correct area is measured!

In through-plane flow imaging, vessels can appear remarkably similar. Ensure that you are measuring the correct part of the image.

Accurate contour placement

Ensure the contours are correct throughout the cardiac cycle. This is particularly the case if copied from an initial image. Otherwise, the flow measurement may miss some of the flow within the region of interest or measure additional flow from an adjacent vessel/chamber.

Avoiding turbulence

Turbulent flow in CMR usually occurs adjacent to high velocity jets (e.g. mitral regurgitation, severe aortic stenosis, VSD), but can also occur at other sites of complex flow, e.g. the edges of valve leaflets, narrowed outflow tracts. It causes random noise in the flow image (due to unpredictable phase shifts) and inaccuracies in flow measurement. The 'noise' is usually distinguishable from normal laminar flow and the contours for flow measurement should avoid the usually small areas of turbulent flow. This is particularly important for identifying peak velocity, which should normally lie towards the centre of the flow jet.

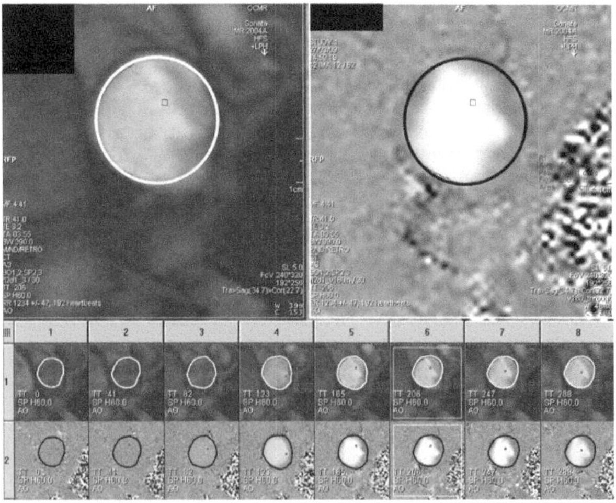

Fig. 4.8 Example of contour placement on flow images – Argus® software (Siemens Medical Systems, Erlangen, Germany). (Top left) Magnitude image. (Top right) Corresponding flow image. The bottom rows show the sequence of magnitude and flow images through the cardiac cycle.

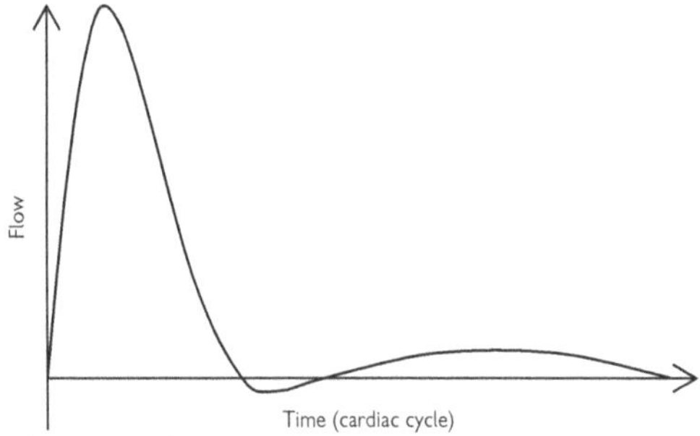

Fig. 4.9 Normal flow-time curve from above the aortic valve. Note the fast upstroke, peak, and rapid fall in late systole, with a small negative dip at the time of aortic valve closure. There is often a small forward flow in mid-late diastole due to movement of the valve ring back towards the base of the heart.

Background correction

Inhomogeneities in the magnetic field can cause phase shifts across a whole image, resulting in inaccurate flow data. Static parts of the image (e.g. the chest wall) should normally be mid-grey (zero velocity), but with a suboptimal field can appear to have a small velocity (higher or lower signal), which can be visible as a linear shift in velocity across the image. This can be overcome at the post-processing stage with 'background correction', which most systems perform automatically. It can also be performed 'manually' by placing multiple points to identify the static parts around the image (e.g. chest wall), from which the software can correct the background phase shift.

Other phase errors from Eddy currents in the magnetic field can be minimized by positioning the flow image at the isocentre of the scanner.

Accurate end-diastolic flow measurement

If prospective triggering is used for flow sequences in valve regurgitation, the latter part of diastolic flow may be missed (📖 p. 52), which could represent a significant proportion of the total regurgitant flow (Fig. 4.10).

Using the flow curve

Assessing the flow-time curve can be helpful in identifying errors in the flow measurement. The flow curve should be smooth (Fig. 4.9) and sudden changes may indicate a measurement error in one or more images, often due to aliasing or incorrect positioning of the region of interest.

For aortic and pulmonary flow, it may indicate if there are gaps in the flow measurement. Flow should start from close to zero at the start of the cycle and if it starts significantly higher than this, this may be an indication of inappropriate data acquisition techniques (e.g. from delayed triggering, Fig. 4.10).

Aliasing

Occurs when the velocity in the image plane exceeds the chosen velocity range. The excess phase shift causes the velocity to appear in the negative range, in much the same way as velocities above the scale do in colour Doppler imaging with echocardiography. The voxels exceeding the velocity range thus appear the opposite colour to the expected flow direction, e.g. several 'black' (low signal) voxels within an area of 'white' high signal from high velocity forward flow (Fig. 4.11), or vice versa for flow in the reverse direction.

Corrective steps

- The best option is avoidance by using the correct velocity range, repeating the acquisition if necessary (if recognized during scanning).
- Moderate degrees of aliasing may be amenable to correction during post-processing. The velocity range can be shifted to raise the upper end of the scale by re-assigning the phase shift towards the forward direction, at the expense of the reverse direction. However, flow in the reverse direction then has a lower velocity range. There is also a limit to the amount of phase shift possible – twice the maximum velocity range originally set, which results in no allowance for reverse flow. Aliasing in the reverse direction can be treated in the opposite way.

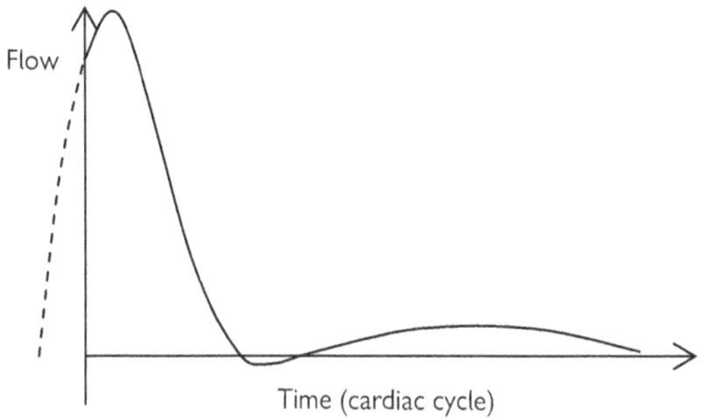

Fig. 4.10 Representative flow curve in a patient using pulse oximetry triggering. Note the 'missing' flow in the upstroke at the start of the graph (dashed section).

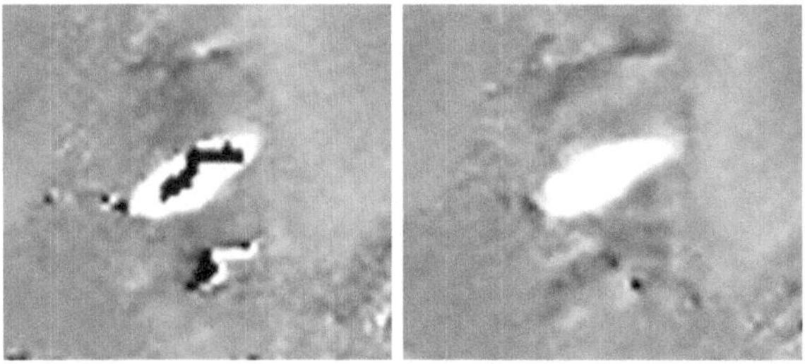

Fig. 4.11 Velocity aliasing on a bicuspid aortic valve with moderately restricted flow. The image on the left has been acquired with a velocity window below the velocity of the flow. Note the 'black' (reverse) flow in the centre of the flow jet, where the highest velocity forward flow would be expected. On the right is the same image acquired with a higher velocity range.

In-plane flow sequences

In-plane flow sequences are good for visualizing flow and velocities in a longitudinal plane (see Fig. 4.12) and are excellent for assessing the location of flow acceleration. The peak velocity in any given area can be assessed by selecting the area, and analysing the data from the software – peak velocity is usually displayed automatically.

Don't rely on data from a single voxel, however, particularly if it is significantly different from surrounding ones, as this is likely to be inaccurate due to turbulence/other effects. Adjacent voxels should have similar velocities, and the 'random' velocity signal from turbulent flow can usually be identified from inspecting the flow images.

Remember, too, that the plane is 5–7mm thick, so partial volume effects can occur if the flow jet is narrow (📖 p. 100).

In-plane flow sequences cannot be used to quantify flow volume, however, as the image only contains data from one plane. It does not contain cross-sectional data from the whole vessel/conduit through which flow quantification is desired.

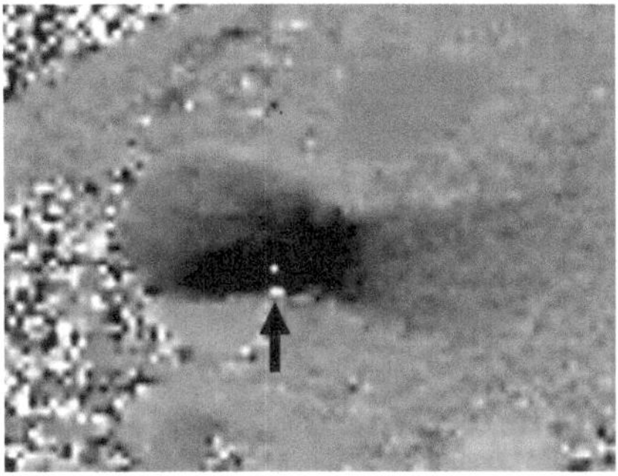

Fig. 4.12 In-plane flow image showing flow across the aortic valve in the standard LVOT view. Note the white voxel of turbulent flow at the periphery of the main flow jet (arrow), and a second white voxel of either turbulent flow or aliasing in the centre of the flow jet. These should be avoided when assessing velocity.

Angiography and other 3D datasets

3D image data is acquired as a large cuboid (or voxel) made up of many smaller voxels, typically 1–3mm in each dimension. The whole dataset is viewed in specialized viewing software, usually part of the manufacturer's software package, and can be processed for viewing in a number of ways:

Unprocessed data

The raw data can be viewed as multiple contiguous (very thin) 2D planes, often in the transaxial, coronal, and sagittal planes for ease of orientation (Fig. 4.13). This has the advantage of no data loss and fine structures can be followed in consecutive images. If required, the views can usually be rotated to any plane to provide the viewing angle required.

2D planes

2D planes can be constructed from the 3D data at the processing stage. If the image planes are processed during scan acquisition, they can be used to plan further images.

Maximal intensity projection (MIP)

Angiographic data can be viewed as a 'maximal intensity projection', or MIP, in which all the data is viewed together, as if the multiple slices are 'projected' on top of each other onto one plane. Although this may be expected to produce a messy image with too much data, the angiographic dataset contains mostly luminal anatomy of the imaged vessels, and combining all the data in fact results in a 3D 'cast' of the imaged vessels. This can be rotated or 'dragged' into any viewing angle, to visualize the vessels concerned. A 3D rotation can also be created, viewing the images from all positions as if rotated on a turntable, although any plane of rotation can be chosen. This has the advantage of excellent fine detail, but has lower 3D spatial visualization than the surface-rendered method below (Fig. 4.13).

Surface rendering

The MIP of an angiographic dataset can also be 'surface rendered' with appropriate software to create a 'shaded' view with better depth perspective. The advantages are clear views of tortuous vessels and the relative location of surrounding vessels in 3D perspective. The disadvantage is that an intensity threshold is required to indicate the included parts of the image, so some data loss occurs. Sections with lower signal intensity, e.g. small vessels or significant stenosis may be under-appreciated and appear smaller, or the stenosis may appear more severe. Optimizing the intensity threshold can help, but if a tight stenosis or small vessel is seen, it is often more accurate to view the MIP or even the unprocessed dataset for confirmation.

Editing

3D datasets can be edited to 'remove' unwanted parts of the image, highlighting key areas for ease of visualization. For example just the pulmonary veins and left atrium can be visualized, without the aorta, LV, or pulmonary arteries (Fig. 4.14). Editing techniques differ according to the software.

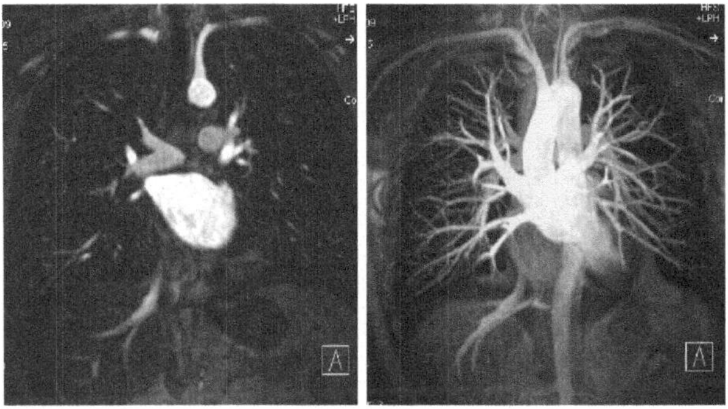

Fig. 4.13 Raw data in 'ultra-thin' slice coronal view (left) and maximal intensity projection (right) of the same dataset, showing normal thoracic vascular anatomy.

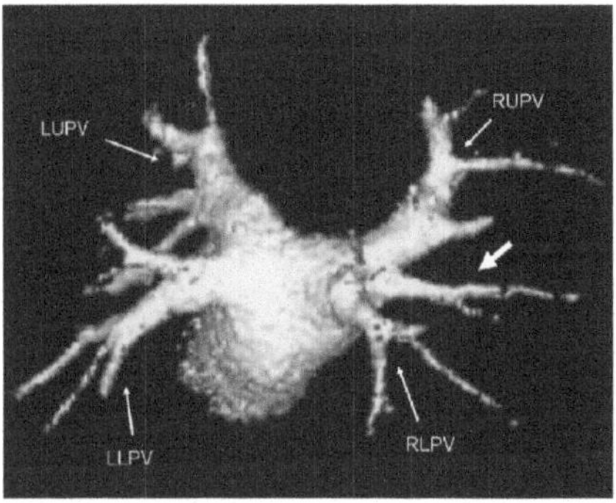

Fig. 4.14 Surface-rendered pulmonary veins, edited to remove other parts of the image and viewed from posteriorly. The greater 3D perspective can be appreciated. LUPV = left upper pulmonary vein; LLPV = left lower pulmonary vein; RUPV = right upper pulmonary vein; RLPV = right lower pulmonary vein. The arrow indicates an accessory right middle pulmonary vein (a common variant).

Chapter 5

Ventricular function assessment

Left ventricular function

Background

Cardiac dilatation, hypertrophy, and dysfunction are a common final pathway for many disease processes, and a good understanding of the normal appearance of the LV is important for reporting CMR scans. The LV is characterized by its muscular wall, papillary muscles, and their chordal attachments. LV trabeculations are typically present, but to a much lesser degree than in the RV.

Quantification of LV volumes, mass, and ejection fraction is one of CMR's major strengths, particularly due to its high reproducibility and accuracy. Hence, it is considered the 'gold-standard' or reference method for these.

Scanning

3 long axis planes (HLA, VLA, and LVOT views)

Look for areas of wall motion abnormalities (normokinesis, hypokinesis, akinesis, dyskinesis).

Short axis cine stack

For measurement of LV mass, volumes, and function.

'Tagging' or other CMR techniques (tissue phase mapping or DENSE) investigate myocardial velocities, strain, or strain-rate. These techniques are mainly used in the research setting for comprehensive assessment of systolic and diastolic function. The clinical importance of these promising techniques is yet to be established.

Reporting should include:

- LV volumes (end-diastolic, end-systolic) and mass ± wall thickness. Normal ranges depend on sequence used (SSFP produces better endocardial definition and slightly larger chamber volumes than older FLASH methods). See Table 5.1 for ranges based on SSFP. These are often normalized (e.g. to height, weight, body surface area), although there is no uniform consensus on the best normalization algorithm.
- Calculated stroke volume and ejection fraction.
- Any unusual anatomy or excessive LV trabeculation (if the latter, assess non-compaction to compaction ratio, 📖 p. 188).
- Comment on overall LV volumes, mass, and function, and whether any regional differences exist (e.g. inferior wall hypokinesis or septal hypertrophy). The long axis views usually provide the best appreciation of function, although asymmetric hypertrophy can be particularly well visualized on short axis views.
- For regional function analysis, long axis views are best to avoid artefactual wall motion defects due to through-plane motion of the LV. The LV may be divided according to the AHA / ACC 17 segment model (Fig. 5.1), with approximate correlation to coronary artery territories.
- For detailed assessment, segmental wall thickening can be measured with several software packages (usually quoted in mm *thickening* and/or % of the original thickness). Normal ranges are currently not available and, thus, this is mainly used for research purposes.

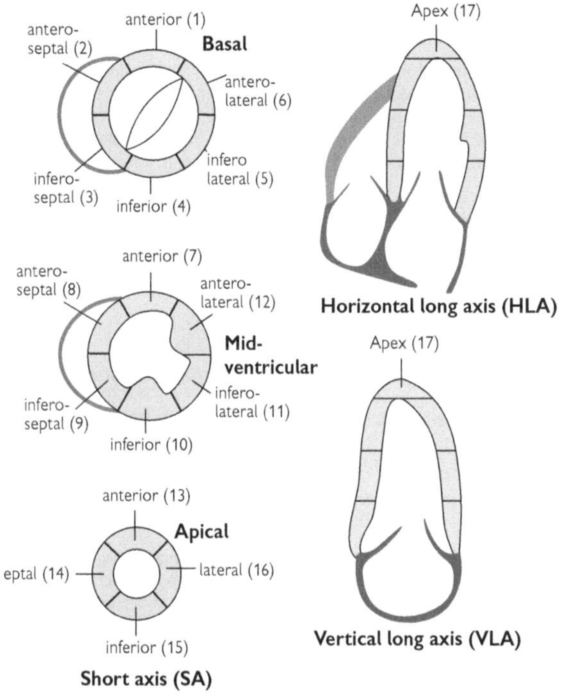

Fig. 5.1 17 segment model modified from the American Heart Association/ American College of Cardiology consensus paper.

Table 5.1 Normal ranges of LV volumes, ejection fraction and mass using steady state free precession cine imaging and inclusion of papillary muscle for LV mass measurement (Data from Hudsmith *et al.*, 2005)

	EDV (ml)	**ESV (ml)**	**SV (ml)**	**EF (%)**	**Mass (g)**	**Mass index (g/m^2)**
Male	102–218	18–82	74–150	57–81	81–165	45–81
Female	83–187	18–66	57–125	57–81	42–150	31–79

Further reading

Hudsmith LE, Petersen SE, Francis JM *et al.* Normal human left and right ventricular and left atrial dimensions using steady state free precession magnetic resonance imaging. *J Cardiovasc Magn Reson* 2005; **7**: 775.

Right ventricular function

Background

The right ventricle forms an 'elongated crescent' on the side of the LV and consists of the free wall, the inter-ventricular septum, and the infundibulum (sub-pulmonary portion of the RV outflow tract). It is much more trabeculated than the LV and usually contains a fused 'bundle' of trabeculations towards the apex called the moderator band, linking the free wall, and septum.

Most RV contraction occurs along its long axis from base to apex, particularly the free wall, with a smaller component from radial contraction. This is in contrast to systolic emptying of the LV, which involves significant radial contraction.

Scanning

3 long axis planes (HLA, RVOT and RV 2-chamber views)

Assess global and regional wall motion (normokinesis, hypokinesis, akinesis, dyskinesis (Fig. 5.2). The ventricular portion of the RVOT (the infundibulum) is particularly muscular and normally contracts vigorously in systole (Fig. 5.3).

Short axis cine stack

Performed for measurement of both LV and RV mass and function.

Transaxial cine stack

This is preferable for assessment of RV free wall function (Fig. 5.4), particularly regional differences, as it avoids wall motion artefacts due to the significant through-plane motion of the RV in the short axis images. RV volumes can be reliably measured with a transaxial stack, though it is usual to use the short axis stack, as (i) LV volumes can be measured too, and (ii) most processing software is designed for use with a short axis stack.

Reporting should include:

- RV volumes (end-diastolic and end-systolic) ± mass as required. See Table 5.2. Normal ranges depend on the sequence, as for LV volumes. See 🕮 p. 130 for processing.
- Calculated stroke volume and ejection fraction.
- Comment on overall RV volumes and function, and whether any regional differences exist. Look for co-ordinated contraction of the RV free wall. Any areas of hypo- or dyskinesis in systole? Assessment of RV free wall function can be difficult and requires significant experience of normal RV contraction with CMR. See also Arrhythmogenic right ventricular cardiomyopathy, 🕮 p. 184).

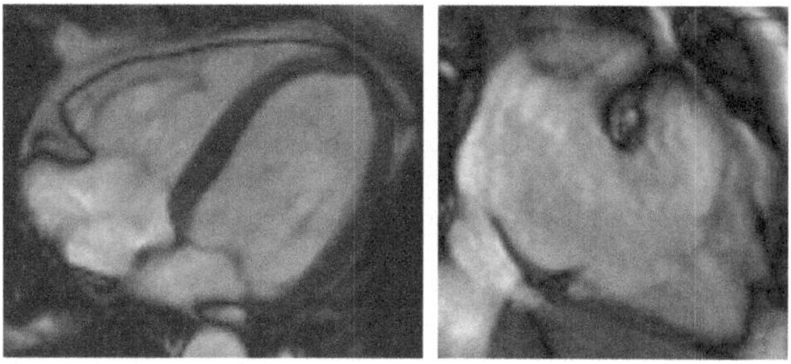

Fig. 5.2 Long axis views for assessing RV function. Horizontal long axis (HLA) view (left), RV 2-chamber view (right).

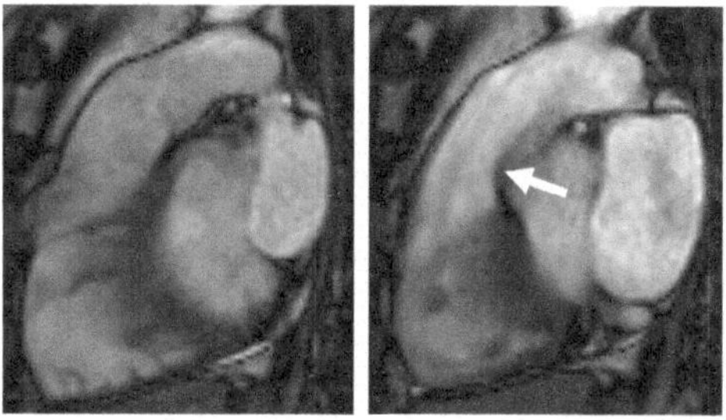

Fig. 5.3 RV outflow tract (RVOT) view in diastole (left and systole (right) showing contraction of the infundibulum (arrowed).

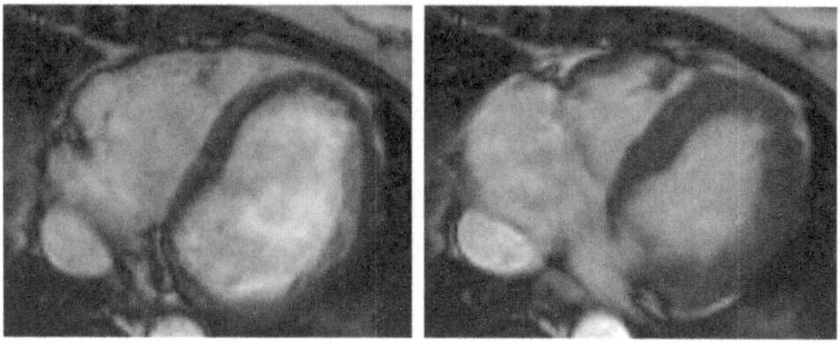

Fig. 5.4 Transaxial SSFP images showing RV free wall contraction. Diastole (left) and systole (right). Note the considerable base to apex motion of the RV free wall.

Table 5.2 Normal ranges of RV volumes, ejection fraction and mass using steady state free precession cine imaging (data from Hudsmith *et al.*, 2005)

	EDV (ml)	**ESV (ml)**	**SV (ml)**	**EF (%)**	**Mass (g)**	**Mass index (g/m^2)**
Male	124–256	38–118	75–151	47–71	25–57	13–28
Female	78–218	20–92	52–128	53–73	21–49	13–27

Further reading

Hudsmith LE, Petersen SE, Francis JM *et al.* Normal human left and right ventricular and left atrial dimensions using steady free precession magnetic resonance imaging. *J Cardiovasc Magn Reson* 2005; **7:** 775–82.

RV volume and pressure overload

The motion of the interventricular septum can help in diagnosing RV volume and pressure overload. Normally, the LV has a circular shape in the short axis view, with the septum 'bowed' towards the RV throughout the cardiac cycle due to higher pressures in the LV.

RV volume overload

Volume overload results in ↑ RV diastolic volumes with normal RV free wall thickness. The excess blood volume also results in rapid filling of the RV in diastole, causing diastolic pressure to rise quickly. This can equal LV diastolic pressure, causing movement of the septum towards the LV and resulting in a 'flattening' of the septum, with the LV assuming a 'D' shape in the short axis view (Fig. 5.5). Near equal diastolic pressures in both ventricles can also cause slight side-to-side or 'wavy' motion of the septum as the pressure in each ventricle changes slightly during filling. During systole, LV pressures exceed those in the RV and the septum returns to its normal position. As the wavy movement occurs in diastole only, this is sometimes referred to as a 'diastolic bounce'.

▶ It is not specific for volume overload however, and a similar diastolic flattening can occur in other conditions, including pericardial constriction (particularly on inspiration; 📖 p. 300). RV volumes may be normal in other situations, or even reduced in pericardial constriction.

Major causes
- Severe tricuspid or pulmonary regurgitation.
- Severe left to right shunt from a large atrial septal defect.

RV pressure overload

Pressure overload results in hypertrophy of the RV free wall and interventricular septum. If RV pressures are severely increased and approach systemic levels, the septum may be 'pushed' towards the LV in both diastole and systole, reflecting the relative pressures in the ventricles. The greater the RV pressure relative to the LV, the greater the shift in the septum (Fig. 5.6). Note this differs from volume overload in which septal shift occurs in diastole only.

This may sometimes be supported by estimating the RV/pulmonary systolic pressure from any tricuspid regurgitation present. Using velocity mapping, the gradient between the RV and RA can be assessed by employing the modified Bernoulli equation:

$$\text{RV systolic pressure} = 4(\text{peak TR velocity})^2 + \text{RA pressure}$$

RA pressure can be estimated from the JVP. In the absence of pulmonary stenosis, RV pressure approximates to pulmonary systolic pressure. In practice, however, the velocity of TR jets is high and these are difficult to measure with CMR, due to their often narrow width and turbulent flow, and are better assessed with echocardiography.

Major causes
- Severe pulmonary hypertension (from any cause).
- Pulmonary stenosis (valvar, sub-valvar, supra-valvar).

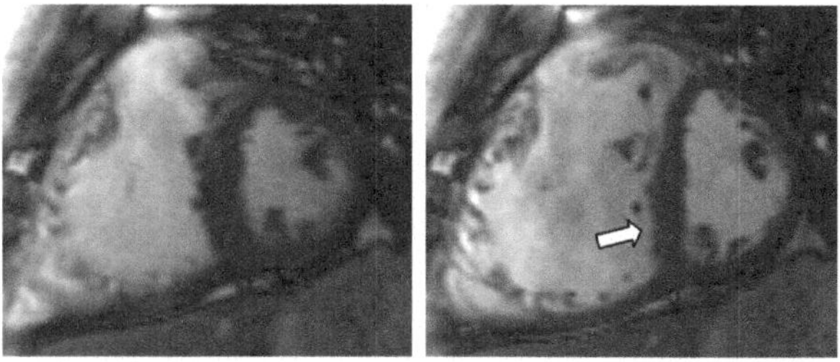

Fig. 5.5. Volume overloaded RV in short axis view (SSFP sequence). Note the enlarged RV, the normal circular shape of the LV in systole (left), and the flattening of the septum in diastole (right, arrowed), creating a more 'D'-shaped LV.

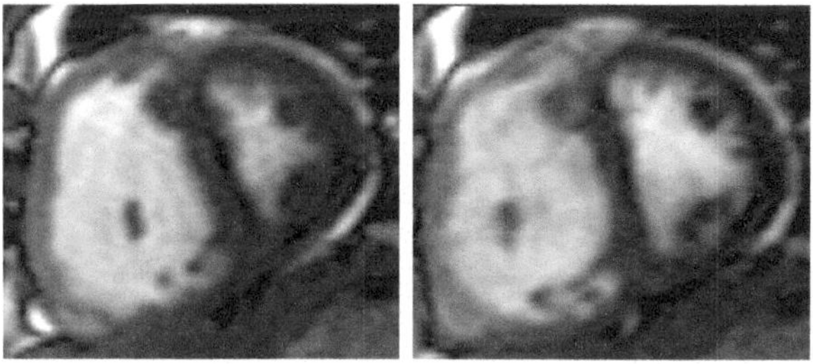

Fig. 5.6. Pressure overloaded RV in short axis view (SSFP sequence). Note the normal-sized RV (relative to the LV), with flattening of the septum in both systole (left) and diastole (right). In this case, only mild RV hypertrophy is present, as the ↑ pulmonary pressure was caused by a large acute pulmonary embolus. The mild hypertrophy may be related to background chronic pulmonary embolic disease.

Causes of RV dilation

- Significant pulmonary or tricuspid regurgitation.
- Left to right shunt from:
  - Atrial septal defect
  - Anomalous pulmonary venous connection.
- ARVC.
- (Idiopathic) dilated cardiomyopathy involving the RV.
- Other inherited cardiomyopathies.
- RV infarction.

Chapter 6

Ischaemic heart disease

Ischaemic heart disease

CMR offers a comprehensive assessment of patients with coronary artery disease (CAD). In a single imaging session, CMR can assess cardiac anatomy and function, myocardial perfusion, and viability (Fig. 6.1). The detection of coronary stenosis is also possible in principle (see Chapter 15 Coronary MRI, 📖 p. 399), but requires further technological advances to improve the resolution and currently is not robust enough for routine clinical practice.

Complications of myocardial infarction, e.g. LV mural thrombus, aneurysmal dilatation, and rupture of the interventricular septum can be readily recognized, and in acute chest pain, CMR can assess myocardial oedema (area at risk) and necrosis (irreversibly injured myocardium). Importantly, because of the absence of ionizing radiation, CMR is an ideal non-invasive modality for the serial follow-up of patients with CAD.

CMR features

- **Contractile dysfunction:** wall motion abnormalities, either at rest or during stress, can indicate CAD, particularly if regional and if these correlate to a coronary artery territory – regional wall motion defects are a hallmark of coronary disease. Dysfunction predominantly relates to the LV, but RV contractile abnormalities should also be noted. Complications of myocardial infarction, e.g. aneurysm formation, can be readily recognized and, if present, mural thrombi can be seen, although further confirmation may be needed on post-contrast images.
- **Oedematous myocardium, in acute coronary events:** On T_2-weighted imaging, areas of acute injury (oedema) may be identified by high signal from excess water. These may be larger than any areas of infarction (necrosis) and this difference may indicate the area at risk. The utility in clinical practice has yet to be determined.
- **Inducible perfusion defects:**
  - See Perfusion imaging, 📖 p. 166.
  - Areas of poor perfusion during vasodilator stress indicate a functionally significant stenosis in the relevant coronary artery(ies). The high resolution of CMR perfusion imaging allows a detailed assessment, with the endocardium affected first, progressing towards a full thickness perfusion deficit with increasing stenosis\ severity. Global hypoperfusion (i.e. triple vessel disease) can also be identified by global endocardial hypoperfusion.
  - Resting perfusion deficits mostly indicate infarction.
- **Infarction (viability imaging):** late gadolinium enhancement imaging (📖 p. 162) is a sensitive and reliable indicator of infarction in the setting of coronary disease, and can be considered the 'gold standard' for *in vivo* imaging. The depth of infarcted myocardium can be visualized and this correlates strongly with the chance of functional recovery post-revascularization. Infarcted myocardium appears bright (white), in comparison to the normal 'black' myocardium, with a similar pattern to perfusion defects, starting at the endocardium and progressing to full thickness infarction with increasing infarction severity. It should correlate with a coronary artery territory.

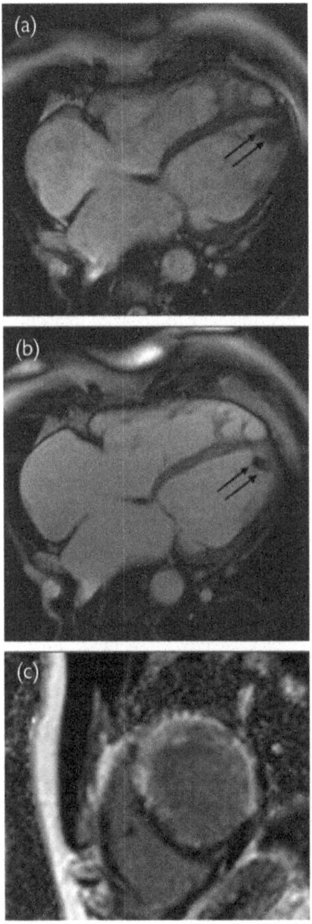

Fig. 6.1 Substantial previous MI due to occlusion of the left anterior descending and right coronary arteries. (A) End-diastolic frame of an HLA cine image (SSFP sequence). Note the small thrombus at the apex (arrows). (B) Early post-contrast image with a segmented inversion recovery gradient echo sequence (long inversion time, 450ms). The apical thrombus appears dark due to absent perfusion (arrows). (C) Short axis late gadolinium enhancement image showing a near transmural infarct of the anterior septum, anterior and lateral walls (white). The inferior septum (<25% wall thickness enhancement) and the inferior wall (no enhancement), are viable.

Scanning

Long axis SSFP cines (HLA, VLA, and LVOT views)
Allows good appreciation of wall motion, and any areas of thinning or aneurysm formation.

Short axis SSFP image stack
Provides detailed regional assessment of LV function, in addition to global volumes and ejection fraction.

± oedema imaging
T_2-weighted turbo-spin echo images in the appropriate long or short axis planes, prior to gadolinium administration (T_2-weighted sequences are sensitive to gadolinium). Look for high signal relative to the surrounding myocardium, particularly adjacent to areas of infarction.

± perfusion imaging
See Perfusion imaging, 📖 p. 120.

Late gadolinium enhancement imaging
See 📖 p. 112).

For viability assessment. Important for decisions on revascularization.

Reporting should include:

- **Global and regional contractile function:**
  - LV (and RV) volumes and ejection fraction
  - Wall motion abnormalities.
- Regional analysis should refer to coronary artery territories, and the AHA 17 segment model can be used (📖 p. 147).
- **Regional myocardial perfusion:** inducible perfusion defects during vasodilator stress that are not present at rest are indicative of significant coronary stenosis(es). Indicate the area involved, the degree of perfusion defect (wall thickness) and the likely coronary artery. Perfusion defects present at stress and rest are likely to be infarcts – can be confirmed with delayed enhancement viability/infarct imaging.
- **Oedema** (in selected acute cases): compare to the area of any infarction for an indication of the differential salvageable area.
- **Viability of the relevant coronary territories/cardiac segments:** the enhancement pattern should be typical for coronary disease. Describe the transmural thickness of any infarction in quartiles, and the likelihood of functional recovery post-revascularization (see Table 6.1). The total amount of infarcted tissue (in grams) relative to the myocardial mass may also be reported.
- **Coronary artery anatomy**: if imaged with sufficient resolution.
- If coronary anatomy is already known (e.g. from invasive angiography), incorporate this in the report and relate to the CMR findings.

► It is important to be logical with reporting and to relate the various components (areas of poor perfusion and/or infarction; contractile abnormalities) to each other. For example, a large full thickness infarction would be expected to have akinetic/dyskinetic wall motion, and a thinned, dyskinetic area would not normally be expected to have full viability. If significant discrepancies occur, question the accuracy of the imaging – are the areas really aligned properly? Is the infarction in a thin wall difficult to visualize?

Table 6.1 Viability assessment with late gadolinium enhancement inversion recovery technique. The extent of infarction in each segment determines the likelihood of functional recovery post-revascularization. (Data from Kim *et al.*, 2000)

% Wall thickness infarction	Likelihood of functional recovery
0	80%
1–25	60%
26–50	40%
51–75	10%
>75	Almost nil

Further reading

Kim RJ, Wu E, Rafael A *et al.* The use of contrast enhanced magnetic resonance imaging to identify reversible myocardial dysfunction. *N Engl J Med* 2000; **343:** 1445–1453.

Differential diagnosis

(Peri-)myocarditis

See 📖 p. 196.

Can present with chest pain, although any late gadolinium enhancement is usually *sub-epicardial* and not in keeping with a coronary territory. The areas of enhancement are usually small. Global LV dysfunction is possible in severe cases, though regional dysfunction is unusual.

Dilated cardiomyopathy

See 📖 p. 182.

Global dysfunction; delayed enhancement pattern can include a thin mid-wall band, but not the typical thicker endocardial enhancement of infarction.

Valve disease

Can cause global cardiac dysfunction if severe, but typically no late enhancement.

Sarcoidosis

See 📖 p. 200.

Regional contractile dysfunction is possible, although this is more often global. Patchy late enhancement can also occur, but this is usually multiple, not related to coronary territories, and occurs anywhere within the myocardial wall.

Hypertrophic cardiomyopathy

See 📖 p. 178.

Can occasionally cause regional dysfunction, though the hypertrophy is usually apparent and any late enhancement is usually mid-wall, in the hypertrophied segment or at the LV/RV junctions in the septum.

Eosinophilic myocarditis

See 📖 p. 204

Can cause global/regional (especially apical) dysfunction and an endocardial delayed enhancement pattern, sometimes with apical thrombus. However, the enhancement is usually circumferential, of uniform thickness and endocardial (not full wall thickness). It spreads from the apex to involve the mid- and, rarely, the basal LV. Although some regional variation can occur, the extent, general uniformity, apical predominance, and ignorance of coronary territories usually allows relatively easy differentiation from coronary disease.

Myocardial viability

There are two methods for viability assessment with CMR – late gadolinium enhancement and low-dose dobutamine stress cine imaging. Late enhancement is the most commonly used, has extensive validation in human and animal studies, and is widely considered the 'Gold-standard' for *in vivo* viability imaging. Low-dose dobutamine stress is much less commonly used and is considered elsewhere (📖 p. 164).

Late ('delayed') gadolinium enhancement (LGE)

Infarcted myocardial tissue contains an expanded interstitial space, either due to cell membrane breakdown in acute infarction or fibrosis (scar) in chronic infarction. Gadolinium diffuses into and out of this space slowly (between 10 and 20min), in contrast to the normal (well perfused) myocardium in which gadolinium washes through rapidly (<1min). Imaging with an inversion recovery technique during the 10–20min time window can maximize the signal differences between normal and irreversibly damaged (necrotic or scarred) myocardium (Fig. 1.16, p. 21) and allow visualization of the non-viable tissue. Late enhancement can occur in other conditions, but the pattern and clinical background are different. CMR voxel resolution is 1–2 orders of magnitude greater than SPECT, allowing visualization of even small subendocardial infarcts (~2g) that cannot be detected by other imaging modalities.

The typical enhancement pattern for infarction is a subendocardial distribution, sometimes spreading to full thickness enhancement (Fig. 6.2).

Link between LGE and viability

The transmural extent of enhancement has been shown to predict functional recovery post-revascularization in both acute and chronic ischaemic heart disease, with the likelihood of improvement directly related to the transmural extent of late enhancement (see Table 6.1).

In practical terms, the key cut-off is a 50% transmural extent of enhancement, with >50% enhancement indicating an overall low chance of recovery, and <50% indicating intermediate or good chance of recovery post revascularization. Some studies have suggested additional diagnostic information from low-dose dobutamine CMR in patients with 1–75% enhancement, although this is not routinely undertaken.

Microvascular obstruction

Occurs in acute infarction, due to a combination of athero-thrombotic debris in the small vessels and tissue oedema, and can account for the 'no-reflow' phenomenon seen on angiography after opening the main coronary artery. It can be detected with CMR using both LGE and first-pass perfusion. On LGE, it is characterized by significant hypo-enhancement (black areas) surrounded by enhanced regions (Fig. 6.3) due to negligible penetration of the contrast to the core of the infarction. Microvascular obstruction on CMR has been linked to aggravated ventricular remodelling and adverse cardiovascular events post-acute myocardial infarction. On first-pass perfusion, it is recognized by the presence of hypo-enhanced regions (perfusion defects) despite successful restoration of coronary flow in the infarct-related artery.

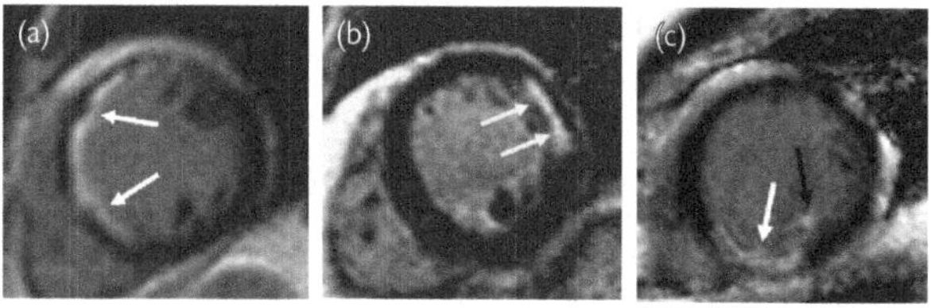

Fig. 6.2 Infarction imaging 10min post-gadolinium injection. (A) Demonstrates ~50% transmural extent LGE in septum and anterior wall (white arrows). (B) Demonstrates a smaller infarct of 25–50% transmural extent in the lateral wall (white arrows). (C) Demonstrates a small transmural inferior infarct (white arrow). Note also the enhancement (infarction) of the posteromedial papillary muscle (black arrow).

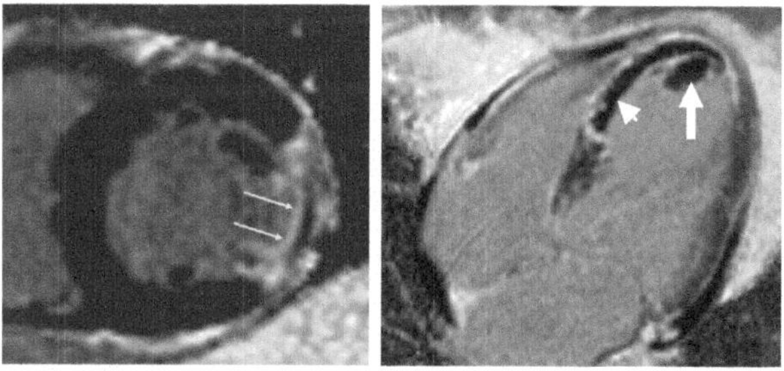

Fig. 6.3 Recent myocardial infarction and microvascular obstruction. (Left) Short axis image showing small area of hypo-enhanced (black) area in the lateral wall (white arrows) completely surrounded by enhanced regions of infarct. (Right) Large area of microvascular obstruction (black, arrowhead) within a large full thickness septal infarct (white). Note also the thrombus at the apex (long arrow).

Thrombus imaging

LGE-CMR can easily differentiate thrombus from surrounding myocardium, due to the absence of contrast uptake in the avascular thrombus. This is especially noticeable when adjacent to the white enhanced myocardium of an infarct (Fig. 6.3). To improve thrombus delineation, the inversion time can be increased (~450ms when gadolinium dose is 0.1mmol/kg). With long inversion times, regions with contrast uptake, e.g. viable myocardium, increase in image intensity (i.e. appear grey rather than black), whereas thrombus appears homogeneously black.

Dobutamine stress CMR

The positive inotropic and chronotropic effects of dobutamine increase myocardial oxygen demand, and can expose haemodynamically significant CAD with new or worsened wall motion abnormalities during stress. Dobutamine stress CMR has good specificity (~86%) and sensitivity (~83%) for detecting CAD, and can be performed with the standard high-dose dobutamine stress protocol used in stress echocardiography (see box High dose dobutamine infusion protocol, 📖 p. 165). The superior spatial resolution and excellent endocardial delineation of CMR provide better diagnostic accuracy compared with dobutamine echocardiography, particularly in patients with poor acoustic windows.

However, there is a small (~2%) risk of ventricular tachycardia with dobutamine and monitoring concerns within the scanner hampers the widespread application of dobutamine CMR in clinical practice. Instead, CMR adenosine stress perfusion imaging is often performed because of its greater safety and also sensitivity in detecting CAD. Dobutamine CMR is usually reserved for patients in whom dobutamine stress is required, but who have suboptimal acoustic windows.

Scanning

See box High dose dobutamine infusion protocol, 📖 p. 165.

Reporting

- Cines should be viewed in a multi-screen format, reviewing rest, intermediate stress, and peak stress levels together for comparison.
- Wall motion in each myocardial segment is graded using the following scoring system. A deterioration in wall motion with stress is regarded as a positive sign of coronary disease in that segment. If initial improvement occurs at an intermediate stage, with deterioration of function at peak stress (a 'biphasic' response), this also indicates coronary disease:
  - 1 – normokinesis
  - 2 – hypokinesis
  - 3 – akinesis
  - 4 – dyskinesis.
- The wall motion score index (sum of wall motion scores divided by the number of segments scored) can be reported at rest and at each level of stress to provide a global score if required.
- Quantitative wall motion assessment (% wall thickening) can be performed, but it is time consuming and mainly applied in research studies.
- Include angiographic data and the correlation to coronary territory.

High dose dobutamine infusion protocol

- The patient should refrain from β-blockers and nitrates for at least 24h prior to the examination due to potential inhibition of the dobutamine effect.
- Acquire rest cines in standard views (HLA, VLA, LVOT, 3 SA – basal, mid-ventricular, and apical).
- IV infusion of dobutamine at 3min stages (10, 20, 30, 40µg/kg/min).
- All standard cine views are acquired at each level of stress.
- Target heart rate [(220-age) × 0.85].
- Atropine in 0.25mg fractions (max 2mg) if target heart rate not reached at 40µg/kg/min dobutamine.
- Stop infusion if:
  - New wall motion abnormality
  - Serious side effect (i.e. deteriorating chest pain, infarction, ventricular fibrillation, sustained ventricular tachycardia)
  - Peak heart rate achieved.

Contraindications

- Severe systemic hypertension (≥ 220/120mmHg).
- Unstable angina.
- Uncontrolled congestive heart failure.
- Significant aortic valve stenosis (peak gradient> 50mmHg).
- Complex cardiac arrhythmias including uncontrolled AF.
- Hypertrophic obstructive cardiomyopathy.
- Myocarditis.
- Endocarditis.
- Pericarditis.

Low dose dobutamine stress CMR

- This can evaluate *viability* by assessing inotropic reserve, though viability is usually assessed by CMR with late gadolinium imaging (📖 p. 162).
- An improvement in regional contractile function with low-dose (5 or 10µg/kg/min) dobutamine is indicative of myocardial viability, with high specificity, although it has moderate sensitivity.
- It has been suggested as an adjunct to delayed gadolinium enhancement, but it is infrequently applied in clinical practice.
- Standard cine views are acquired at each level of stress. The images are projected side by side and graded for each stage of the protocol.

Advantages of delayed gadolinium enhancement over low-dose dobutamine CMR for viability

- Better diagnostic accuracy, particularly in segments with severe dysfunction at rest.
- No stress imaging involved. Superior patient comfort and safety.
- Technically easier.
- Interpretation is less observer-dependent.

Perfusion imaging

Myocardial perfusion CMR involves a 'first-pass' imaging technique, in which a sequence of images is obtained during the passage of the contrast through the heart. This is in contrast to nuclear imaging techniques, which rely on the accumulation of radioisotope in the heart over a short time period. The heart is 'stressed' with a vasodilator (e.g. adenosine), and the stress images compared to those acquired after a period of rest.

CMR perfusion imaging has excellent sensitivity (80-90%) and good specificity (70-80%) for detecting myocardial ischaemia, and its diagnostic performance is at least equivalent to that of nuclear perfusion imaging.

Perfusion imaging benefits substantially from the higher signal-to-noise ratio at 3T, with greater confidence and improved diagnostic accuracy.

Scanning summary

(See 📖 p. 120 for acquisition details).

- Ensure adequate coverage of the left ventricle (at least 3 short axis slices in basal, mid & apical positions).
- The stress perfusion scan is acquired after a 3–6min infusion of a vasodilator (adenosine is the most widely used) and requires a rapid intravenous bolus of gadolinium contrast.
- At least 10min is required before the perfusion imaging is repeated at rest, to allow equilibration of the contrast agent within the myocardium. Other imaging can be acquired during this time.
- Rest imaging is important for distinguishing true defects from artefacts on the stress images (see Table 6.2), though the value of rest perfusion is limited if the stress images are normal, and some centres do not proceed to perfusion imaging at rest in this case.

Analysing a CMR perfusion scan

Qualitative analysis ('eyeball' assessment) is usually performed in the clinical setting. Quantitative measurements (either quantification of myocardial blood flow or calculation of perfusion reserve) are more time consuming methods, and are mainly used for research purposes.

Qualitative analysis

- This is performed by visual comparison of the contrast enhancement during first-pass perfusion in different myocardial regions.
- Myocardial areas subtended by a severely stenosed coronary artery show delayed arrival of the contrast and appear hypo-intense in stress images compared with the normal myocardium, which shows a homogeneous ↑ in signal intensity (Figs 6.4 and 6.5). The extent of any perfusion deficit (both across regions and transmuraliy) is indicative of the severity.

Suggested routine

- View stress and rest images simultaneously (displayed side by side).
- Examine the images initially without zooming to gain a good general impression, although images are smaller, the picture quality is better.
- Then zoom and concentrate on the stress image looking for any areas of regional hypo-enhancement. Differentiate between true perfusion defects and artefacts (see Table 6.2). Compare with the rest image.
- Repeat the process for each of the acquired slices.

Artefacts

- **Blurred images:** may be related to ECG mis-triggering (the saturation recovery sequence used for perfusion has a significant effect on the ECG) or to breathing artefact due to the long scan length (30–45s).
- **Dark rim artefact:** these appear as a hypointense subendocardial rim (Fig. 6.6) and can mimic true perfusion defects, leading to false positive results. They are attributed to several effects, including susceptibility differences between blood pool and endocardium, Gibbs ringing due to inadequate spatial resolution and cardiac motion. Diagnostic accuracy can be increased by including all data from both stress and rest perfusion, cine and delayed enhancement imaging.

Table 6.2 Tips for identifying susceptibility artefacts

True perfusion defects	Susceptibility artefacts
The area of hypo-enhancement usually corresponds with typical coronary artery perfusion territories	Do not always follow the typical territories – tend to be more circumferential
Last several cardiac cycles (>5) and usually appear at second pass as well	Appear mostly during peak LV contrast concentration and disappear quickly (<5 cardiac cycles)
Usually present in several slices depending on how proximal the location of the disease is	May be more pronounced in one slice, but disappear on the next one
Present only during stress, if ischaemia is reversible (inducible perfusion defects). If an infarct is present, perfusion defect may be present at both stress and rest	Present at stress and rest even in the absence of myocardial scar

In equivocal cases, semi-quantitative analysis (time-signal intensity curves) may help.

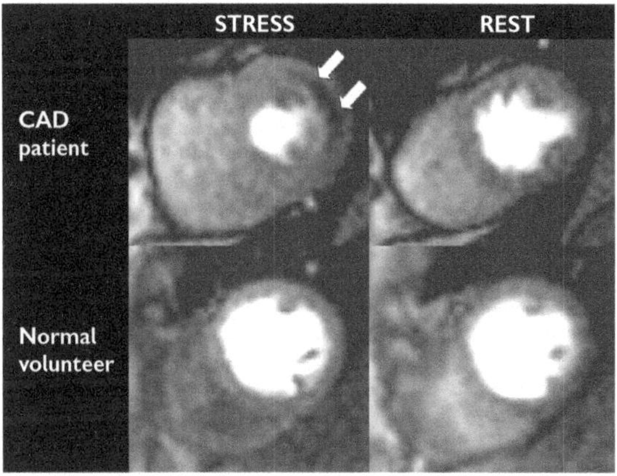

Fig. 6.4 CMR perfusion scans during adenosine stress (left panels) and rest (right panels). The top panels show a patient with a significant left circumflex stenosis. Note the reversible perfusion deficit in the lateral segments (white arrows).

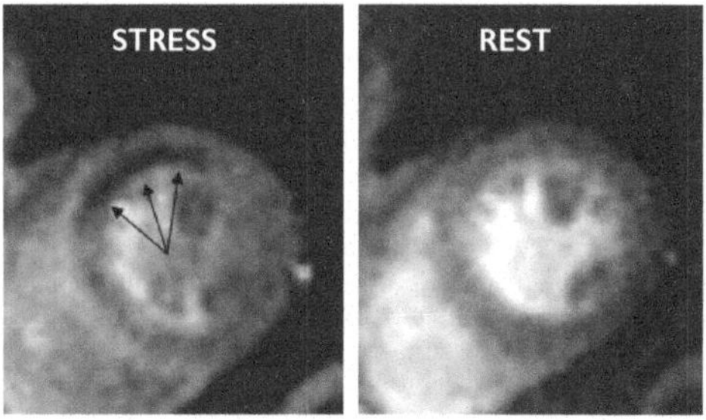

Fig. 6.5 True perfusion defect in a patient with significant LAD stenosis. Note the reversible perfusion deficit in the anterior segment (black arrows).

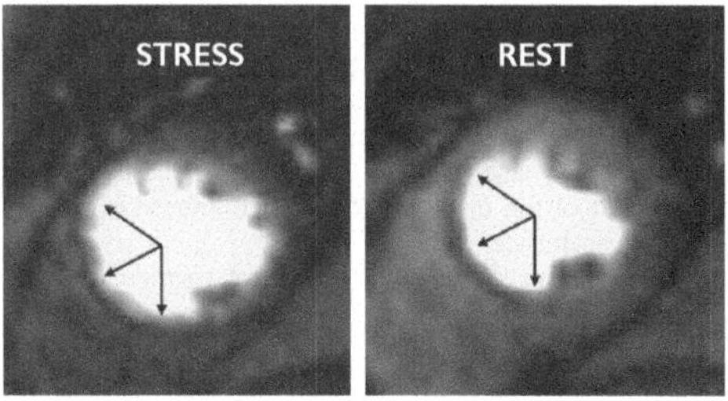

Fig. 6.6 Susceptibility artefact in a subject with normal coronary arteries. Note the hypo-enhanced area in the septum (black arrows) in both stress and rest images.

Semi-quantitative perfusion assessment

Relative perfusion can be assessed by comparing the signal intensity in each region as the contrast passes through the myocardium. A low contrast dose is required (0.025–0.05mmol/kg) to preserve the linearity in relationship between myocardial contrast concentration and signal intensity. The AHA 16-segment model (📖 p. 147) is used for dividing the myocardium into segments – 6 for the basal and mid-ventricular slices, and 4 for the apical slice. Time signal intensity curves are measured from each region and several parameters of perfusion can be derived:

- Maximal signal intensity.
- Contrast appearance time.
- Time to maximal signal intensity.
- Up-slope of the signal intensity curve (corrected for arterial input function by dividing the up-slopes of the myocardial segments by the up-slope of the left ventricular signal intensity curve).

Calculation requires careful tracing of the endo- and epicardial contours, and is time-consuming, especially with respiratory motion or ECG mis-triggering. Automatic registration methods exist, but manual correction is usually needed.

Myocardial perfusion reserve index

This can be calculated by dividing the up-slope values obtained during stress imaging by the upslope values at rest. There is no clear consensus on the 'normal' threshold index, however, which ranges from 1.2 to 2.0, with values below this suggesting a perfusion defect.

Standard process for calculating relative perfusion parameters

- Identify the phase with the maximum intensity of contrast in the LV cavity (and ideally some residual contrast in the RV cavity).
- View the cine sequence in each slice to get an idea of where the contours may be best situated. Optimize the contrast/windowing.
- The epicardial contour should be placed at least 1–2mm inside the actual epicardial border, ensuring no epicardial fat or RV blood pool is included. The endocardial contour should exclude the blood pool, with its high intensity signal, which will affect the results. Place the contour at least 1–2mm outside the actual endocardial border.
- Draw a region of interest in the centre of the LV cavity, avoiding papillary muscles. This is required for the blood pool signal intensity curve.
- Copy the three contours (epicardium, endocardium, blood pool) to the other images, adjusting for breathing motion or mis-triggering.
- Divide the myocardium into the relevant segments, using a reference point at the inferior/anterior LV–RV junction (depending on the software). The remaining segments are usually automatically assigned.
- Identify the start of the up-slope of the time-intensity curve in the LV blood pool for each slice.
- The time-intensity curve for each myocardial segment can be viewed (Fig. 6.7). Spikes in the curve usually indicate an incorrectly placed contour – these should be corrected.
- The parameters for each segment can be assessed and compared with other segments. Some software provides an automated comparison.

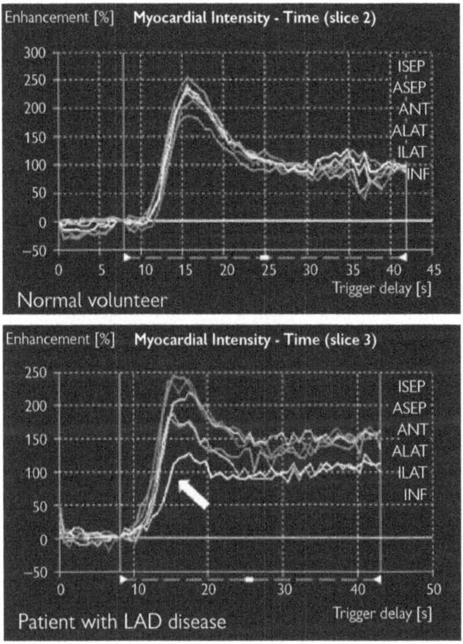

Fig. 6.7 Myocardial time-intensity curves from a normal volunteer (top) and a patient with significant left anterior descending coronary artery disease (bottom). Note for the normal volunteer: all six curves have a similar up-slope, while the patient with LAD stenosis has a significantly reduced anterior wall signal intensity curve (white arrow).

Absolute quantification of myocardial blood flow

First pass perfusion images may be used to measure absolute myocardial blood flow in ml/min/g. This is more objective than qualitative (visual) assessment and is better able to demonstrate global reductions in blood flow (i.e. 3-vessel disease). However, it involves complex mathematical analysis, is very time-consuming, and dedicated software is needed. Currently it is only used in research.

A low contrast dose is required (0.025–0.05mmol/kg) to maintain the linear relationship between changes in the signal intensities and contrast concentration, both in the blood pool and myocardial tissue. Calculation uses the mathematical process of model-independent deconvolution and myocardial perfusion reserve can also be calculated as the ratio of hyperemic and resting blood flow. A detailed discussion of the process is beyond the scope of this book, but references are included at the end of this Chapter.

Perfusion reporting

This should include the following.

Physiological indicators

- Duration of pharmacological stress.
- Symptoms during stress.
- Heart rate and blood pressure at both baseline and peak stress.

Perfusion images

- The presence and myocardial extent of *Inducible* perfusion deficits the AHA 16-segment model is recommended and/or correlation to coronary territories.
- The transmural extent of the perfusion deficit can be graded visually:
    - 0 – no regional hypoenhancement
    - 1 – transmural extent <25%
    - 2 – transmural extent 25%–50%
    - 3 – transmural extent 51–75%
    - 4 – transmural extent >75%.
- Appearances of the rest perfusion images, to confirm the inducible nature of the perfusion deficit.
- Include all the information available from the CMR scan. Assess cine images for wall motion abnormalities and late enhancement images for evidence of myocardial scar, in comparison with perfusion images.
- Final conclusion on whether the scan is abnormal (true perfusion defect) or not (artefact or entirely normal).

Coronary artery imaging

The small size, tortuous course and rapid motion of the coronary arteries makes MR coronary angiography a demanding technique. Very high spatial and temporal resolution is required for this, and although some progress has been made, reliable assessment of coronary stenoses by CMR remains challenging and requires further improvements in MR technology. In current clinical practice, the main application of MR coronary angiography is the identification of anomalous coronary artery origins. For further details see Chapter 15, Coronary magnetic resonance imaging, 📖 p. 399).

Multiparametric CMR approach to ischaemic heart disease

The techniques described in this chapter can be combined in a single comprehensive study for patients with known or suspected IHD (Fig. 6.8). In everyday practice, cine imaging, first-pass (stress and rest) perfusion assessment, and LGE are the key aspects in CMR evaluation of these patients. Oedema imaging may become a valuable tool for the assessment of patients with acute coronary disease. As described above, coronary imaging needs further improvement to be used in routine clinical practice.

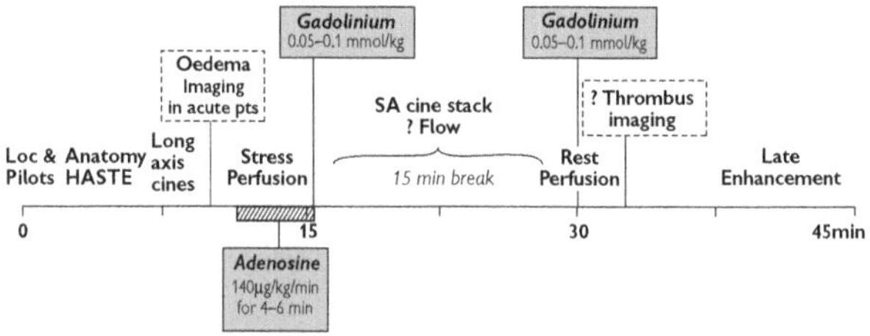

Fig. 6.8 Fully time-optimized protocol for a multi-parametric CMR study in IHD. The central components of this protocol are cine imaging, first-pass perfusion at stress and rest, and LGE. The full short-axis cine stack is acquired during the break between stress and rest perfusion. During this break flow imaging can also be performed (e.g. if the patient has concomitant valvular disease). The second short break after rest perfusion can be used for early post contrast images (thrombus imaging) or additional flow imaging. If needed, T_2-weighted oedema imaging can be added to this protocol (before contrast administration), extending its duration by 5–10min.

Useful references for CMR in IHD

Aletras AH, Tilak GS, Natanzon A *et al.* Retrospective determination of the area at risk for reperfused acute myocardial infarction with T_2-weighted cardiac magnetic resonance imaging: histopathological and displacement encoding with stimulated echoes (DENSE) functional validations. *Circulation* 2006; **113:** 1865–70.

Jerosch-Herold M, Swingen C, Seethamraju RT. Myocardial blood flow quantification with MRI by model-independent deconvolution. *Med Phys* 2002; **29:** 886–97.

Kim RJ, Wu E, Rafael A *et al.* The use of contrast-enhanced magnetic resonance imaging to identify reversible myocardial dysfunction. *N Engl J Med* 2000; **343:** 1445–53.

Nagel E, Lehmkuhl HB, Bocksch W *et al.* Noninvasive diagnosis of ischemia-induced wall motion abnormalities with the use of high-dose dobutamine stress MRI: comparison with dobutamine stress echocardiography. *Circulation* 1999; **99:** 763–70.

Schwitter J, Wacker CM, van Rossum AC *et al.* MR-IMPACT: comparison of perfusion-cardiac magnetic resonance with single-photon emission computed tomography for the detection of coronary artery disease in a multicentre, multivendor, randomized trial. *Eur Heart J* 2008; **29:** 480–9.

Selvanayagam JB, Kardos A, Francis JM *et al.* Value of delayed-enhancement cardiovascular magnetic resonance imaging in predicting myocardial viability after surgical revascularization. *Circulation* 2004; **110:** 1535–41.

Chapter 7

Inheritable cardiomyopathies

Hypertrophic cardiomyopathy

Background

The commonest inheritable cardiomyopathy (prevalence 1 in 500), often with autosomal dominant inheritance. Typically asymmetric hypertrophy, particularly in the basal septum, which may lead to outflow tract obstruction (about 25% of patients). Can present with predominantly apical thickening [apical hypertrophic cardiomyopathy (HCM)] and concentric hypertrophy is also possible. Progressive LV dilatation can occur late in the disease process.

CMR features

- **Increased wall thickness:** significant LV hypertrophy (wall thickness >15mm or >13mm if a family history of HCM present), in the absence of other causes. LV mass should be measured with CMR, although there are no criteria for HCM, particularly as many cases involve regional hypertrophy, which may increase total LV mass only slightly.
- **Regional 'asymmetric' hypertrophy:** this often occurs in the septum (see Fig. 7.1), but not exclusively, and the apex and anterior wall are common alternative sites. Compare the thickest and thinnest myocardial segments in a single slice to obtain the diastolic wall thickness ratio (thickest/thinnest wall thickness). A wall thickness ratio >2.0 may be considered abnormal.
- **LV outflow or mid-cavity obstruction:**
  - Occurs in 25% of cases. The hypertrophied septum thickens, maximally in late systole, and may obstruct the LVOT, with visible narrowing and turbulence (see 📖 p. 254). There may also be anterior motion (towards the LVOT) of the anterior mitral valve leaflet, from the suction or 'Venturi' effect of the high velocity jet in the LVOT, which exacerbates the obstruction
  - Obstruction may occur in the mid-cavity as the opposing walls meet, if the hypertrophy is predominantly in the mid ventricle.
- **Obliteration of the LV cavity in systole:** can occur due a combination of the much thickened myocardium and reduced chamber size. It is not a feature of hypertensive heart disease, which helps the differentiation.
- **Late gadolinium enhancement:**
  - Typically mid-wall enhancement, often where wall thickness is greatest
  - Also commonly occurs in the basal septum at the junction with the RV free wall, either the superior or inferior junction (Fig. 7.2)
  - The enhancement is likely to represent areas of fibrosis and limited post-mortem studies have supported this
  - May be absent, but if present, is strongly suggestive of HCM, and aids the differentiation from pressure overload LVH (e.g. aortic valve disease, hypertension)
  - There is little prognostic data on the presence of enhancement, but it is frequent in HCM patients with multiple clinical risk factors of sudden cardiac death and is a strong indicator of abnormal pathology

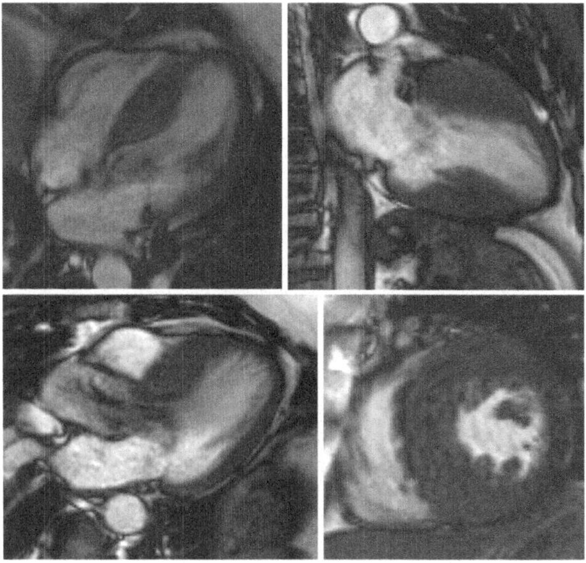

Fig. 7.1 End-diastolic cine images in standard views (HLA – top left, VLA – top right, and SA – bottom right) demonstrating marked asymmetric LV hypertrophy typical of HCM. The LVOT view (bottom left) is in late systole and shows significant turbulence in the LVOT indicative of obstruction.

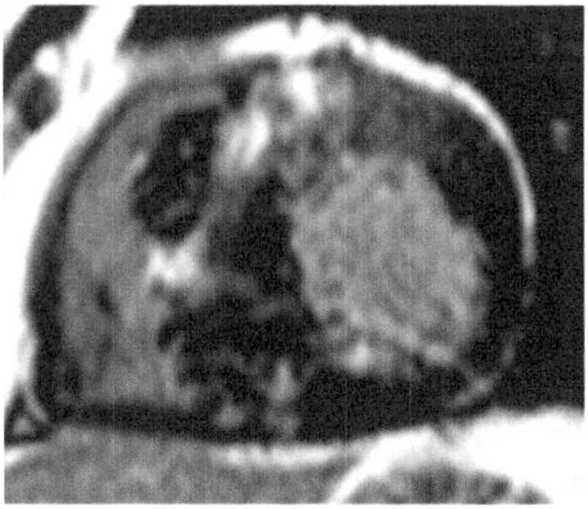

Fig. 7.2 Late gadolinium image in the mid-ventricular short axis plane demonstrating the typical enhancement pattern seen in HCM. Enhancement is present at both the superior and inferior septal LV/RV junctions and in the mid-wall of the hypertrophied segment.

Scanning

3 long axis planes (HLA, VLA, and LVOT views)
Look for abnormal wall thickness (particularly regional hypertrophy), LVOT/mid-cavity obstruction, obliteration of the LV cavity in systole, and systolic anterior motion of the anterior mitral valve leaflet.

Short axis cine stack
For measurement of LV mass and function (both regional and global). Short axis images are often the best planes for measuring wall thickness and judging the degree of asymmetry.

In-plane ± through-plane flow
If LVOT or mid-cavity obstruction is present, acquire an in-plane flow sequence in the appropriate plane to measure peak velocity. Through-plane flow may be more accurate in high velocity, narrow jets. Note that this is the resting gradient and could rise significantly on exertion.

Late gadolinium enhancement
Image 3 long axes and all short axis slices to cover whole ventricle. Any questionable areas of enhancement should have the image repeated with a 'phase swap' (Avoiding artefacts, 🕮 p. 114). Aim also to confirm in a second imaging plane positioned through the enhanced area on the short axis view.

Reporting should include:

- LV volumes and mass (comment on degree of hypertrophy).
- Location of hypertrophy – septum, apex, generalized.
- Degree of asymmetry – compare thickest to thinnest wall (e.g. septum and lateral wall).
- Any mid-cavity or LVOT obstruction? Provide peak velocity/gradient in LVOT (peak gradient = 4 × (peak velocity)^2.
- Systolic anterior motion of the anterior mitral valve leaflet.
- Any areas of late gadolinium enhancement. Examine the pattern of enhancement.
- Evidence of mitral regurgitation.

Differential diagnosis

Consider other forms of (mostly diffuse) LV hypertrophy:

- Hypertension.
- Aortic stenosis (valve disease should be clear from CMR scan/echo).
- Infiltrative myocardial disease (e.g. amyloid, sarcoid, iron overload) (🕮 p. 202, 204).
- Fabry disease (Anderson-Fabry disease, 🕮 p. 190).
- Eosinophilic myocarditis (🕮 p. 204).
- Left ventricular non-compaction ('hypertrophy' is really hyper-trabeculation; 🕮 p. 188).

Further reading

Maron MS, Hauser TH, Dubrow E *et al.* Right ventricular involvement in hypertrophic cardiomyopathy. *Am J Cardiol* 2007; **100:** 1293–8.

Moon JC, McKenna WJ, McCrohen JA *et al.* Toward clinical risk assessment in hypertrophic cardiomyopathy with gadolinium cardiovascular magnetic resonance. *J Am Coll Cardiol* 2003; **41:** 1561–7.

Petersen SE, Selvanayagam JB, Francis JM *et al.* Differentiation of athlete's heart from pathological forms of cardiac hypertrophy by means of geometric indices derived from cardiovascular magnetic resonance. *J Cardiovasc Magn Reson* 2005; **7:** 551–8.

Dilated cardiomyopathy

Background

Characterized by ventricular chamber dilatation and global systolic dysfunction. Idiopathic dilated cardiomyopathy is a diagnosis of exclusion of 2° causes, and is familial in 20–50% of cases, often with an autosomal dominant inheritance pattern.

CMR features

- **LV ± RV dilatation with impaired global systolic function:**
  - Some degree of regional dysfunction is possible
  - Increased LV mass may be seen, in proportion to the increased volumes, but wall thickness is usually normal (<12mm) or even decreased.
- **± LV thrombus:** if ↓ LV function; best seen on early gadolinium images.
- **Late gadolinium enhancement:**
  - Typically a thin band of mid-wall enhancement (Fig. 7.3). Seen in ~30%
  - This likely represents fibrosis, but is not specific for any aetiology
  - Its presence is also a predictor of mortality and hospitalization.

Scanning

3 long axis planes (HLA, VLA, and LVOT views)

Look for LV and RV dilatation, and global systolic dysfunction. Are there regional wall motion abnormalities that suggest coronary disease?

Short axis cine stack

For LV and RV volumes, mass, and function.

T_2-weighted black blood imaging

This may be helpful to document acute necrosis or oedema (myocarditis).

Early and late gadolinium enhancement

- **Early:** 3 long axes only.
- **Late:** 3 long axes and all short axis slices.

Reporting should include:

- LV and RV volumes, function (global and regional), and mass (including wall thickness as required).
- Evidence of mitral regurgitation.
- Any areas of late gadolinium enhancement.
- Evidence of LV thrombus.

Differential diagnosis

Consider other forms of LV dilatation and systolic dysfunction:

- Ischaemic heart disease.
- Aortic/mitral regurgitation (should be clear from CMR scan/echo!).
- End-stage hypertensive heart disease.
- Left ventricular non-compaction (📖 p. 188).
- Alcoholic cardiomyopathy.
- Iron-overload cardiomyopathy (📖 p. 210).

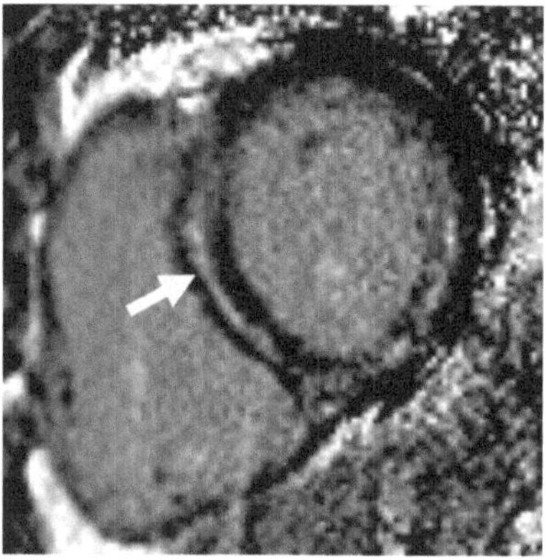

Fig. 7.3 Late gadolinium enhancement image in the mid-ventricular short axis view showing a thin band of mid-wall enhancement in the septum (arrowed). The pattern is distinct from the endocardial enhancement seen in coronary artery disease.

Further reading

Assomull RG, Prasad SK, Lyne J *et al.* Cardiovascular magnetic resonance, fibrosis, and prognosis in dilated cardiomyopathy. *J Am Coll Cardiol* 2006; **48**: 1977–85.

McCrohon JA, Moon JC, Prasad SK *et al.* Differentiation of heart failure related to dilated cardiomyopathy and coronary artery disease using gadolinium-enhanced cardiovascular magnetic resonance. *Circulation* 2003; **108**: 54–9.

Arrhythmogenic right ventricular cardiomyopathy

Background

Degenerative disease mostly affecting the right ventricle, but which may also involve the LV. Typical pathological findings are an enlarged RV with regional wall thinning and fibro-fatty replacement of the myocardial tissue. Complications include malignant arrhythmias and right heart failure.

CMR features

- The diagnosis is made according to task force criteria, taking into account several aspects, some of which can be assessed with CMR (see Table 7.1).

► Note that a diagnosis of ARVC is very difficult to make solely on CMR findings.

- **Global RV dilatation and systolic dysfunction:** if severe, this is a major criterion, if mild, a minor criterion (Fig. 7.5).
- **Segmental RV dilatation and dysfunction:** look for areas of regional RV thinning (see Fig. 7.4), dilation and poor systolic contraction relative to adjacent segments. Commonly occur in the RVOT, the basal inferior wall and close to the moderator band. If regional RV abnormalities are severe, these are a major criterion; if mild, a minor criterion.
- **RV 'micro-aneurysms':** these are localized areas of *dyskinesis* during *systole*. When present, these represent a major criterion (Fig. 7.6).
- **Fibro-fatty infiltration of the RV free wall:** either on T_1-weighted imaging (fat) or late gadolinium enhancement (fibrous tissue). In practice, this is rarely seen, due to the diffuse nature of the infiltration, the mixed signal from fibro-fatty tissue, the late stage of the disease in which it occurs, and the difficulties in reliably imaging the thin RV free wall. It is usually only seen in advanced cases where other diagnostic features are grossly evident.
- **± LV involvement:** regional/global wall motion abnormalities ± late gadolinium enhancement. Consider other diagnoses if LV is significantly involved (e.g. sarcoid, other infiltrative diseases).

Challenges in interpreting RV wall motion

- The abnormalities can be very subtle.
- Be careful not to over-call minor abnormalities. Experience is required to recognize normal RV contraction. In particular, there is considerable through-plane motion from the longitudinal contraction of the RV, and an apparently akinetic or dyskinetic segment may be due to a larger, more basal, segment entering the imaging plane.
- Interpreting wall motion near the moderator band is difficult. The contraction of the band can make adjacent segments appear relatively hypokinetic.

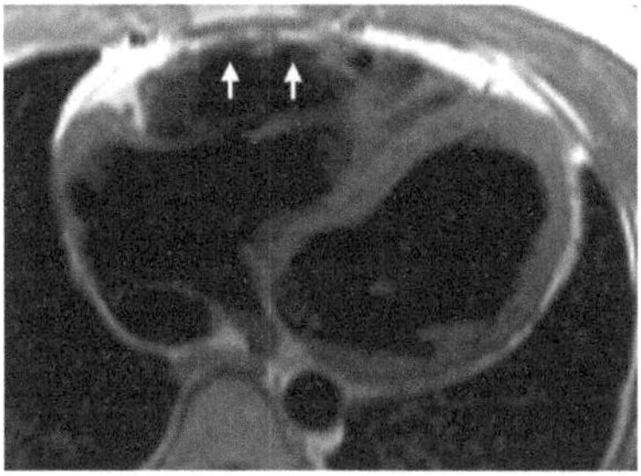

Fig. 7.4 Transverse turbo-spin echo image showing thinning of the RV free wall (arrowed) in a patient with ARVC.

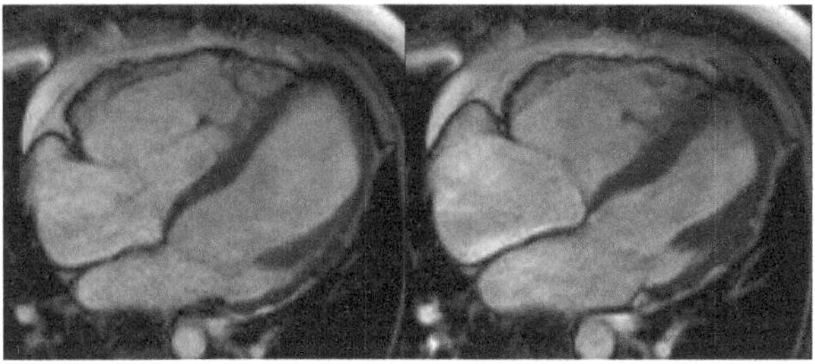

Fig. 7.5 HLA cine images in diastole (left) and systole (right) of patient with ARVC, showing reduced global RV function.

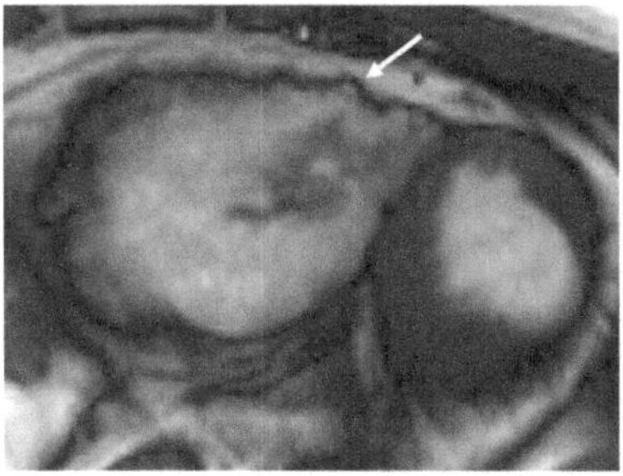

Fig. 7.6 Low transverse cine image in systole showing RV micro-aneurysm (arrowed).

Scanning

Cines of 3 long axis planes (HLA, VLA and LVOT views)

Look for LV and RV dilatation, and global systolic function. Are there regional wall motion abnormalities?

Short axis cine stack

For measurement of LV and RV mass and function.

RV outflow and RV 2-chamber cines

See 🕮 p. 92.

The RVOT allows detection of wall motion abnormalities of the anterior RV wall and outflow tract (infundibulum). The inferior RV wall below the tricuspid valve is best seen on the RV 2-chamber view.

Transverse cine stack

Transverse views are excellent for visualizing RV free wall motion abnormalities. Image from the RV outflow tract down to the inferior RV wall, at 1cm intervals with a small gap between slices. If these images look suspicious, use contiguous slices without a gap in the relevant areas.

Black blood images (e.g. turbo spin echo) with and without fat saturation

For imaging myocardial tissue characteristics. Short axis and transverse planes, as for cine imaging. If the heart rate allows (typically <90bpm), a saturation band over the anterior chest wall creates better contrast by removing the high signal from the subcutaneous fat.

Late gadolinium enhancement

Same imaging planes as above.

Reporting should include:

- LV and RV volumes, ejection fractions and mass.
- Any RV wall thinning (often difficult due to the already thin RV wall!).
- Regional RV wall motion abnormalities.
- RV micro-aneurysms.
- Fibro-fatty infiltration of RV wall (if seen).
- Evidence of LV involvement.
- Presence, extent, and location of any late gadolinium enhancement.

Differential diagnosis

- RV dilatation and impairment secondary to other causes, e.g. pulmonary or tricuspid regurgitation, atrial septal defect, RV infarction.
- Dilated cardiomyopathy involving the RV.
- Other inherited cardiomyopathies.
- Cardiac sarcoidosis.

Table 7.1 Diagnostic criteria for ARVC (adapted from Task Force criteria). Diagnosis requires the presence, from different categories, of:
- 2 major criteria *or*
- 1 major and 2 minor criteria *or*
- 4 minor criteria.

► NB the diagnosis can rarely be made on CMR findings alone!

Category	Major criteria	Minor criteria
RV structural/ dysfunctional alteration	Severe dilation and reduction of RV function with no or mild LV involvement Localized RV aneurysms Severe segmental dilation of RV	Mild global RV dilation or reduction in function with normal LV Mild segmental dilation of RV Regional RV hypokinesia
Myocardial tissue	Fibro-fatty replacement of myocardium on endomyocardial biopsy	
12-lead ECG	Epsilon waves or localized prolongation (>110ms) of QRS duration in right precordial leads (V1-3)	Inverted T waves in right precordial leads (V2, V3) if aged >12 years and in the absence of RBBB Late potentials on signal averaged ECG
Arrhythmias		LBBB-type ventricular tachycardia (sustained or non-sustained) Frequent ventricular extra-systoles (>1000/24h)
Family history	Family disease confirmed at necropsy or surgery	Family history of premature sudden death (<35 years) due to suspected ARVC Family history (clinical diagnosis)

LBBB = left bundle branch block; RBBB = right bundle branch block.

Further reading

McKenna WJ, Thiene G, Nova A *et al.* Task Force Criteria of the Working Group on Myocardial and Pericardial Disease of the European Society of Cardiology. *Br Heart J* 1994; **71:** 215–18.

Tandri H, Macedo R, Calkins H *et al.* Role of magnetic resonance imaging in arrhythmogenic right ventricular dysplasia: insights from the North American arrhythmogenic right ventricular dysplasia (ARVD/C) study. *Am Heart J* 2008; **155:** 147–53.

Left ventricular non-compaction

Background

Characterized by extensive trabeculation of the endocardial layer of the myocardium and a thinned epicardial layer. It resembles the early foetal heart and may represent arrest of this stage of development. It is not currently classified as a cardiomyopathy by the World Health Organization and its underlying pathophysiological mechanisms remain controversial. Familial forms are increasingly recognized. Potential complications include cardiac failure, thrombo-embolism, and malignant arrhythmias, but definitive prognostic data, especially in asymptomatic patients, are lacking.

CMR features

- **Increased trabeculation:** left ventricular non-compaction (LVNC) involves an *excess* of normal trabeculation, so experience of the normal variation is important. There is a spectrum of severity, with some patients having ↑ trabeculation, but not to a clearly pathological degree.
  - Look for an increase in the trabeculated layer in diastole (see Fig 7.7). The adjacent compacted layer may appear thin and the ratio of thicknesses (non-compacted to compacted myocardium) should be measured. A ratio >2.3 seems to be a useful indicator of abnormal trabeculation
  - Failure of the trabeculated layer to compact in systole should raise suspicions. This doesn't apply however to those with ↓ systolic function, in whom the trabeculations may not compact fully anyway.
- **LV ± RV dilatation with impaired systolic function.**
- **LV thrombus:**
  - Thrombus may form due to slow flow in the trabeculated layer
  - Early gadolinium imaging should be used.
- **Late gadolinium enhancement:** limited experience in non-compaction.

Scanning

See Dilated cardiomyopathy, Scanning, 📖 p. 182.

Reporting should include:

- Location and degree of excess trabeculation – include RV.
- Thickness of trabeculated (non-compacted) to compacted myocardial layers in diastole (normal ratio <2.3).
- LV and RV volumes, function, and mass.
- Any evidence of mitral regurgitation.
- Any areas of late gadolinium enhancement.
- Evidence of LV thrombus.

Differential diagnosis

- DCM.
- Apical HCM.
- Pronounced trabeculation in poorly contractile segments.
- Variation of normal, particularly in the absence of symptoms, LV dilatation, or systolic dysfunction.

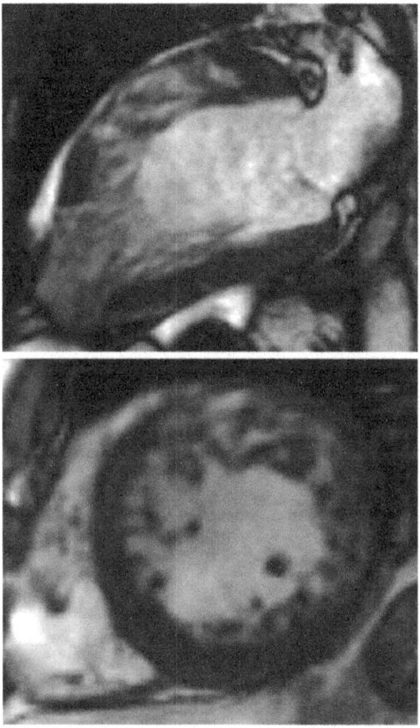

Fig. 7.7 SSFP image from a patient with significant non-compaction. VLA view (top), short axis view (bottom). Note the marked trabeculation of the LV with thinning of the anterior wall, and a non-compaction to compaction ratio >2.3.

Anderson-Fabry disease

Background

X-linked recessive deficiency of the enzyme alpha-galactosidase A, one of the lysosomal storage diseases. Cardiac features include hypertrophy, conduction abnormalities, and aortic and mitral valve thickening.

Most patients with this condition are male, but there have been cases of female carriers with typical features.

CMR features

- CMR features are not specific enough for diagnosis. If Anderson-Fabry disease is suspected, this can be confirmed by reduced serum levels of alpha-galactosidase A.
- **LV hypertrophy:** usually concentric and moderate to severe, but can be asymmetrical and mimic HCM.
- **Late gadolinium enhancement:** small series have shown enhancement in the basal infero-lateral wall (see Fig. 7.8), but the pattern is not well defined.

Scanning

See Hypertrophic cardiomyopathy, Scanning, 📖 p. 180.

Reporting should include:

- LV volumes and mass (comment on degree of hypertrophy).
- Location of hypertrophy.
- Degree of asymmetry – compare thickest to thinnest wall (e.g. septum and lateral wall).
- Any features that more typical for HCM, e.g. LVOT obstruction, systolic anterior motion of the anterior mitral valve leaflet.
- Any areas of late gadolinium enhancement.

Differential diagnosis

- HCM.
- Hypertensive heart disease.
- Infiltrative heart diseases (e.g. amyloid, sarcoid).

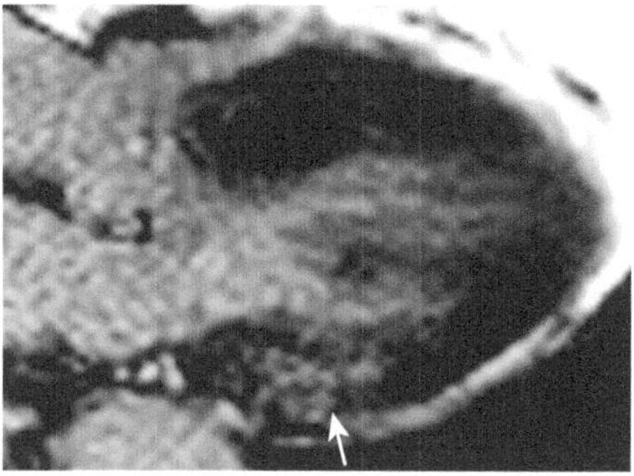

Fig. 7.8 Delayed enhancement image in the LVOT plane in a patient with Anderson-Fabry disease. There is mid-wall enhancement in the infero-lateral wall (arrowed). Reproduced with kind permission from Dr Oliver Strohm, University of Calgary.

Further reading

Moon JC, Sachdov B, Elkington AG *et al.* Gadolinium enhanced cardiovascular magnetic resonance in Anderson-Fabry disease. Evidence for a disease specific abnormality of the myocardial interstitium. *Eur Heart J* 2003; **24**(23): 2151–5.

Chapter 8

Myocardial inflammation and infiltration

Myocardial tissue characterization

The unique CMR ability of non-invasive tissue characterization is invaluable in the investigation of inflammatory and infiltrative diseases of the heart. It provides a comprehensive assessment of the severity of myocardial dysfunction, and the acuity and reversibility of the disease process.

Acute inflammatory changes include:

- **Oedema** (increased water content): visible on T_2-weighted images.
- **Capillary leak** (ongoing inflammation): detectable on T_1-weighted images by increased contrast uptake early after gadolinium injection ('early enhancement').
- **Necrosis/fibrosis** (irreversible myocardial damage): visible on delayed gadolinium enhancement imaging.

General scanning technique

LV and RV volumes and function

3 standard long axes cine images and a short axis cine stack for assessment of the global and regional effect of the disease.

T_2-weighted imaging

For oedema assessment. Increased water content results in high signal on T_2-weighted imaging {T_2-WI). Use fast spin echo or hybrid sequences with strong T_2-weighting. Regional oedema and delayed enhancement often occur together. Global oedema may be difficult to see, but can be verified by normalizing myocardial signal intensity to skeletal muscle - a SI-ratio ≥ 2.0 is considered abnormal (Fig. 8.1).

T1-weighted imaging pre- and post-gadolinium

- Increased uptake of gadolinium (an extra-cellular contrast agent) is a typical finding in acute inflammation, reflecting ↑ capillary leak and extracellular volume. Acquire T_1-weighted images pre- and immediately post-contrast ('early' gadolinium enhancement, Fig. 8.2).
- An increase in post-contrast myocardial signal intensity >45% from baseline is considered abnormal. In global myocardial inflammation, the skeletal muscle can be used to normalize myocardial enhancement, and an early enhancement ratio is suggested (see box Scanning suggestions for T_1-weighted imaging, 📖 p. 195), although this is not currently standard clinical practice; a ratio ≥ 4.0 is abnormal. If significant muscle enhancement is seen, however, the ratio may be falsely negative – report on the increase in myocardial enhancement instead.
- Newer sequences are being developed for improved image quality and compatibility with multi-element coils.

Late gadolinium enhancement

- Indicates expansion of the interstitial space, due mainly to necrosis (breakdown of cell membranes), or severe infiltration. This usually represents irreversible myocardial damage, though the area of enhancement can reduce with time in some inflammatory conditions (e.g. myocarditis, sarcoidosis), predominantly due to fibrotic contraction.
- The distribution of enhancement in inflammatory and infiltrative conditions is significantly different from coronary disease, and it is usually easy to distinguish non-ischemic damage from infarction.

Scanning suggestions for T_2-weighted imaging

- Use body coil to avoid signal intensity inhomogeneity from the surface coil.
- Obtain images prior to contrast application.
- Consider fat suppression.
- Breath-hold, segmented fast spin-echo with dark blood prep (double or triple-inversion recovery).
- Time acquisition to mid-diastole.
- TE >60ms, TR >2000ms.
- Slice thickness >8 mm, or even thicker (up to 15mm) if SNR inadequate.
- Calculate T_2 ratio for global assessment (normal <2.0):

$$T_2 \text{ ratio} = SI_{\text{myocardium}} / SI_{\text{skeletal muscle}}$$

Scanning suggestions for T_1-weighted imaging

- Use body coil to avoid signal intensity inhomogeneity from the surface coil.
- Non-breath-hold fast spin-echo without fat suppression. Carefully instruct patients to breathe regularly.
- Start post-contrast scanning within 15s after contrast injection.
- Slice thickness 8–10mm.
- Consider prior β-blocker administration if heart beat very irregular.

Calculation of early myocardial enhancement

Myocardial enhancement (norm ≤45%):

$$(SI_{\text{myocardium}}\text{ post} - SI_{\text{myocardium}}\text{ pre})/SI_{\text{myocardium}}\text{ pre} \times 100\%$$

Skeletal muscle enhancement:

$$SI_{\text{skeletal muscle}}\text{ post} - SI_{\text{skeletal muscle}}\text{ pre})/SI_{\text{skeletal muscle}}\text{ pre} \times 100\%$$

Early enhancement ratio (norm <4.0). NB this is not currently a standard clinical measurement, but may become more widely accepted in the future):

$$\text{Enhancement}_{\text{myocardium}}/\text{Enhancement}_{\text{skeletal muscle}}$$

Myocarditis

Background

Myocarditis is typically caused by viral agents, although many may not be identified in clinical practice. Myocardial inflammation has various other causes, however, including toxic or autoimmune mechanisms. The clinical diagnosis is frequently difficult to establish because of non-specific or subtle symptoms and the lack of other specific non-invasive diagnostic criteria. The 'Gold standard' for diagnosis, endomyocardial biopsy, is often not appropriate, unless patients suffer from severe heart failure, and the patchy nature of the inflammation can reduce the sensitivity of the technique. CMR can provide valuable information on myocardial inflammation, regional or global wall motion abnormalities, pericardial effusion, and regional necrosis/fibrosis that significantly aids the diagnosis.

CMR features

- **Global/regional dysfunction:** globally reduced function occurs in ~50% of cases and LVEDV may be increased (depending on the severity of inflammation). Regional wall motion abnormalities, if present, are most often seen in the lateral segments. Pericardial adhesion may be noted on tagged cine images.
- **Myocardial oedema:** oedema identifies acute injury and can be seen as a global or regional increase in signal intensity on T_2-weighted images. Occasionally, regional swelling (↑ wall thickness) is apparent. Sensitivity for myocarditis is high in the acute phase (70–85%) with good specificity (~75%).
- **± Pericardial effusion:** T_2-weighted or SSFP images visualize pericardial effusions well.
- **Increased early myocardial contrast uptake:** usually indicates acute inflammation. Myocardial enhancement is best normalized to skeletal muscle (📖 p. 194), but can also be apparent on visual inspection of the post-contrast images (Fig. 8.2).
- **Late gadolinium enhancement:**
  - Indicates areas of necrosis ± severe oedema, and usually represents irreversible myocardial damage, though the extent is often limited. The area of enhancement can reduce with time, although the process is unclear. Small necrotic areas during the acute phase may disappear due to scar contraction and the limited spatial resolution of CMR.
  - The pattern is mid-wall or sub-epicardial enhancement, usually in the basal lateral wall or septum (Fig. 8.3). Although the inflammation in myocarditis is often patchy, the reason for this localization is unclear.
  - This pattern of late enhancement has high specificity for myocarditis (80–95%), although it is not always present, so sensitivity is lower (~40%).

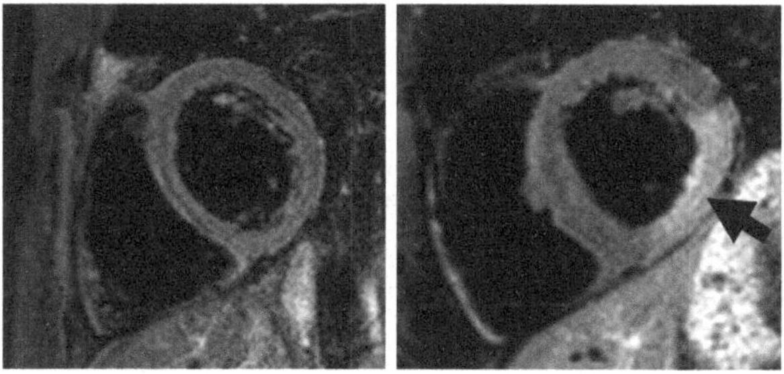

Fig. 8.1 Short axis T_2-weighted STIR sequence. Normal patient (left) and patient with acute oedema in the inferolateral wall (right). Note increased wall thickness and regionally increased SI.

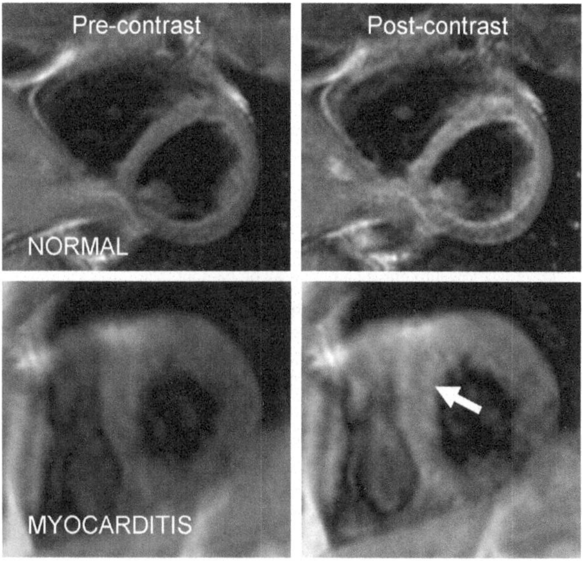

Fig. 8.2 Mid-ventricular short axis T_1-weighted spin echo images pre-contrast (left) and post-gadolinium contrast (right) in a normal volunteer (top) and patient with acute myocarditis (bottom). There is no regional myocardial contrast uptake in the normal study (early enhancement ratio 2.6), while the patient with myocarditis shows regional uptake of gadolinium consistent with acute inflammation (early enhancement ratio 6.4).

Scanning

- As for standard technique.
- Other sequences may address valvular function as required.

Reporting should include:

- **Cardiac volumes, function, para-cardiac findings:**
  - LV and RV volumes, mass, and regional and global function; atrial volumes
  - Any regional increase in wall thickness (suggesting oedema)
  - Pericardial and/or pleural effusion; pericardial adherence (Pericardial effusion, 📖 p. 298).
- **Evidence of inflammation:**
  - Location and regional distribution of oedema on T_2-weighted imaging. Report the calculated T_2 ratio and note if pathologic (≥2.0)
  - *Early enhancement* – describe any visible foci of enhancement and include the global early enhancement ratio. Report if pathologic (≥4.0)
  - *Late enhancement* – extent, location, and intramural distribution, including any enhancement of the RV. Correlate with wall motion abnormalities.
- **Conclusion**
  Summarize findings. Two or more positive criteria provide good evidence for myocarditis, with ~80% sensitivity and ~90% specificity in the acute phase. The chronic phase is less well evaluated.

Indicators of acute injury:

- Oedema.
- Regional or global wall motion abnormalities.
- Inflammation (↑ early gadolinium enhancement).
- Delayed gadolinium enhancement may be present.

Indicators of chronic injury (inflammatory activity resolved):

- Lack of oedema or early enhancement.
- Persistent regional or global LV dysfunction.
- Late enhancement may persist, if scars sufficiently large.

Differential diagnosis

Consider other conditions with localized myocardial damage:

- Ischaemic heart disease: delayed enhancement pattern is usually subendocardial, and oedema/inflammatory changes absent.
- Sarcoidosis: discrete foci of inflammation; pulmonary disease may be present.
- Inheritable cardiomyopathies (Chapter 7, 📖 p. 177).
- Anthracycline or other chemotherapeutic cardiomyopathy – may represent a myocarditis.
- Systemic disease with myocardial involvement.
- Other infiltrative disorders.

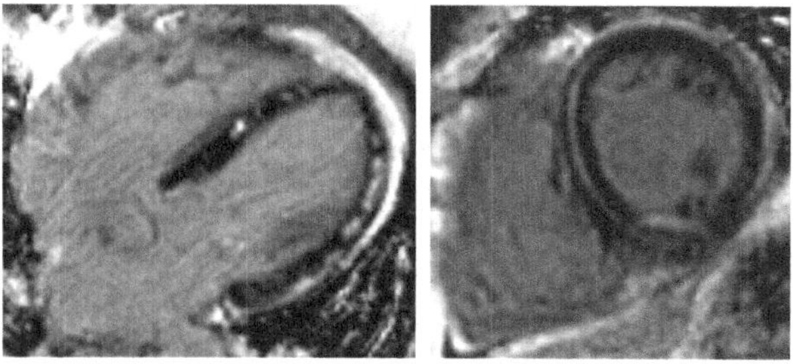

Fig. 8.3 Late gadolinium enhancement images in a patient with acute myocarditis; HLA view (left) and short axis view (right). Note the distribution of enhancement, in the mid-wall to sub-epicardium, sparing the endocardial layer, and crossing several coronary territories.

Further reading

Abdel-Aty H, Boyé P, Zagrose KA *et al.* Diagnostic performance of cardiovascular magnetic resonance in patients with suspected acute myocarditis: comparison of different approaches. *J Am Coll Cardiol.* 2005; **45:** 1815–22.

Friedrich MG, Strohm O, Shulz-Menger J *et al.* Contrast media-enhanced magnetic resonance imaging visualizes myocardial changes in the course of viral myocarditis. *Circulation* 1998; **97:** 1802–9.

Gutberlet M, Spors B, Thoma T *et al.* Suspected chronic myocarditis at cardiac MR: diagnostic accuracy and association with immunohistologically detected inflammation and viral persistence. *Radiology* 2008; **246:** 401–9.

Mahrholdt H, Goedecke C, Wagner A *et al.* Cardiovascular magnetic resonance assessment of human myocarditis: a comparison to histology and molecular pathology. *Circulation* 2004; **109:** 1250–8.

Skouri HN, Dec GW, Friedrich MG *et al.* Noninvasive imaging in myocarditis. *J Am Coll Cardiol* 2006; **48:** 2085–93.

Cardiac sarcoidosis

Background

Sarcoidosis is a systemic disease of unknown origin, characterized by non-caseating granulomas. Nearly all organs can be affected, although pulmonary involvement is common. Cardiac sarcoidosis has a significant impact on prognosis and requires more aggressive treatment, but is difficult to detect *in vivo*. CMR is able to provide diagnostic information in a number of patients and aid the clinical management.

CMR features of cardiac sarcoidosis

- **Global/regional dysfunction:** regional wall motion abnormalities are more likely than homogeneous global dysfunction, but global hypokinesis and dysfunction may occur in severe cases, when LV volumes may also be increased. Mildly increased LV mass may sometimes be present, possibly due to oedema.
- **Foci of oedema/inflammation:**
  - Patchy foci of inflammation can occur in an almost random distribution in the myocardium
  - Localized increases in T_2-weighted SI (indicating oedema) and early gadolinium enhancement ± increased wall thickness may be seen in cases with acute cardiac involvement
  - Global enhancement ratios may be less helpful, due to the small myocardial foci and the involvement of skeletal muscle in the disease.
- **Late gadolinium enhancement:** sarcoid lesions are usually mid-wall or sub-epicardial, although these can be sub-endocardial or trans-mural (associated with regional dys/akinesis). Often located in the septum, lateral wall, or involving the papillary muscles, and can involve the RV (Figs 8.4 and 8.5). The pattern is usually differentiated from ischaemic damage (i.e. infarction) by the multiple foci, mid-wall or epicardial location, and non-adherence to coronary artery territories.

Scanning

As for standard sequences (📖 p. 194)

Reporting should include:

- LV and RV volumes, mass, and function.
- Any areas of oedema/inflammation and transmurality. Describe visible foci of enhancement and global enhancement (with ratios) if present.
- Location and nature of any foci of delayed enhancement.
- If applicable, comment on the presence of hilar lymph nodes or pulmonary features of sarcoidosis (📖 p. 430).
- Follow-up imaging post-treatment may show some resolution.

Differential diagnosis

- Myocardial infarction (if sub-endocardial or transmural delayed enhancement). Usually conforms to a coronary territory(ies).
- Other cardiomyopathies with regional fibrosis, e.g. HCM (📖 p. 178).
- Myocarditis can be difficult to differentiate.

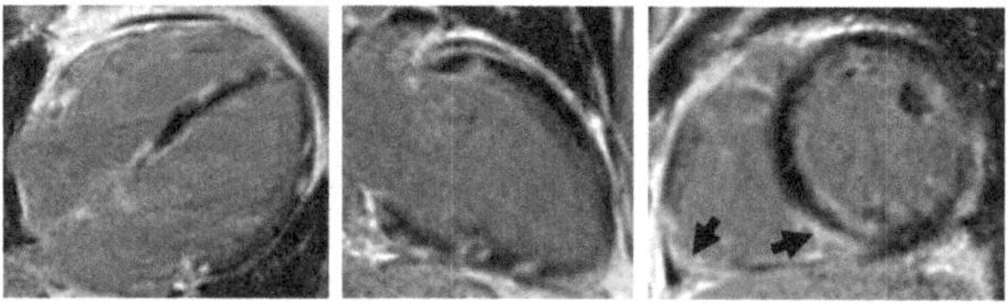

Fig. 8.4 Late enhancement images from a patient with moderate cardiac sarcoidosis. (Left) HLA. (Middle) VLA. (Right) Mid-ventricular short axis view. Note the widespread distribution of multiple patchy areas of enhancement, as well as the tendency to involve the mid-wall ± the sub-epi and endocardium. The RV is involved, appreciated best on the short axis view (right, arrows).

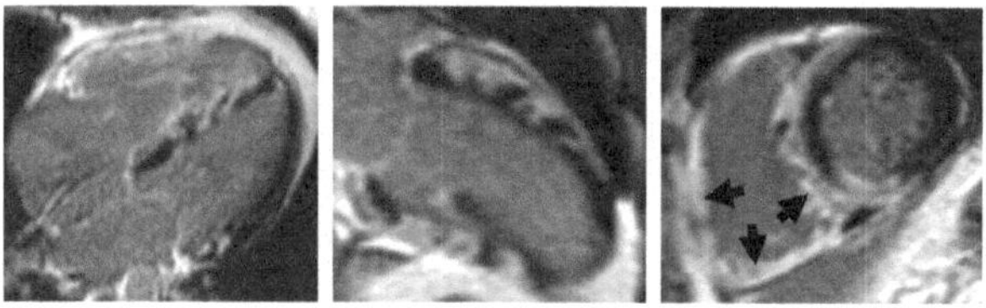

Fig. 8.5 Late enhancement images from a patient with severe cardiac sarcoidosis. (Left) HLA. (Middle) VLA. (Right) Mid-ventricular short axis view. Again, multiple areas of enhancement are seen, often involving the full thickness of the myocardium, although with a tendency towards sub-epicardial regions. The RV is extensively involved (right, arrows), and there is some papillary muscle enhancement (short axis view, right), Both LV and RV function were significantly reduced.

Further reading

Borchert B, Lawrenz T, Bartelsmeir M *et al.* Utility of endomyocardial biopsy guided by delayed enhancement areas on magnetic resonance imaging in the diagnosis of cardiac sarcoidosis. *Clin Res Cardiol* 2007; **96:** 759–62.

Schulz-Menger J, Wassmuth R, Abdel-Aty H *et al.* Patterns of myocardial inflammation and scarring in sarcoidosis as assessed by cardiovascular magnetic resonance. *Heart* 2006; **92:** 399–400.

Smedema, JP, Snoep G, Van Kroonenburgh MP *et al.* Evaluation of the accuracy of gadolinium-enhanced cardiovascular magnetic resonance in the diagnosis of cardiac sarcoidosis. *J Am Coll Cardiol* 2005; **45:** 1683–90.

Cardiac amyloidosis

Background

A systemic disease involving deposition of amyloid protein in any organ, with both acquired and hereditary forms. Cardiac involvement is common with AL ('primary') amyloid, related to β-cell dyscrasias including myeloma and lymphoma. Cardiac amyloidosis is rare in AA amyloid (secondary to chronic systemic inflammation). An endomyocardial biopsy is the 'gold standard' for diagnosis, but increasingly, CMR can identify patients non-invasively.

CMR features

- **LV hypertrophy ± globally reduced function:** amyloid protein is deposited in the myocardium, increasing LV wall thickness, and resulting in concentric hypertrophy. Right ventricular and interatrial septum thickness may also be increased. Systolic function may be normal until late in the disease, but a restrictive diastolic filling pattern and atrial enlargement is common.
- **No myocardial oedema/inflammation:** normal T_2 signal and early gadolinium enhancement is expected.
- **Late gadolinium enhancement:** there are some characteristic features of cardiac amyloidosis on delayed enhancement imaging (Figs 8.6 and 8.7). Amyloid deposits cause a significant expansion of the interstitial space, and a diffuse uptake of gadolinium can be seen on delayed imaging, predominantly in a subendocardial 'ring', although in some cases, LV enhancement can be more variable. Enhancement may also be seen in the RV and atrial walls. In addition, gadolinium binds to amyloid protein, causing a more rapid 'emptying' of gadolinium from the blood pool, which appears darker than normal (Fig. 8.6). Relatively early imaging (~5min post-injection) ± an extra dose of gadolinium can help improve image quality.
- **Pericardial and/or pleural effusions.**

Scanning

- Standard scanning sequence for infiltrative diseases (📖 p. 194).
- T2 and early post-contrast T1-imaging can be used to exclude other diagnoses but may not always be required.

Reporting should include:

- LV volumes, mass (?concentric hypertrophy) and function.
- RV thickening, dilated/thickened atria, pericardial, or pleural effusions.
- Pattern of late enhancement.
- Other organ involvement, e.g. hepato-splenomegaly.

Differential diagnosis

- **Hypertrophic cardiomyopathy:** usually asymmetric hypertrophy, normal systolic function, and different delayed enhancement pattern.
- **Other storage diseases**: e.g. Fabry's disease.
- **Hypertensive and other causes of LV hypertrophy.**

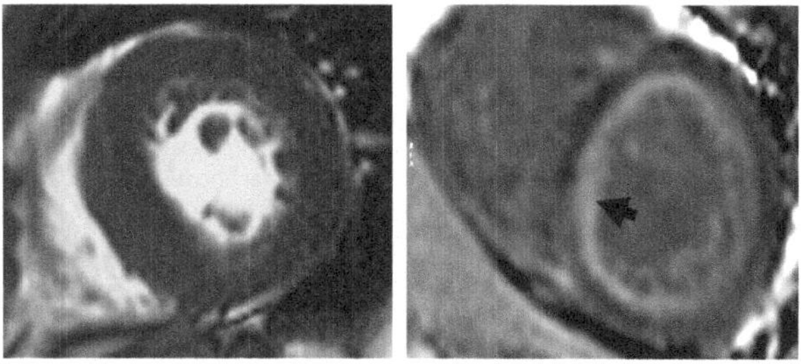

Fig. 8.6 Cardiac amyloidosis. Short axis cine in diastole (left) showing severe LV, mostly concentric, hypertrophy. Late enhancement image of a different patient (right) shows diffuse, mostly sub-endocardial, enhancement (arrowed) with a relatively dark blood pool.

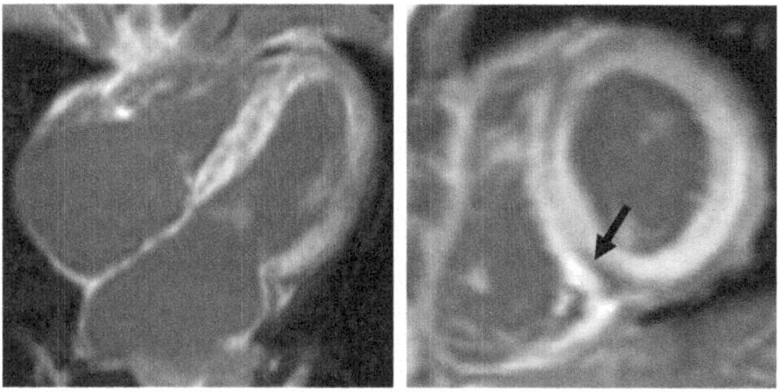

Fig. 8.7 Severe cardiac amyloidosis. Late enhancement pattern in HLA view (left) and short axis view (right). There is extensive enhancement of both ventricles, although predominantly sub-endocardial with relative sparing of the mid-wall (arrowed). The atrial walls also show enhancement.

Further reading

Maceira AM, Joshi J, Prasad SK *et al.* Cardiovascular magnetic resonance in cardiac amyloidosis. *Circulation* 2005; **111:** 186–93.

Selvanayagam JB, Hawkins PN, Paul B *et al.* Evaluation and management of cardiac amyloidosis. *J Am Coll Cardiol* 2007; **50:** 2101–10.

Vogelsberg H, Mahrholdt H, Dalvigi CC *et al.* Cardiovascular magnetic resonance in clinically suspected cardiac amyloidosis: noninvasive imaging compared to endomyocardial biopsy. *J Am Coll Cardiol* 2008; **51:** 1022–30.

Eosinophilic myocarditis

Background

Eosinophilia can be associated with endomyocardial inflammation, often leading to fibrosis, and ultimately a restrictive cardiomyopathy. It occurs in various conditions, including eosinophilic myocardial fibrosis, Loeffler's endocarditis, and Churg-Strauss syndrome, although the precise mechanism is unclear. The inflammation occurs in the endocardium around the apex, spreading to the mid-ventricle and papillary muscles. Apical thrombus formation is common. Endomyocardial biopsy provides a definitive diagnosis, but CMR features strongly support a non-invasive diagnosis.

CMR features

- **LV hypertrophy ± globally reduced function:** concentric hypertrophy can occur, although apical thrombus can appear as thickened myocardium, and specific thrombus imaging is recommended. LV function is reduced in severe disease, and RV involvement is possible.
- **Endomyocardial oedema/inflammation:** increased T_2 signal and early gadolinium enhancement can occur throughout the myocardium, but particularly in the endocardial layer towards the apex and in the papillary muscles (Fig. 8.9).
- **Apical thrombus:** thrombus often forms at the apex and can appear as apical hypertrophy. Early imaging post-gadolinium is required for differentiation (Fig. 8.8b).
- **Late gadolinium enhancement:** a characteristic pattern is seen of circumferential sub-endocardial enhancement, mostly towards the apex, and often including the papillary muscles (Figs 8.8 and 8.9). Thrombus can also be seen, appearing dark against the enhanced endocardium. Some regression of enhancement can occur with treatment, suggesting a reduction in inflammation or fibrotic contraction.

Scanning

- **Standard protocol** (📖 p. 194): LV function (long and short axes), and early and late gadolinium imaging are the most important components.
- Thrombus imaging early after gadolinium, with either a T1-WI or inversion recovery sequence with a long inversion time (400–500ms). It appears dark (low signal) against the intermediate signal of the blood pool and myocardium.

Reporting should include:

- LV volumes, mass, and function.
- Any thrombus identified.
- Sub-endocardial circumferential pattern of late enhancement.

Differential diagnosis

- Any restrictive cardiomyopathy, but the sub-endocardial enhancement pattern is characteristic for eosinophilic myocarditis.
- **Cardiac amyloidosis:** hypertrophy is usually more severe and the late enhancement more diffuse (although greatest in the sub-endocardium).

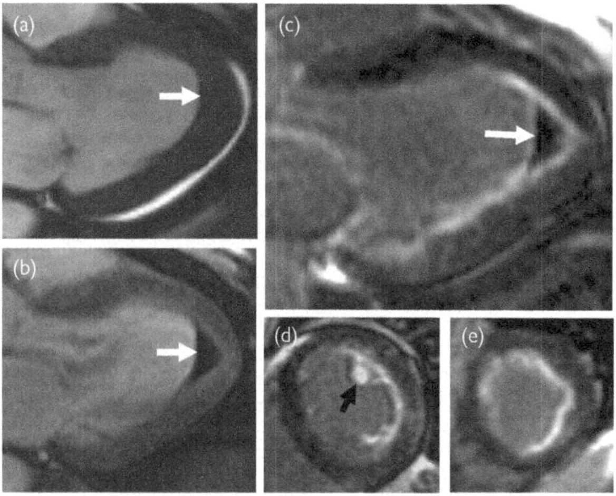

Fig. 8.8 Eosinophilic endocardial myocarditis. Note the apical thickening (white arrow), which appears as hypertrophy on the SSFP LVOT cine (a), but the laminated thrombus is clearly seen on both early (b) and late (c) gadolinium enhancement images. Short axis late enhancement images are shown from the mid ventricle (d) and apex (e). There is almost circumferential, sub-endocardial enhancement, particularly towards the apex, and involving the papillary muscles (black arrow).

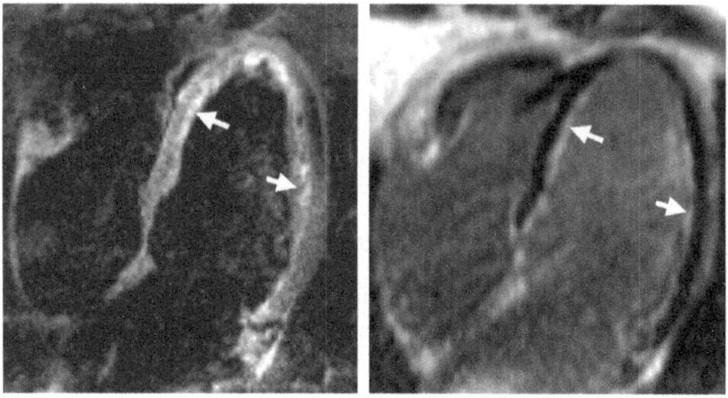

Fig. 8.9 HLA views in a patient with eosinophilic endocardial fibrosis. T_2-weighted (STIR) image (left), late gadolinium enhancement image (right). Note the widespread, predominantly sub-endocardial, increased signal on both images.

Muscular dystrophies

Background

Muscular dystrophies (MD) are a group of hereditary muscle diseases that cause progressive muscle weakness, with the commonest being Duchenne, Becker, and limb girdle muscular dystrophies. Improvements in life expectancy in recent years has resulted in a greater awareness of associated cardiomyopathy, and this has become a major factor in prognosis. Duchenne muscular dystrophy (DMD) is the more severe of the two and both skeletal and cardiac muscle involvement occurs at a younger age than Becker muscular dystrophy (BMD). Patients with DMD are less likely to survive into adult life, but patients with BMD are now surviving into their fifth or sixth decade. Cardiac involvement can be subtle.

CMR features

- **Global and regional function:** left ventricular dysfunction can be global or regional, and can develop slowly over time, or may sometimes have rapid onset.
- **Myocardial oedema and inflammation:** regional or global oedema and inflammation may be noted in patients with acute involvement, and may appear similar to myocarditis (Fig. 8.10). Increased wall thickness, regionally increased SI on T_2-weighted images and increased early gadolinium enhancement.
- **Late gadolinium enhancement:** regional fibrosis may be noted as enhancement, predominantly in the lateral and inferolateral wall – again, a similar pattern to myocarditis. (Fig. 8.11).

Scanning

As for dilated cardiomyopathy (📖 p. 182).

Reporting should include:

- LV volumes, mass, and function. Comment on regional wall thickness and extent of hypokinetic areas.
- Oedema and late enhancement.
- Comment on relation between late enhancement and function.

Differential diagnosis

- The skeletal muscle dystrophy is often obvious.
- Myocarditis.
- Other non-ischaemic cardiomyopathies with fibrosis.

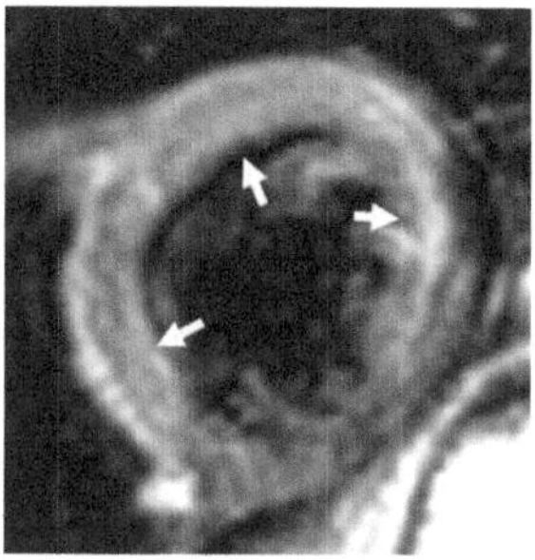

Fig. 8.10 Short axis T_2-weighted sequence (STIR) in a patient with muscular dystrophy. Note increased SI in the septum and anterolateral regions (arrowed).

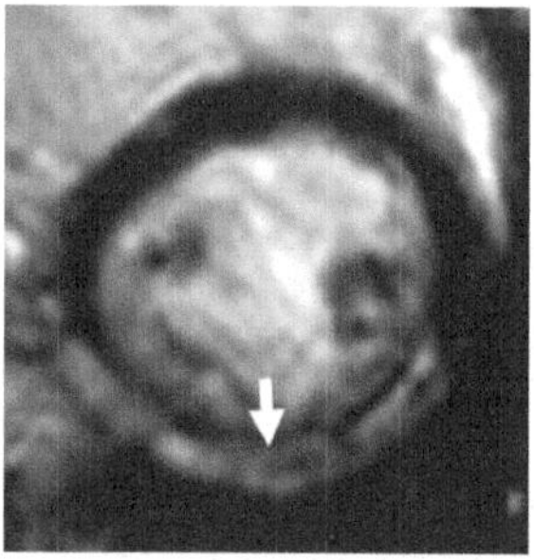

Fig. 8.11 Short axis late gadolinium enhancement image in a patient with muscular dystrophy. Note enhancement in the infero-lateral walls in a non-ischemic pattern (arrowed).

Further reading

Gaul C, Deschauer M, Templemann C *et al.* Cardiac involvement in limb-girdle muscular dystrophy 2I: conventional cardiac diagnostic and cardiovascular magnetic resonance. *J Neurol* 2006; **253:** 1317–22.

Silva MC, Meira ZM, Gurgel Gianetti J *et al.* Myocardial delayed enhancement by magnetic resonance imaging in patients with muscular dystrophy. *J Am Coll Cardiol* 2007; **49:** 1874–9.

Smith GC, Kinali M, Prasad SK *et al.* Primary myocardial dysfunction in autosomal dominant EDMD. A tissue Doppler and cardiovascular magnetic resonance study. *J Cardiovasc Magn Reson* 2006; **8:** 723–30.

Myocardial iron overload

Background

Excess body iron can occur due to hereditary or acquired conditions, most commonly from the regular blood transfusions required for haematological disorders, such as thalassemia or myelodysplasia. The accumulated iron cannot be excreted and is deposited in many organs, often causing a deterioration in function. The liver is commonly affected, but cardiac deposition is the major determinant of prognosis. The iron can be chelated, but the subcutaneous infusions are cumbersome and expensive. Liver biopsies were used to gauge the level of iron loading, but there is little correlation between liver and myocardial iron deposition, and significant cardiac loading can be missed. Cardiac biopsies are hazardous, and serial measurements are required for monitoring.

CMR can detect myocardial iron deposition using T_2* imaging (see box opposite) and is the only non-invasive method for this. Combined with its accurate cardiac function measurement and safety for serial studies, CMR is the optimal tool for myocardial iron assessment.

CMR features

- **LV dilatation and dysfunction:** increased LV volumes and globally decreased LV function occur with increasing iron deposition.
- **Reduced T_2* measurement:** iron loading reduces tissue T_2*, resulting in lower signal intensities on T2-WI with longer echo times. A series of T_2-weighted images with increasing echo times is used to plot the drop-off in signal (Fig. 8.12).

Scanning

Standard long axis cines

Look for abnormal wall motion. The myocardium may appear darker than usual, due to the T_2*-shortening effect of iron.

Short axis cine stack

For measurement of LV mass, volumes, and function.

Myocardial T_2 mapping*

- Choose a mid-ventricular short axis plane and use a dedicated T_2* mapping sequence to acquire multiple T_2-weighted images at different echo times (ranging from 2 to 18ms). Either a single breath-hold multi-echo sequence, or multiple acquisitions can be performed.
- Measure the T_2* from the septum to avoid artefacts (see Fig. 8.13).
- Liver T_2* can also be measured – choose a transaxial image plane through the mid-portion of the liver and image without ECG gating. Avoid any vessels in the analysis, to avoid errors.

T_2* measurement

How it works

Tissue iron causes localized magnetic field inhomogeneities, resulting in a shorter T_2 relaxation time (termed T_2*), which is relative to the degree of iron loading. T_2* is measured by acquiring several T_2-weighted images with different echo times. Shorter relaxation times (from iron loading) cause a more rapid decrease in myocardial SI with increasing echo time, and this rate of decline can be plotted (Fig. 8.14).

Clinical correlation

Liver T_2* measurements correlate well with liver iron loading on biopsy, and although cardiac T_2* measurements have not yet been compared with cardiac biopsies (due to the risks involved), they have a strong association with the degree of cardiac function and have been shown to improve prognosis from heart failure when used to guide chelation therapy.

Myocardial T_2* values below 20ms (on a 1.5T system) indicate significant iron deposition in the myocardium.

Applying the technique

- Multiple images in the same LV short axis plane are acquired with different echo times.
- An area for analysis is chosen in the septum (Fig. 8.13) – this avoids errors from susceptibility artefacts at lung/myocardium interfaces. Care should be taken to avoid the blood pool and the coronary arteries in the interventricular grooves, to avoid signal intensity errors.
- The SI at each echo time can be plotted and the rate of decline measured, which provides the T_2*. Some software applications automate this process, e.g. CMRtools ©Imperial College, London (Figs 8.13 and 8.14).

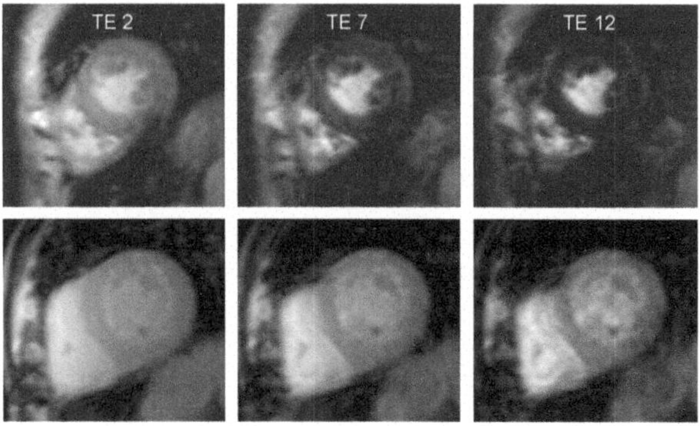

Fig. 8.12 T_2-weighted short axis images with different echo times (TE 2, 7 and 12ms). (Top) Patient with significant iron loading, showing rapid fall in signal intensity at longer echo times. (Bottom) Normal subject with only mild fall in signal intensity with increasing echo time.

Reporting should include:

- LV volumes and function.
- Myocardial T_2* and indication of severity of iron loading - values <20ms (on a 1.5T system) indicate significant iron deposition; <10ms indicate severe iron loading.
- Appearance of the liver (±T_2*) and spleen – enlarged? ↓ SI due to iron loading? Normal liver T_2* values are >6.3ms, with severe liver iron loading indicated by T_2* <1.4ms.

Differential diagnosis

Other non-ischaemic cardiomyopathies, although T_2* values should be normal in these.

Further reading

Anderson LJ, Holden S, Davis B *et al.* Cardiovascular T_2-star (T_2*) magnetic resonance for the early diagnosis of myocardial iron overload. *Eur Heart J* 2001; **22:** 2140–1.

He T, Kirk P, Firmin DN, *et al.* Multi-center transferability of a breath-hold T2T_2 technique for myocardial iron assessment. *J Cardiovasc Magn Reson* 2008; **10:** 11.

Lam, WW, Au WY, Chu WC, *et al.* One-stop measurement of iron deposition in the anterior pituitary, liver, and heart in thalassemia patients. *J Magn Reson Imaging* 2008; **28:** 29–33.

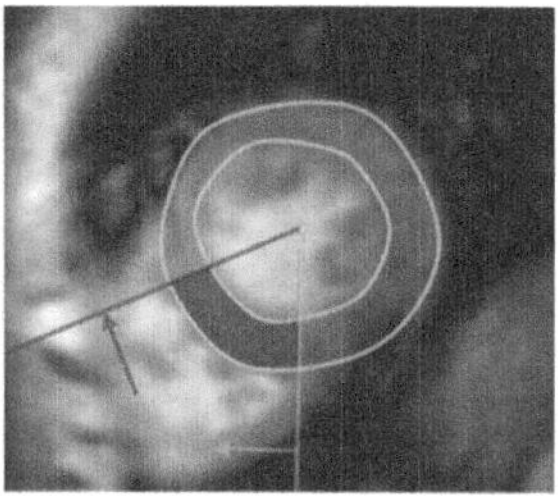

Fig. 8.13 Selection of region for T_2* analysis using CMRtools ©Imperial College London.

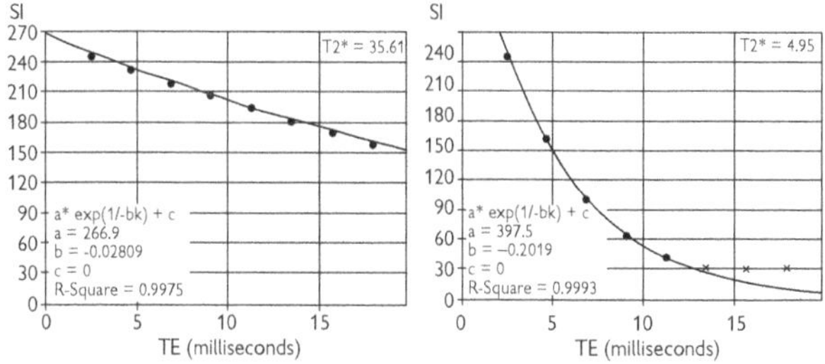

Fig. 8.14 Myocardial T_2* plot for a normal patient (left) and one with severe iron loading (right), showing the rapid rate of decline in signal intensity (SI) at longer echo times.

Chapter 9

Tumours and masses

Introduction

Cardiac tumours are rare – ~0.1–0.3% at autopsy, many of which may be incidental findings. Benign tumours and other masses are far more common than malignant tumours, and of the malignancies, metastases are many times more common than primary cardiac tumours. Masses in or around the heart can be seen on echocardiography or CT and further investigation is required to separate artefact and innocent structures from true masses potentially of concern to the patient and clinician.

CMR is highly valuable in the assessment of cardiac masses, due to its versatility in image planes and excellent ability to discriminate tissue types based on their MR properties, and their response to gadolinium contrast. CMR can differentiate normal from abnormal myocardium, identify the size, location, and anatomy of a mass, and can often provide a likely diagnosis. While CMR may not always provide a definitive pathological diagnosis, it can usually identify abnormal tissue and determine the likelihood of a tumour based on the characteristics of the mass. It may also guide surgery and/or biopsy, if this is deemed appropriate.

General scanning technique

A high degree of adaptability is required when imaging cardiac masses, given their wide variation in size and location, and several non-standard imaging planes are often required. Gadolinium contrast is important for characterizing any mass and should be given unless contra-indicated. If assessment of calcification is needed, consider CT.

Basic scanning protocol

There will be significant variability in what images are needed, depending on the nature of the mass. A general scheme is provided here (see also Fig. 9.1).

- **Standard orthogonal thoracic imaging:** standard body planes (e.g. with a HASTE sequence), covering the entire mediastinum. This provides a good overview of the anatomy and can identify larger masses.
- **LV and RV function assessment:** long axes plus a short axis stack (SSFP cine sequences), provides full coverage of both ventricles, and also an assessment of the functional consequences of any mass. Look for motion of the mass, impairment of myocardial contraction, or obstruction to flow.
- **± Thin-slice transaxial cine images:** imaging the specific region where a mass is identified/suspected can be helpful in determining the presence of a mass and its motion. Use thin slice (4–6mm) transaxial (±coronal/sagittal) cine images, without a gap. If necessary, the entire heart can be covered, checking for additional findings (e.g. metastases).
- **± Other cine images as required:** non-standard image planes are commonly required, to fully visualize the anatomy and extent of a mass. Plan these from existing images demonstrating the mass, ensuring at least two (preferably three) perpendicular planes through the mass to visualize the extent in all directions.
- **Turbo spin echo images:** acquire T_1-weighted (with or without fat sat), as well as T_2-weighted images (preferably triple inversion recovery, with blood and fat suppression) in the same slice positions as SSFP or in representative slices.
- **± Tagging:** tagging may be applied to further characterize the functional consequences of tissue infiltration (lack of mobility), if required.
- **± Perfusion imaging or angiography:** administering gadolinium using a perfusion technique can determine the blood supply/vascularity of a suspected cardiac mass. Choose 2 or 3 representative image positions that best demonstrate the mass. 3D MR angiography can be helpful if infiltration of nearby vascular structures is suspected or for characterizing any feeding vessels.
- **Early gadolinium imaging:** good for identifying thrombi (either adherent to the mass, or may also be the mass itself; Fig. 9.2). T_1-weighted imaging may also be used to characterize any uptake of gadolinium by the mass.
- **Late gadolinium enhancement:** identifies areas of sequestration of the contrast within the mass and/or fibrosis/necrosis.

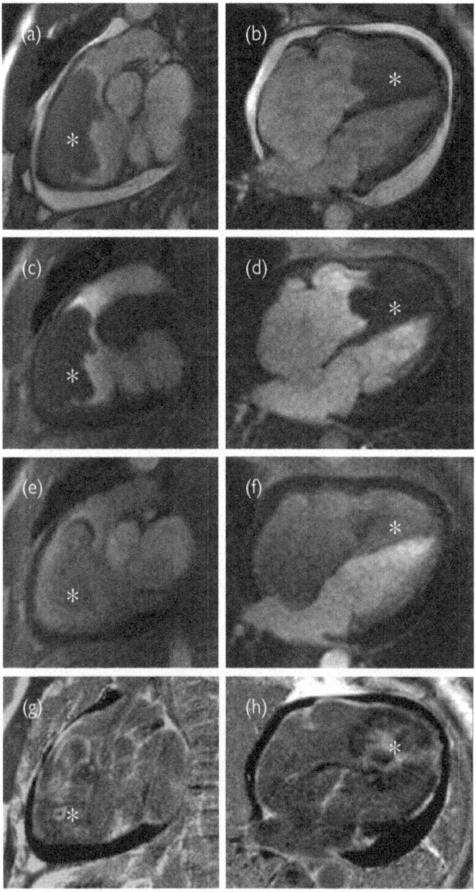

Fig. 9.1 Example of an approach to imaging masses. A large RV tumour is present (a malignant melanoma metastasis), imaged in the RVOT view (left: a,c,e,,g) and the HLA view (right: b,d,f,h). Top panels (a,b) show SSFP sequences; the tumour (*) is almost isointense to myocardium and can be seen obstructing the RVOT (a). There is a moderate pericardial effusion - a marker of malignancy. (c,d) Early images from the perfusion sequence, with contrast in the blood pool outlining the mass (*). (e,f) Later images from the perfusion sequence demonstrating uptake of contrast in the mass, though heterogenous in part. (g,h) Late gadolinium enhancement images showing patchy persistence of gadolinium, particularly in the centre of the mass, suggestive of central necrosis.

Reporting should include:

- Confirmation of the presence or absence of a mass.
- Description of the anatomical relationships of the mass, and whether there is infiltration into adjacent tissues or pericardium.
- Whether the mass appears to arise from the heart/myocardium or elsewhere in the mediastinum? See 📖 p. 440 for mediastinal masses.
- Any additional masses or lung metastases.
- The motion of the mass and its functional significance, e.g. valve or pulmonary artery obstruction.
- Description of the signal characteristics on differing sequences, and contrast enhancement patterns (perfusion, early, and late).
- Assessment of likely diagnoses and criteria that may suggest malignancy, taking into account the whole picture. CMR cannot offer a histological diagnosis, but can provide strong clues to guide further management.

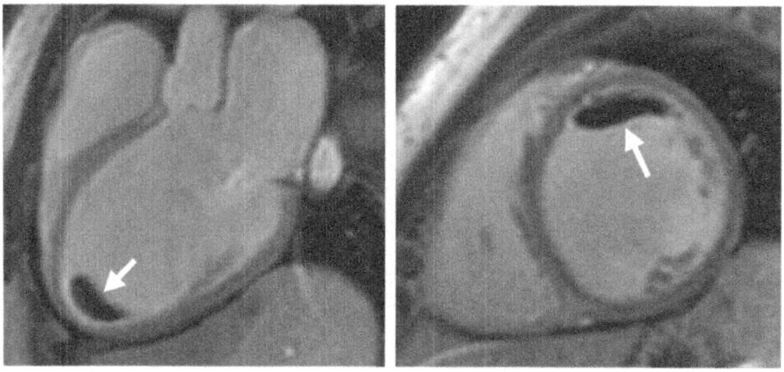

Fig. 9.2 Early gadolinium imaging images in the LVOT view (left) and short axis view (right) demonstrating two separate thrombi (arrowed) in the same patient. The low signal intensity of the thrombus is highlighted by the intermediate to high signal from the blood pool and myocardium.

Identifying cardiac masses

When assessing cardiac masses, a consideration of the full differential diagnoses is important, particularly given the rarity of cardiac tumours. Normal cardiac structures should be differentiated from abnormal masses, and non-neoplastic diagnoses for the latter should be explored - the most common non-tumourous mass is cardiac thrombus, which can usually be easily differentiated with CMR. Cardiac 'masses' can be categorized into three groups:

- **Normal structures**
- **Benign masses:**
  - Non-tumourous masses (e.g. thrombus, infective vegetation)
  - Benign cardiac tumours.
- **Malignant:**
  - Cardiac metastases (30–40 times more likely than 1° tumours)
  - Primary malignant cardiac tumours.

The following are considered in separate chapters:

- Mediastinal masses, 📖 p. 440.
- Pericardial masses, 📖 p. 304.

Normal cardiac structures commonly confused with masses

Moderator band in the RV

This can appear as an apical mass, especially if a degree of RV hypertrophy is present. The proximity of the apex to the echocardiographic transducer on an apical 4-chamber view increases the echogenicity of the moderator band, which can appear as a mass. It should be recognized by its location, connecting the RV free wall to the septum and the relatively uniform thickness along its length.

The 'warfarin' ridge in the left atrium

This rim, between the left upper pulmonary vein and left atrial appendage, can be prominent in some subjects (Fig. 9.3). It is known as the 'warfarin' ridge (due to its possible misinterpretation as thrombus on echocardiography), and can appear as a mass, especially if viewed in cross-section. It can usually be recognized by its elongated nature, sometimes with a rolled tip (the 'Q-tip' sign, after the brand of cotton buds this resembles) and by its continuity with the left atrial wall.

Eustachian valve/Chiari network/crista terminalis in the right atrium

The Eustachian 'valve', a vestigial remnant from *in utero* life, is a ridge of tissue attached to the inferior right atrial wall just above the inferior vena cava (IVC), directing blood from the IVC towards the foramen ovale (Fig. 9.4). It can be mistaken for a vegetation or mass, though can usually be recognized by its elongated nature and location of attachment.

A Chiari network of fine web-like strands can be attached to the tip of the Eustachian valve or to the adjacent RA wall. It is highly mobile, with a whip-like motion, and is sometimes mistaken for an infective vegetation.

The crista terminalis is a ridge of tissue between the SVC and right atrial appendage.

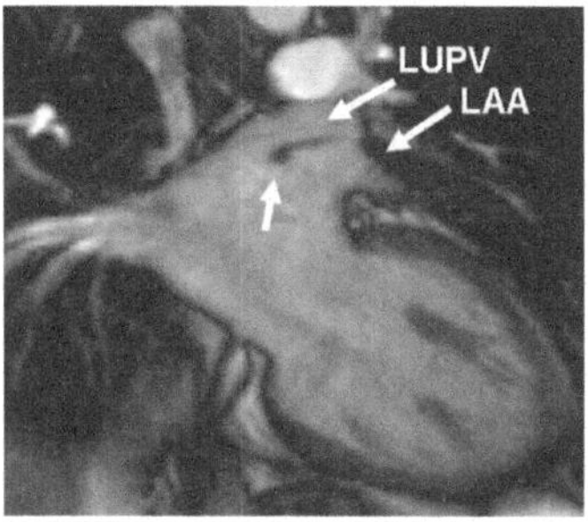

Fig. 9.3 Oblique coronal SSFP image showing a prominent warfarin ridge (thick arrow) between the left upper pulmonary vein (LUPV) and the left atrial appendage (LAA). The tip is bulbous, exhibiting the 'Q-tip' sign.

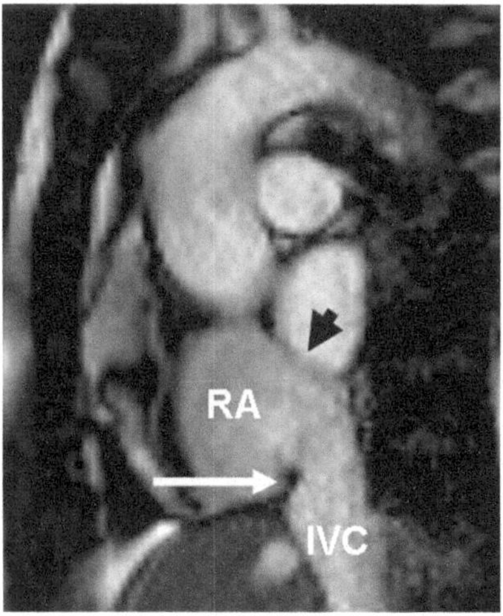

Fig. 9.4 Oblique coronal view through the right atrium (RA), showing the IVC, and a prominent Eustachian valve (long arrow) directed towards the atrial septum (arrowhead).

CMR features suggesting malignancy

There are no specific features diagnostic of malignancy, but several aspects visualized well with CMR can suggest malignancy is more likely (below). Some tumours also have typical features, which are covered in subsequent sections.

Tumour characteristics

- Large size.
- Extension beyond one cardiac chamber.
- Pericardial involvement: nodular thickening, effusions.
- Invasion through tissue planes.
- Multiple lesions (within the heart, pericardium, or lungs).
- Location (can be typical for individual masses).

MR characteristics

- Regional cardiac dysfunction.
- Signal heterogeneity, especially if areas of:
  - Haemorrhage (variable signal depending on the age of haemorrhage)
  - Necrosis (low signal on T1-WI and high on T2-WI).
- Haemorrhagic pericardial effusion (high T_1 signal).

Specific signal characteristics

- Most cardiac masses share a common pattern, limiting the diagnostic value of the signal pattern:
  - Low to intermediate on T1-WI
  - Intermediate to high signal on T2-WI.
- Some masses differ from this, however:
  - *Low T_2 signal* – fibroma/fibroelastoma, metastatic malignant melanoma
  - *High T_1 signal* – lipoma, haemorrhage in a malignant mass, metastatic malignant melanoma.

Non-tumourous masses

Thrombus

- Commonest benign cardiac mass.
- Two common sites:
  - Atrial, especially LA appendage (associated with AF; Fig. 9.5)
  - Ventricular (related to infarcted segments, frequently apical).
- T_1/T_2 signal pattern depends on thrombus age (Table 9.1).
- Usually easily identifiable by the lack of enhancement (very low signal) on early gadolinium imaging; similarly on first pass perfusion and late gadolinium enhancement.
- Can be adherent to tumours!
- Differential diagnosis: atrial myxoma (📖 p. 226), infective vegetation.

Cysts

Typically well circumscribed, rounded lesions with homogenous signal intensity (high signal on T2-WI).

Pericardial

See Pericardial cysts, 📖 p. 302.

Usually well circumscribed, encapsulated, homogenous, and rounded (Fig. 9.6). High signal on T2-WI; almost no signal on phase-sensitive LGE.

Hydatid

Rare. Hydatid disease occurs mostly in Mediterranean countries, the Middle East, and South America, but cardiac involvement is unusual. Cysts are usually located in the LV, but can occur elsewhere, including the pericardium. Often asymptomatic, but can cause obstruction, or rupture to cause anaphylaxis, embolization of cystic/thrombotic material, or occasionally cardiac rupture. Surgical removal is often required.

Other differential diagnoses

Cardiac sarcoidosis

See Cardiac sarcoidosis, 📖 p. 200.

Multiple cardiac lesions can appear in a pattern similar to metastases. Sarcoid lesions are usually mid-wall/epicardial and often have a more linear shape. Do not generally show mass effect or local invasion.

Hypertrophic cardiomyopathy

See Hypertrophic cardiomyopathy, 📖 p. 178.

Localized myocardial hypertrophy may mimic an intramyocardial tumour, although it usually has a typical distribution and characteristic mid-wall late enhancement pattern ± other features (e.g. LVOT obstruction).

Prominent apical fat pad

Can mimic a cardiac mass, particularly at the apex.

Infective vegetation

Mostly attached to a valve, on the up-stream side. Unless large, these are difficult to see with CMR. Usually do not enhance post-contrast.

Table 9.1 T_1/T_2 signal pattern for thrombus

	T_1-weighted	T_2-weighted
Acute	High	High
Subacute	High	Low
Chronic	Low	Low

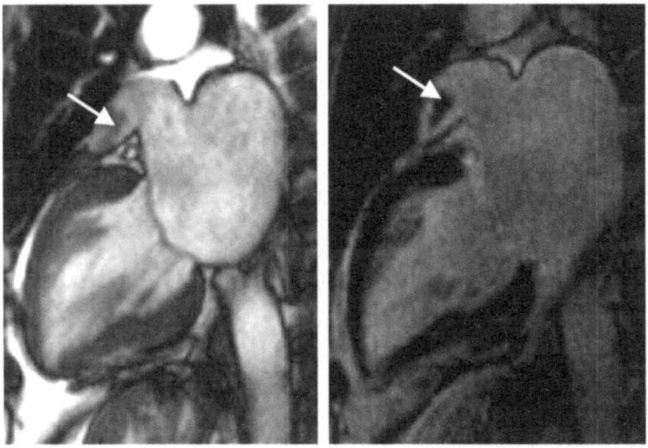

Fig. 9.5 Thrombus in the left atrial appendage (arrowed). SSFP image (left) and late enhancement image (right) in the VLA view. The location within the appendage and lack of contrast enhancement were important features aiding the diagnosis.

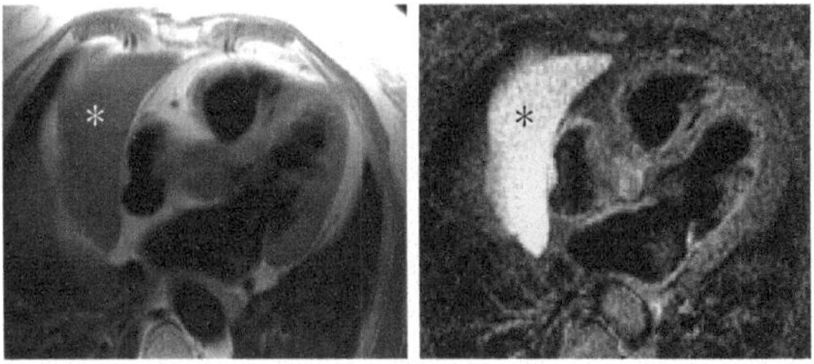

Fig. 9.6 Pericardial cyst in the typical location of the right cardio-phrenic angle. Note the well circumscribed mass with typical signal characteristics of homogenous low signal on T_1-WI (left) and high signal on T_2-WI (right, triple inversion recovery with fat saturation). The cyst is not septated and does not displace or infiltrate surrounding structures.

Benign cardiac tumours

Myxoma

Most common primary cardiac tumour (Fig. 9.7), with 75% being left atrial, 20% right atrial, and 5% ventricular. Clinical presentation is variable, but may include inflow/outflow obstruction, embolization, and systemic symptoms. Cardiac problems occur due to mass effect. Surgical resection is the main treatment.

- Usually a large (>1–2cm) atrial mass at presentation, with a predilection for the atrial septum, particularly close to the fossa ovalis.
- Often pedunculated, with a well-defined, smooth, lobular or oval shape.
- Can be highly mobile and even prolapse through cardiac valves (a characteristic of myxomas).
- Signal pattern and contrast enhancement are heterogenous due to the complexity of tissue types, and frequent central cystic degeneration, haemorrhage, or calcification.
- Needs to be differentiated from thrombus, although thrombus can also occur on a myxoma. Early gadolinium imaging is usually diagnostic.

Rhabdomyoma

- Most common cardiac mass in infants and children ~50% of cases are associated with tuberous sclerosis.
- Multiple, mostly ventricular, fairly well defined, variably sized, intramural lesions that may protrude into the chamber cavity.
- Isointense to myocardium on T1-WI and iso- to hyperintense on T2-WI. May enhance after contrast injection.

Fibroma

- Paediatric/young adults.
- Usually ventricular (intramural); can cause a mass effect.
- Low to intermediate homogenous signal on T2-WI (Fig. 9.8). Characteristic of fibromas and helps to differentiate them from other masses in which high T_2 signal is common.
- Can have diffuse central enhancement on late gadolinium imaging.

Papillary fibroelastoma

- Common with older age; rarely seen with CMR due to their size.
- Small, elongated, polyp-like masses usually attached to the downstream side of valves.
- Similar T_1/T_2 characteristics to fibromas.

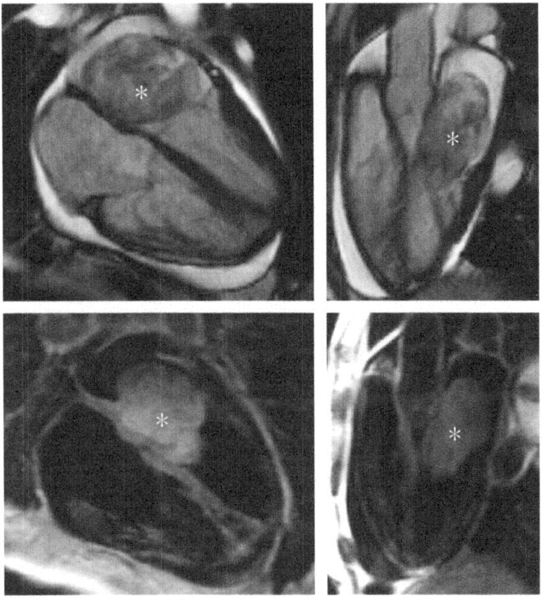

Fig. 9.7 Large left atrial myxoma attached to the inter-atrial septum (*). (Top) SSFP cine sequence in the HLA (left) and LVOT (right) views. The myxoma prolapses through the mitral valve in diastole, causing significant obstruction to flow and mimicking mitral stenosis. (Bottom) T1-weighted TSE images with fat saturation, highlighting the tumour against the low signal of the moving blood.

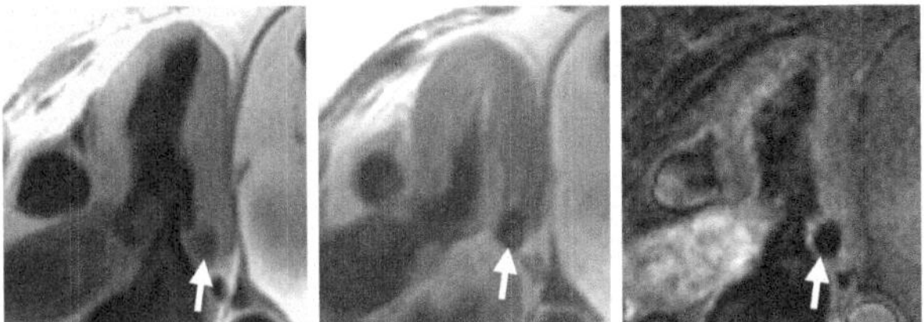

Fig. 9.8 Fibroma. T1-WI in the LVOT view pre-contrast (left) and post-contrast (middle). (Right) T2-WI (triple inversion recovery with fat and blood signal suppression) in the same image position. The well-defined, round mass (arrow) is close to the mitral valve and exhibits low signal on both T1-WI and T2-WI imaging, and does not enhance after contrast injection.

Lipoma

- Well defined ± encapsulated, broad-based, sessile, or pedunculated.
- Vary considerably in size, from tiny to huge.
- Homogenous high signal on T1-WI and suppressed signal with fat saturation (often the key diagnostic test).
- Do not enhance with contrast.

Cardiac lipomatous hypertrophy

- Benign expansion of adipose tissue, usually in the inter-atrial septum, but can include the pericardial space (Fig. 9.9).
- Common with increasing age and is the most likely cause of a thickened atrial septum.
- Non-capsulated.
- Similar MR characteristics to lipomas; does not enhance with contrast.

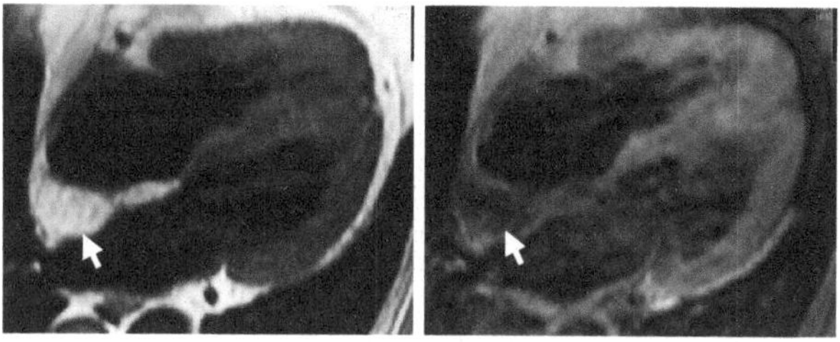

Fig. 9.9 Lipomatous hypertrophy of the inter-atrial septum, HLA views. Note the high signal of the fat in the inter-atrial septum on T1-WI (left, arrowed) and the disappearance following a fat-saturation sequence (right).

Malignant cardiac tumours

Metastases

Cardiac metastases are 30–40 times more likely than primary cardiac tumours and are discovered in ~12% of cancer patients at autopsy, although many may be asymptomatic. The most common primary sites are lung, breast, lymphoma, and malignant melanoma. Some tumours have a particular predilection for the heart, with a high proportion with cardiac metastases (melanoma ~50%, germ cell ~40%, leukaemia ~30%), even though their overall incidence may be lower. Metastatic spread is by:

- **Direct invasion:** e.g. lung, breast.
- **Haematological:** e.g. melanoma, lymphoma, leukaemia.
- **Transvenous via great veins:** renal cell carcinoma, hepatoma.

MR characteristics

- Commonly located on the epicardial surface. The LV myocardium is the second most likely location (it has the greatest blood supply). See Fig. 9.10.
- Pericardial effusions are common (See Fig. 9.11). May be haemorrhagic (high signal on T1-WI).
- Multiple lesions, nodular pericardial thickening and a pericardial effusion are helpful clues to the diagnosis.
- Signal pattern and contrast enhancement are usually heterogeneous, due to the frequent foci of necrosis (low in T1-WI and high in T2-WI) and haemorrhage.
- May mimic the characteristics of the primary tumour, e.g. melanomatous lesions have high T_1 signal, while lymphomatous lesions are solid, infiltrative and non-enhancing.

Primary cardiac tumours: general

These are nearly all sarcomas, although some may be poorly differentiated. The remaining few tend to be lymphomas. Primary cardiac tumours commonly protrude into the cardiac chambers (Fig. 9.12).

Angiosarcoma

- Most common primary cardiac malignancy.
- There are two patterns.

Focal

Characteristically originating in the right atrium and can cause intracavity obstruction. There are no specific MR characteristics – generally heterogenous signal intensity and can have other features of malignancy (📖 p. 222).

Diffuse/infiltrative

Spreads over the pericardium with pericardial thickening/enhancement and haemorrhagic effusion.

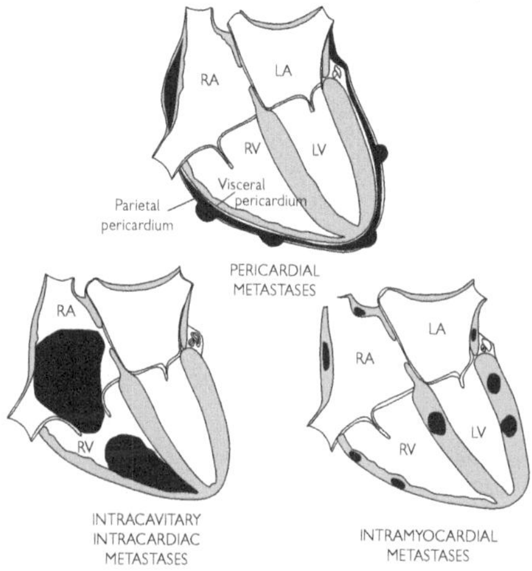

Fig. 9.10 Cardiac locations for metastases. Reproduced from Roberts WC (1997) Primary and secondary neoplasms of the heart. *Am J Cardiol* **80:** 671–682, copyright 1997 with permission from Elsevier.

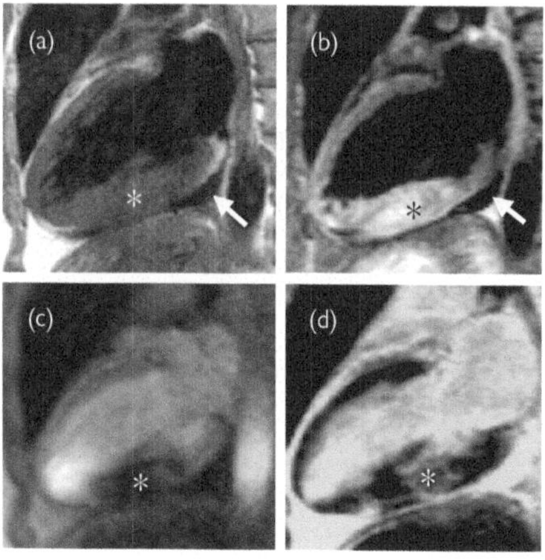

Fig. 9.11 VLA views of an intramyocardial metastasis from a cervical carcinoma. (a) T_1-weighted imaging – only a thickened inferior wall is visible (*). (b) T_2-weighted image showing heterogeneous high signal (*). (c) First-pass perfusion showing a perfusion deficit (*) and (d) enhancement on late gadolinium imaging suggest central necrosis within the mass (*). Note the pericardial effusion (arrow) exhibits a low signal on both T1-WI and T2-WI, suggesting old haemorrhage that, together with the infiltrative pattern and central break down, provides important clues to malignancy.

Rhabdomyosarcoma

- Most common cause of 1° cardiac malignancy in infants and children.
- Multiple neoplasms may be present, in different cardiac chambers.
- No particular cardiac chamber is more frequently affected.
- More likely to involve the valves than other sarcomas.
- Can be predominantly cystic.

Leiomyosarcoma

- Left atrial preference (especially posterior wall). Can cause mitral valve obstruction.
- Can involve intense contrast enhancement.
- Pericardial involvement with nodular enhancement and effusion are common.
- The location and invasive nature help differentiate it from myxoma.

Osteosarcoma

- Occur more frequently in the left atrium.
- May be calcified.
- Invasive features, a broad base, and location distant from the fossa ovale help differentiate it from myxoma.

Liposarcoma

- Very rare.
- Mainly atrial.
- Large, multilobulated with areas of haemorrhage and necrosis.

Primary cardiac lymphoma

- Very rare. Cardiac metastases are present, however, in ~¼ of patients with non-cardiac lymphoma.
- Frequently involve the right atrium (see Fig. 9.13), but other chambers can also be involved and multiple lesions are common.
- Heart failure and pericardial involvement are common.
- Nodular, infiltrative masses, with typical MR characteristics for tumours (📖 p. 222). They generally lack large areas of central necrosis or haemorrhage, however, which can help to differentiate them from other cardiac tumours, such as angiosarcoma.
- Central areas of persistently dark signal on T1-WI and T2-WI should make the diagnosis of lymphoma less likely. These areas usually indicate calcification or dilated vascular structures, neither of which are typical of lymphoma.
- Contrast enhancement is variable – may be heterogeneous, homogenous or minimal.

Further reading

Luna A, Ribes R, Caro P *et al*. Evaluation of cardiac tumors with magnetic resonance imaging. *Eur Radiol* 2005; **15:** 1446–55.
Roberts, W. Primary and secondary neoplasms of the heart. *Am J Cardiol* 1997; **80:** 671–82.
Sparrow, PJ, Kurian, JB, Jones, TR, Sivananthan, MU. MR imaging of cardiac tumors. *Radiographics* 2005; **25:** 1255–76.

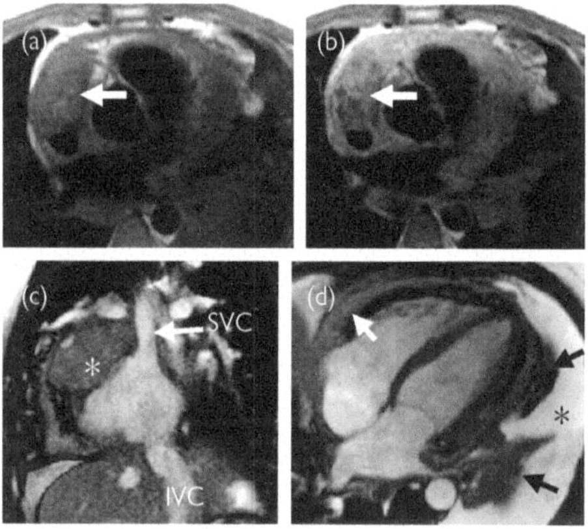

Fig. 9.12 Large right atrial tumour. (a) Transaxial view with T1-WI showing mildly heterogenous signal intensity (arrow). (b) Same image post-gadolinium contrast, demonstrating heterogenous contrast uptake. (c) Right atrial inflow-outflow view (oblique sagittal) on SSFP imaging showing the mass (*) just anterior to the SVC, but with no SVC obstruction. (d) SSFP sequence in the HLA view demonstrating significant pericardial infiltration (white arrow), a large pleural effusion (*) and two tumourous deposits on the pericardial surface (black arrows). Histology showed a poorly differentiated tumour, possibly thymic or teratoma in origin.

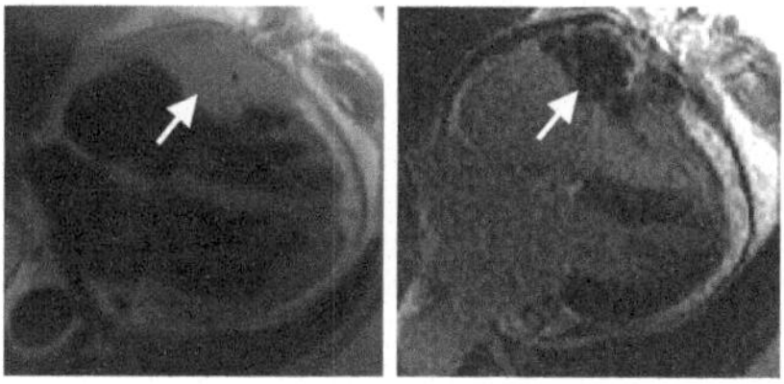

Fig. 9.13 Primary cardiac lymphoma (arrowed) on T1-WI (left) and late gadolinium imaging (right). The mass exhibits a mostly homogenous signal on T1-WI, in contrast to typical malignant tumours, and has minimal contrast enhancement. The irregular outline and infiltrative nature of the mass (seen invading the pericardium) suggests malignancy.

Chapter 10

Valve disease

CMR in valvular heart disease

CMR has great utility in the assessment of valve disease, as the range of imaging techniques (anatomy, function, flow quantification, effect on the LV and RV) allows a comprehensive assessment of the whole picture, including not just the valve itself, but the consequences for the heart and any associated lesions. Accurate visualization of all valves is feasible, including those that can be difficult to visualize with echocardiography (e.g. pulmonary valves, aortic valves with angulated roots). It also provides clear differentiation of valvar from sub- and supravalvar stenosis, accurate assessment of post-stenotic dilation of both aortic and pulmonary arteries, and the quantification of regurgitation, which is a unique and important advantage, adding considerably to the broad assessment available with CMR. Although transoesophageal echocardiography offers higher image resolution, its scope is more focused, and the range and flexibility of CMR adds significant complimentary information.

General approach

- All valve assessments should include LV and/or RV volumes and function to appreciate the effect of the valve(s) on the heart.
- Standard SSFP cine sequences in the usual long axis planes are good for visualizing valve function.
- Image planes may need to be modified slightly to visualize the valve or jet more clearly – don't be afraid to repeat the acquisition with a slightly modified position to achieve a better view of the valve throughout the cardiac cycle.
- Direct planimetry of a stenotic valve area is recommended, and easy to achieve with CMR. Estimation of the valve area using the continuity equation is unnecessary when the area can be measured directly. Moreover, the continuity equation calculates area from three different measurements and relies on certain assumptions, all of which increase the potential for error.

The aortic valve

Normal anatomy

The aortic valve has three cusps – a left and right coronary cusp (with respective coronary arteries arising from these) and a non-coronary cusp (without coronary artery). They are roughly equal in size and, when closed, overlap by 2–3mm to form a commissure between each cusp (Fig. 10.1).

The cusps are intimately associated with the aortic sinuses of the same name (left, right, and non-coronary sinuses), which merge into the tubular aorta at the sino-tubular junction ~2cm above the valve.

Imaging

Standard and coronal LVOT views are good for imaging the aortic valve, outflow tract, and proximal ascending aorta. A short axis (*en-face*) view through the valve is especially good at demonstrating the cusps. These form a triangular shape when open, and a 'Y' shape when closed (see Fig. 10.1). The coronary artery origins can sometimes be seen.

Bicuspid aortic valves

Relatively common (2% of population) and occur in several forms:

- One larger and one smaller cusp (most common). May be formed due to fusion of two of the three cusps *in utero*, and a 'raphe' of fused leaflet tissue can sometimes be seen in the larger cusp.
- Two cusps of equal size.

Imaging

Best visualized in the *en-face* view of the valve, where the classic 'fish mouth' appearance of the open orifice is apparent (see Fig. 10.2). If difficult to see due to turbulence, a through-plane flow sequence can help to visualize the orifice shape

Aortopathy and coarctation

Bicuspid valves have a strong association with aortic coarctation, and ~50% of patients with coarctation have a bicuspid valve. The aorta should, therefore, be imaged whenever a bicuspid valve is identified, to exclude coarctation.

There is good evidence for an aortopathy associated with bicuspid valves, of which coarctation may be one aspect. The proximal aorta can also be affected, with dilation even in the absence of significant stenosis. The mechanism of this is unclear, but may involve an underlying pathology affecting the aortic wall, causing dilation and/or coarctation, and the bicuspid valve (which is derived from the aorta embryologically).

Quadricuspid aortic valves

These are rare and may lie undetected. Aortic regurgitation can occur, due to the difficulties of adequate coaption with 4 cusps and this may lead to their discovery. See Fig. 10.2.

Quinticuspid (5-leaflet) valves have also been reported, but are exceedingly rare.

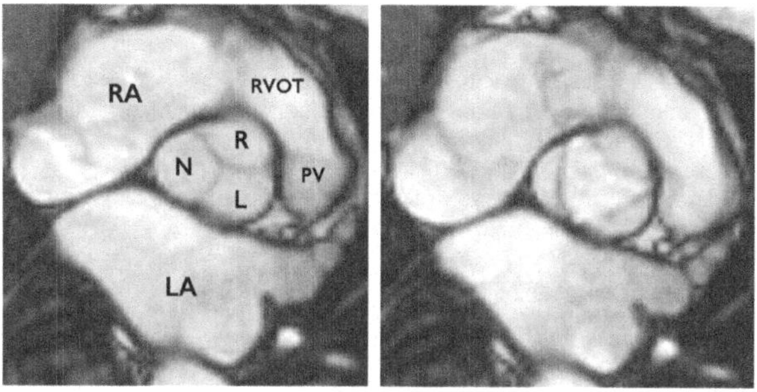

Fig. 10.1 Through-valve view of normal aortic valve in diastole (left) and systole (right). The right coronary cusp (R) is most anterior, adjacent to the RV outflow tract (RVOT). The left coronary cusp (L) lies between the pulmonary valve (PV) and the left atrium (LA) and the non-coronary cusp (N) lies adjacent to the inter-atrial septum.

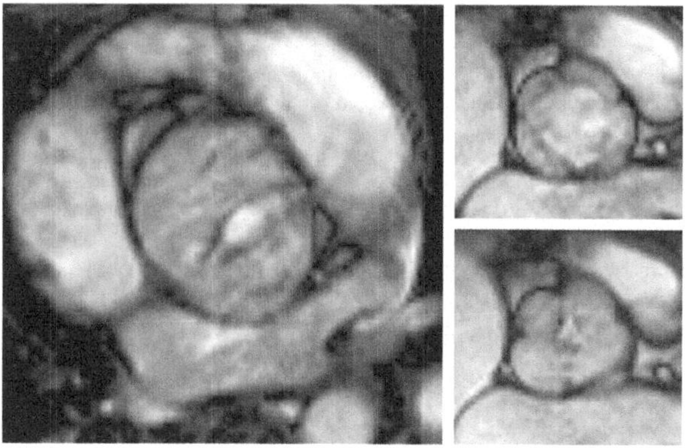

Fig. 10.2 Bicuspid aortic valve with moderate restriction (left). Note the two equal sized leaflets. Quadricuspid aortic valve (right). Note the rare 4 sinuses; the valve opens normally (top), but fails to coapt properly in diastole and the gap can be seen (bottom).

Aortic regurgitation

Background

Small amounts are common with increasing age. Causes of significant aortic regurgitation (AR) include:

- Degenerative.
- Dilated aortic root (e.g. hypertension, Marfan syndrome, inflammatory – any cause of aortitis).
- Bicuspid aortic valve.
- Previous infective endocarditis or rheumatic fever.
- Aortic dissection.

The regurgitation can be *quantified* accurately with CMR and a proper assessment should include this. Very small amounts of AR may be difficult to detect, however, due to a lower sensitivity than echocardiography for small jets.

CMR features

- **Regurgitant aortic jet:** the regurgitant jet can be seen as a flow void (due to turbulence) arising from the aortic valve in diastole and entering the LV (Fig. 10.3). The width of the jet and size of the flow void have a modest correlation with the degree of regurgitation, but this is highly variable, depending on the sequence used, and should not be relied upon. Proper quantification should be performed.
- **± dilated LV/reduced LV function:** secondary to significant chronic regurgitation (acute regurgitation does not cause significant dilation).
- **± dilated aortic root:** identifies a potential cause.

Scanning

Both standard and coronal LVOT views

To visualize AR jet and position aortic flow slice.

Through-plane flow mapping above aortic valve

To quantify the AR. Place image slice as close to the valve as possible to minimize underestimation of regurgitation (See 🕮 p. 242).

LV volumes and mass ± RV volumes

To determine effect on LV, and provide alternative method of quantification by comparison of LV and RV stroke volumes (see 🕮 p. 242).

Further aortic root imaging

E.g. transverse view through sinuses, if dilated. See Imaging the aorta, 🕮 p. 356).

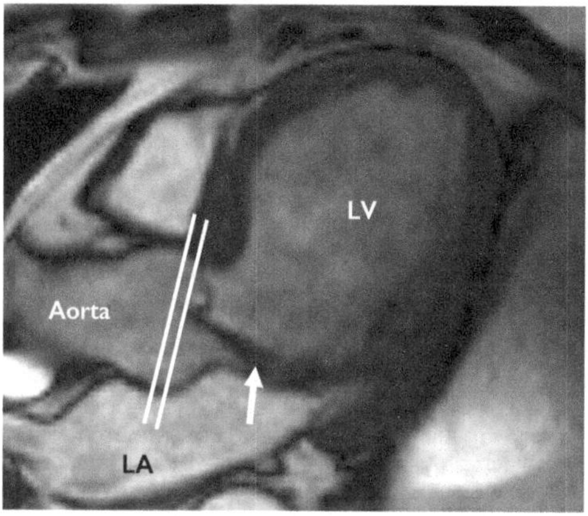

Fig. 10.3 LVOT view showing aortic regurgitant jet (arrowed) and position of the flow mapping slice (parallel lines).

Quantification of aortic regurgitation

A major advantage of CMR is the ability to quantify aortic regurgitation, and this should be used when performing and reporting the scan. Through-plane flow (both forward and reverse; 📖 p. 102) should be measured above the aortic valve (Fig. 10.4) and is normally expressed as:

Regurgitant volume – ml/cardiac cycle

Regurgitant fraction – % (the proportion of forward flow through the aortic valve that returns to the LV:

= (regurgitant volume/aortic forward flow in systole) × 100%

Potential for underestimation (see opposite and Fig. 10.5)

CMR quantification may slightly underestimate the true volume of AR, due to the motion of the valve annulus during the cardiac cycle (see box opposite). Very small amounts of AR are thus difficult to measure, even though a small jet can be seen. The underestimation is reduced (but not eliminated) when the image plane is close to the valve.

Alternative method of quantification

If flow imaging is unavailable/unreliable, AR can still be quantified using the difference between LV and RV stroke volumes, if no other regurgitant valve is present, this should equal the aortic regurgitation. This method may also be used to corroborate the flow data if necessary.

Reporting should include:

- **Anatomy of aortic valve and root:**
  - Look for any clear cause of AR
  - Bicuspid valve
  - Dilated root
  - Any degree of aortic stenosis.
- **Quantification and severity of regurgitation:** Best quantified as regurgitant fraction: see Table 10.1.
- **Effect on LV – mass, volumes, and function:**
  - If significant LV dilation/dysfunction is present, the degree of aortic regurgitation should be severe, otherwise an alternative cause should be sought
  - LV mass is often in proportion to LV volume (roughly a 1:1 ratio, i.e. mass in g = volume in ml); if excessive increase in LV mass is present, other causes of hypertrophy should be sought.

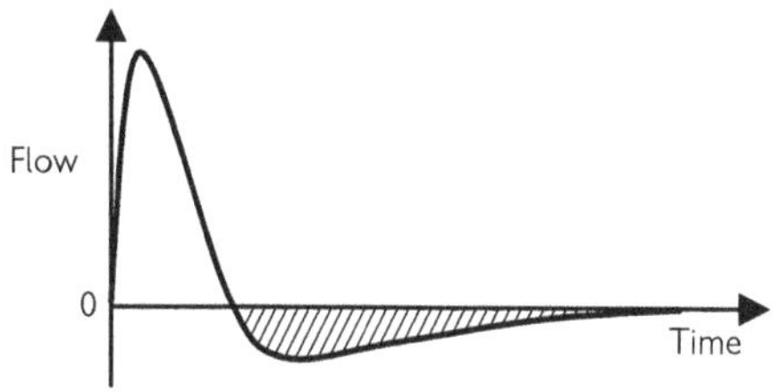

Fig. 10.4 Through-plane flow graph of moderate aortic regurgitation over one cardiac cycle. The hatched area represents the volume of regurgitation.

Table 10.1 Assessment of severity in aortic regurgitation

	Mild	Moderate	Severe
Regurgitant fraction (%)	0–20	21–40	>40
Regurgitant volume (ml/cycle)	<30	30–60	>60

Potential underestimation of aortic regurgitation – mechanism

The gap between the valve and the image plane for flow mapping expands in systole from a combination of:

- Movement of the aortic valve towards the apex.
- Elastic expansion of the aortic sinuses and root

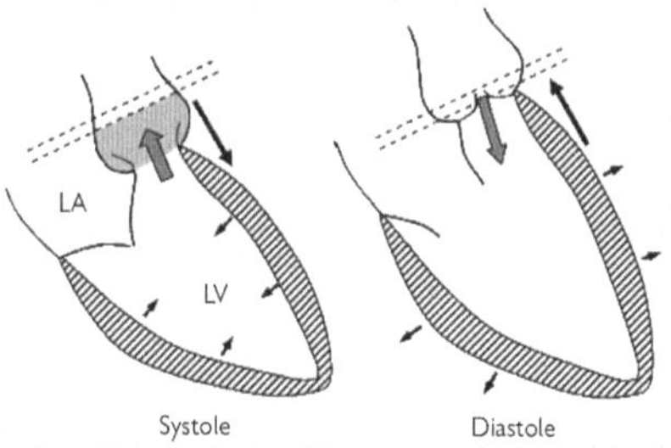

Fig. 10.5 Blood entering this space in systole (grey stippled area) returns to the LV in diastole (via a regurgitant valve) without passing through the image plane (dashed lines), and thus may not be measured.

Exacerbating factors (all increase the volume of the gap):

- Greater distance between valve and image plane for flow.
- Vigorous longitudinal contraction of LV (common in severe AR!).
- Dilated aortic sinuses (common cause of AR!).

Relieving factors

- Position image plane for flow as close to the valve as possible.
- 'Slice tracking' in which the flow image plane moves with the valve annulus – only available on some MR systems.

Aortic stenosis

Background

Common in the older generation (2% of the population over 65 years). The cause is usually degenerative; rarely rheumatic. Bicuspid aortic valves are a more common cause in the young (<40 years), although the mechanism may involve a process of accelerated degeneration.

CMR features

- **Stenotic aortic valve:**
  - May be thickened ± calcified, with restricted movement and a reduced opening area (Figs 10.6, 10.7). Easy to visualize, even with an angulated outflow tract and short axis views through the valve allow good visualization of the orifice. Congenital aortic stenosis in young adults may involve mobile leaflets, but fused tips, with a characteristic appearance (Fig. 10.8)
  - May be bicuspid (esp. if young age).
- **Narrow, high velocity jet:** High signal from linear flow in the jet core, surrounded by low signal from turbulent flow (Fig. 10.6). Some jets are too narrow or turbulent for the MR images to contain any high signal from linear flow and only turbulence (low signal) may be seen.
- **± Concentric LV hypertrophy:** Seen if valve stenosis is severe enough. Significant asymmetry in hypertrophy suggests other diagnosis, e.g. hypertrophic cardiomyopathy, which can exist in combination.
- **Dilation of the proximal ascending aorta:** Occurs in a proportion of cases. The mechanism is debated.

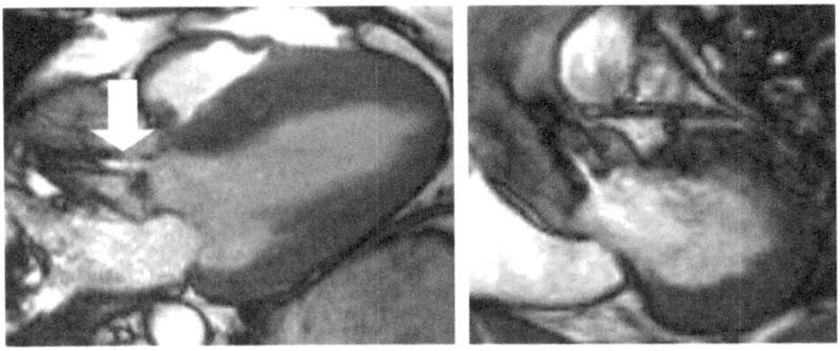

Fig. 10.6 Standard LVOT view (left) and coronal LVOT view (right) in aortic stenosis, showing a high velocity jet (arrowed) of linear flow (high signal) surrounded by turbulence (low signal or black).

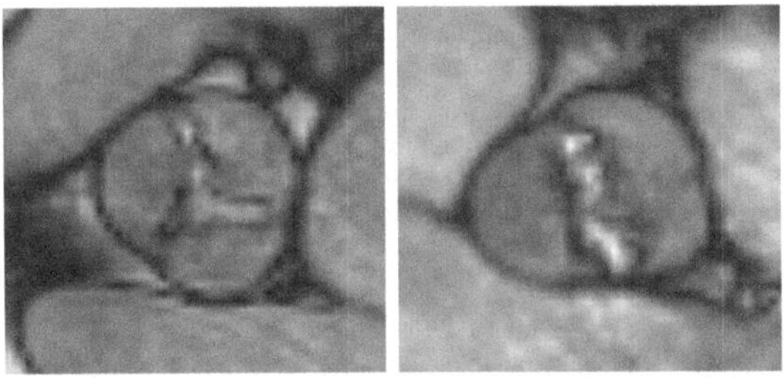

Fig. 10.7 En-face view of tricuspid aortic valve (left) and bicuspid valve (right), both with significant stenosis (valve area 1.0cm^2). Calcification at the rim tips, combined with turbulent flow, creates the dark signal at the leaflet edges.

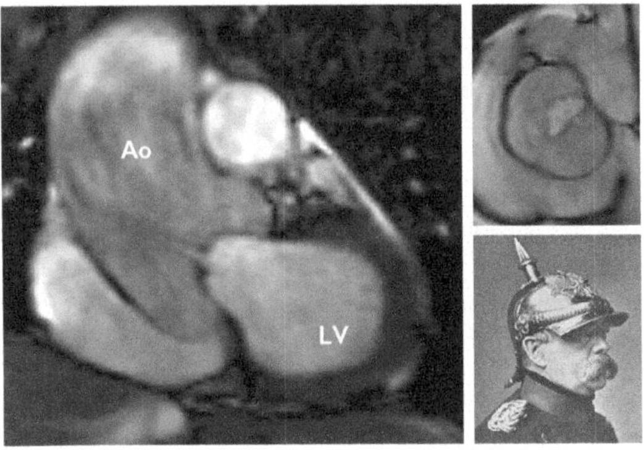

Fig. 10.8 The classic 'Prussian helmet' sign in congenital aortic stenosis (left), with mobile valve leaflets, but fused tips, creating the resemblance to the helmet (bottom right) with a 'spike' formed by the high velocity jet. (Top right) Through-plane view of the bicuspid aortic valve showing the reduced area at the tips. Reproduced with permission from *J Am Coll Cardiol* 2008; **51**(2) (Cover image), copyright 2008 with permission of Elsevier.

Scanning

LVOT cine

Visualize the outflow tract throughout the whole cardiac cycle. You should see the high-velocity jet arising from the restricted valve. Be sure it is aortic stenosis, rather than sub-/supravalvar stenosis or outflow tract obstruction, where the origin of the high velocity jet differs.

*Coronal LVOT cine (**📖 p. 86**)*

Perpendicular to the LVOT view, but aligned with the *jet* rather than the aortic root. The emphasis is on identifying the stenotic jet rather than visualizing the whole ascending aorta.

Aortic valve 'en-face' view

- Good images can be obtained with an '*en-face*' view through the tips (Fig. 10.10). The valve area can be measured directly, which gives a better indication of stenosis severity than velocity using CMR
- Position the cine image through the aortic valve tips in systole, using both LVOT images for alignment. Care should be taken to ensure you are at the tips, and not below, as this would cause over-estimation of the valve area. If difficult to obtain with a single image, multiple parallel cine slices with no gap can be obtained in this orientation.
- Either cine or through-plane flow images may be used (both the magnitude and flow images give good imaging of the open valve).

Velocity mapping

To measure the peak ± mean velocity. CMR can assess angulated roots and valves that are difficult to assess with echocardiography, but has a tendency to underestimate the peak velocity due to partial volume effects (the vena contracta can be very small) and lower temporal resolution. (See 📖 p. 100 for more on flow measurement).

In-plane

Gives good visualization of the origin of the high velocity jet, and allows optimal placement of the through-plane flow image.

Align the flow direction with the jet, starting with the LVOT view that best demonstrates it, and using the other LVOT view to ensure true alignment (Fig. 10.9). Set the velocity window just above the most likely value (usually 4–5m/s for severe aortic stenosis). Repeat with a higher velocity if significant aliasing occurs. Alternatively, a velocity scout sequence can be used to determine the optimal velocity window.

Through-plane

Better resolution across the stenotic jet and especially useful if the jet is narrow, to minimize partial volume effects, and any underestimation of true velocity. Also quantifies any aortic regurgitation.

Similar to the *en-face* valve view, but placed just distal to the valve tips, at the vena contracta (highest velocity on the in-plane flow images), and perpendicular to the flow jet (to minimize partial volume effects; Fig. 10.10).

Using the magnitude (anatomical) component of the flow sequence

Can be useful for visualizing the valve itself, due to the short TE of the sequence minimizing the turbulence.

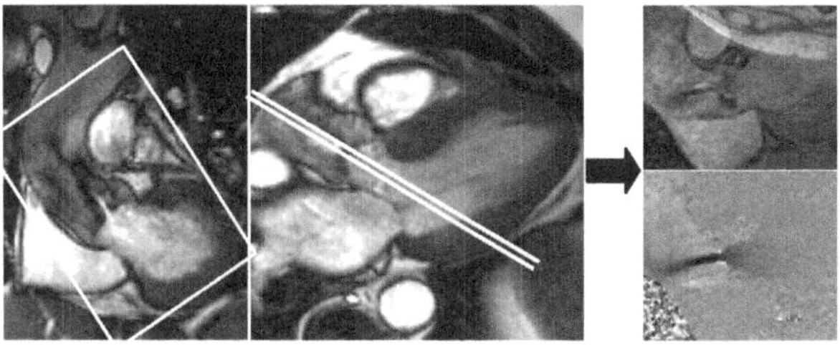

Fig. 10.9 In-plane flow mapping. Based on the coronal LVOT view in this case (left), rotated within this plane to align the direction of flow measurement with the jet and also aligned with the jet in the standard LVOT view (middle). The resulting images are shown on the right: magnitude (top) and velocity (bottom). Image wrap is present from an inappropriately small field-of-view.

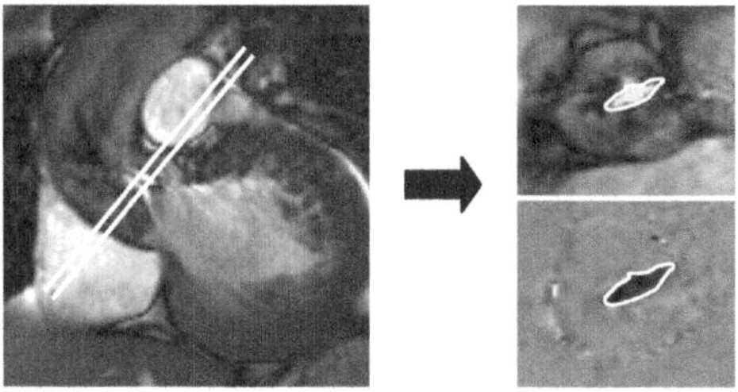

Fig. 10.10 Through-plane flow mapping. Aligning a through-plane flow image (left), resultant magnitude image (top right) and flow image (bottom right), with planimetry of the valve tips. In this case, a bicuspid valve with severe stenosis (0.7 cm^2).

Unable to image flow properly?

- The flow direction may be incorrect (examine the image).
- Small and turbulent jet in very severe stenosis, resulting in negligible signal from the jet. In this case, no accurate measurement of velocity can be obtained and aortic valve planimetry alone should be used. The severe degree of stenosis is usually clear from the images.

Reporting should include

- Anatomy of valve/outflow:
  - Bicuspid or tricuspid
  - *Mechanism of stenosis* – immobile leaflets/mobile leaflets + fused tips
  - LV outflow tract to ensure no sub-valvar stenosis.
- Severity of valve stenosis (see Table 10.2, p. 249):
  - Valve area by direct planimetry
  - Stenotic jet velocity (and calculated gradient across the valve).
- *Effect on LV* – mass, volumes, and function.
- Any associated aortic regurgitation or ascending aortic dilation.

Differential diagnosis

- Sub-valvar or supravalvar stenosis.
- LVOT obstruction (📖 p. 254).
- Consider other forms of LV hypertrophy, especially if the hypertrophy is out of proportion to degree of stenosis (aortic stenosis is common and may co-exist with other conditions):
  - Hypertension.
  - Hypertrophic cardiomyopathy (📖 p. 178).
  - Infiltrative myocardial disease (e.g. amyloid, sarcoid, iron overload).
  - Fabry disease (Anderson-Fabry disease, 📖 p. 190).
  - Endomyocardial fibrosis (📖 p. 204).

Assessing the severity of aortic stenosis with CMR

- Valve area is the most accurate method, being measured directly by planimetry, rather than estimated from the continuity equation (as with echocardiography). The potential errors with velocity measurements by CMR in aortic stenosis reduce their accuracy
- Trans-valvar gradients are estimated using the modified Bernoulli equation. Note this assumes the subvalvar velocity is close to 1m/s. Although mean transvalvar gradient can be calculated, the lower temporal resolution of CMR velocity mapping reduces its accuracy and it is not usually included in software packages:

  Gradient (mmHg) = 4 × (peak velocity)^2

Table 10.2 Guide to severity of aortic stenosis

	Mild	Moderate	Severe
Valve area (cm^2)	1.6–2.0	1.0–1.5	<1.0
Peak velocity (m/s)	2.0–2.9	3.0–3.9	>4.0
Estimated gradient (mmHg)	20–35	36–63	>64

Sub-aortic stenosis

Background

Due to congenital membrane in the LVOT 0.5–1cm below the aortic valve. Often mis-diagnosed as aortic stenosis due to the proximity to the valve, but the valve can be seen to open normally. Surgical resection is the usual treatment if severe enough to warrant intervention.

CMR features

- **Membrane in LVOT:**
  - May be seen just beneath the aortic valve (Fig. 10.11).
  - Circumferential, although often more severe on the septal side.
- **High velocity jet originating from just below the valve:** Systolic anterior motion (SAM) of the anterior mitral leaflet is NOT usually present.
- **Normal aortic valve opening.**
- **± Aortic regurgitation:** due to valve damage from high velocity jet.
- **± LV hypertrophy.**

Scanning

Standard and coronal LVOT cine imaging

Examine carefully – the membrane can usually be seen below the aortic valve causing turbulent flow. Sometimes the turbulent flow obscures the aortic valve in systole, but the valve position is seen in diastole.

Velocity mapping

- In-plane mapping can identify the origin of the high-velocity jet (if not already seen) and provide the peak velocity.
- Through-plane velocity mapping just distal to jet (may be at the valve annulus level). Can measure the velocity if not already obtained on in-plane mapping.

± Short axis view of LVOT

Planned in a similar way to the *en-face* aortic valve view, but positioned through the membrane. May image the circumferential membrane and area of stenosis, (see Fig. 10.12) although partial volume effects can sometimes prevent good visualization of the thin structure.

± En-face view of aortic valve

To visualize leaflet opening and exclude aortic stenosis.

Reporting

As for aortic stenosis.

Differential diagnosis

- Aortic stenosis (valve usually restricted in opening; 📖 p. 244).
- LVOT obstruction (no membrane and SAM more common; 📖 p. 254).

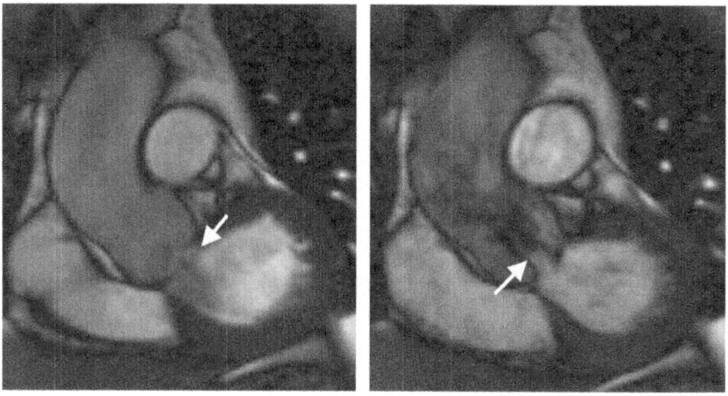

Fig. 10.11 Sub-aortic membrane in coronal LVOT view. The membrane can be seen 0.5cm below the aortic valve in diastole (left, arrowed); there is mild aortic regurgitation. Right: in systole the high velocity jet (arrowed) originates from the membrane, just below the valve.

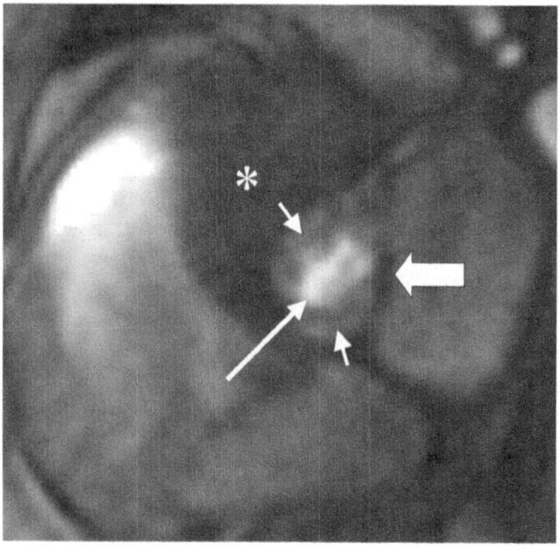

Fig. 10.12 Short-axis view of membrane. Short axis view through the LVOT in the same patient as above. The boundaries of the septal myocardium (*) and anterior mitral leaflet (block arrow) define the area. The circumferential nature of the membrane can be visualized as the mid-grey signal (short arrows) surrounding the orifice area (higher signal, long arrow).

Supra-aortic stenosis

Background

A narrowed aorta just above the aortic valve, usually associated with other congenital conditions, e.g. Williams syndrome (Fig. 10.13). Mostly mild, but if severe, aortic root replacement/reconstructive surgery may be required.

CMR features

- **Narrowed aorta above aortic valve:** Usually at the level of the sino-tubular junction.
- Turbulent jet arising from the narrowed section.
- Normal aortic valve opening.

Scanning

See Aortic stenosis, 📖 p. 244.

± Short axis view through narrowest section of aorta

May allow measurement of true minimum diameter.

Reporting should include:

- Description of aortic root anatomy and minimum aortic diameter.
- Maximum velocity of jet.
- LV mass and function (to indicate effect on LV).

Differential diagnosis

- Aortic stenosis.
- Previous aortic root surgery (e.g. for dissection).
- Relative stenosis (e.g. if aortic sinuses dilated in Marfan syndrome).
- Congenital hypoplasia of the aortic arch – rare, but can affect the ascending aorta.

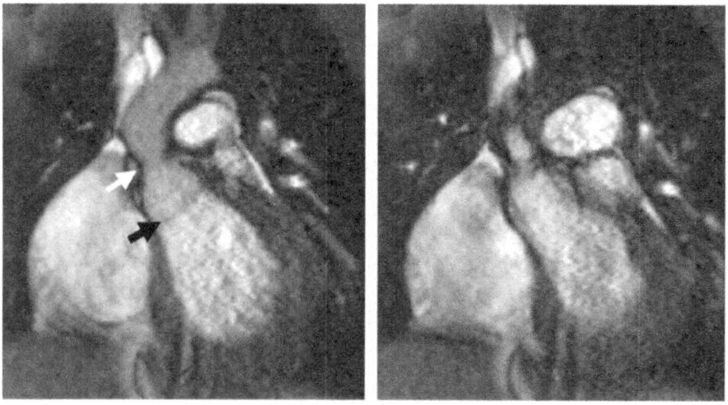

Fig. 10.13 Coronal LVOT view of supravalvar stenosis. The narrowed sino-tubular junction can be seen in diastole (left, white arrow) above the aortic valve (black arrow). The high velocity jet arising from here can be seen in systole (right), above the widely open aortic valve. The patient has Williams syndrome and had difficulty with breath-hold instructions, hence the lower image quality.

Dynamic LV outflow tract obstruction

Background

Dynamic LVOT obstruction occurs in systole, due to narrowing of the outflow tract as the septum thickens ± anterior mitral leaflet movement. Note the multiple listed, although suspicious for hypertrophic cardiomyopathy, LVOT obstruction can occur from other mechanisms.

Causes

- Hypertrophic cardiomyopathy.
- Hypertrophy of the basal septum (e.g. senile sigmoid septum or associated with severe concentric hypertrophy).
- Hyperdynamic LV contraction (can be accentuated by afterload-reducing drugs, dehydration, or positive inotropes).
- Elongated ± floppy anterior mitral valve leaflet.

CMR features

- **Narrowing of LVOT in systole.**
- **Turbulence ± high velocity jet in LVOT (Fig. 10.14):**
  - Arises from below aortic valve and may be very narrow
  - Peak narrowing/turbulence/velocity occurs in late systole.
- **Thickened septum**: if HCM or basal septal hypertrophy present.
- **± SAM of the anterior mitral valve leaflet:**
  - Due to Venturi effect of high velocity jet in LVOT 'pulling' leaflet towards septum and further accentuating the obstruction
  - May cause mitral regurgitation (usually late systolic, coinciding with peak LVOT obstruction).

Scanning

See Sub-aortic stenosis, 📖 p. 250.

- Turbulent jet may be too narrow for accurate velocity measurement.
- Short axis cine of narrowest part of LVOT can show area of stenosis and allow direct planimetry (Fig. 10.15).
- Dobutamine stress can be used to accentuate any LVOT obstruction, but care should be taken in the MR environment (see 📖 p. 120).
- Late gadolinium enhancement may demonstrate features of HCM.

Reporting should include:

- **Location and severity of obstruction:** may be qualitative description if velocity inaccurate, but short axis LVOT area is often helpful – use aortic stenosis for guide to severity.
  ► Remember that the severity seen at rest may be significantly greater when the patient is exercising – it is a *dynamic* obstruction!
- **LV mass and function:** ?regional or global hypertrophy.
- **Any specific features of HCM**: 📖 p. 178

Differential diagnosis

- Aortic stenosis (📖 p. 244).
- Sub-aortic membrane (📖 p. 250).

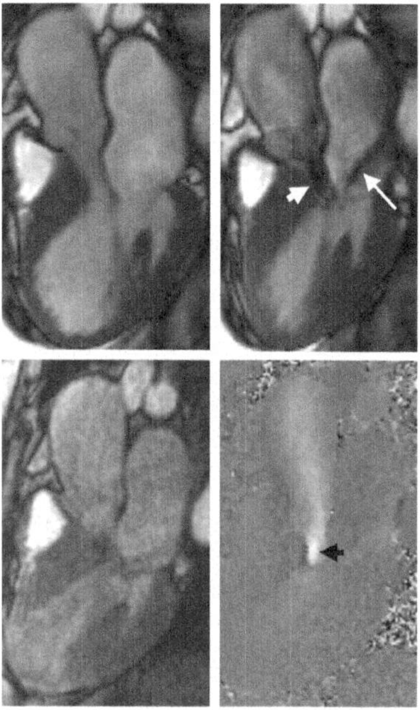

Fig. 10.14 LVOT obstruction. SSFP images (top). Note the narrowed LVOT between the hypertrophied septum and the anterior mitral leaflet (diastole, top left). In systole (top right), there is turbulence in the LVOT (short arrow) and mild mitral regurgitation (long arrow). In-plane flow images (bottom), slightly rotated from SSFP images to align flow direction with jet. Magnitude image (left) and flow image (right), with high velocity flow (4.6m/s) visible in LVOT; velocity window ± 5m/s.

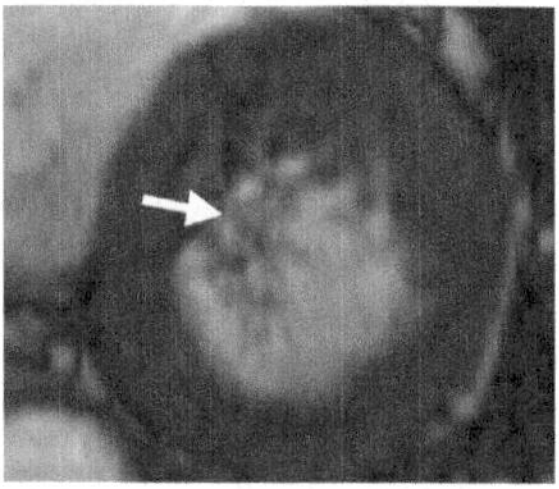

Fig. 10.15 LVOT obstruction (short axis view). The small area of the LVOT in systole (arrowed) can be seen, bordered by the septum and anterior mitral leaflet. The area can be measured by direct planimetry.

The mitral valve

Normal anatomy

The mitral valve is a large and complex valve, which relies on many components to function correctly – leaflets, annulus, sub-valvar apparatus (chordae and papillary muscles), and LV wall contraction. Any component may be involved in dysfunction of the valve and all should be imaged.

Leaflets and segments

The mitral valve has two leaflets; an anterior tongue-shaped one and a posterior crescent-shaped one, which almost surrounds the anterior leaflet, forming a crescentic coaption line (see Fig. 10.16). Each leaflet has 3 'scallops' or segments (according to the Carpentier classification), labelled A1–3 and P1–3 for anterior and posterior leaflets, respectively. The A1 and P1 scallops are located close to the anterolateral LV wall, while the A3 and P3 segments are close to the posteromedial wall (nearer the septum) (Fig. 10.17).

Papillary muscles and chordae

There are two papillary muscles – a larger anterolateral one, and a smaller posteromedial one (which may be comprised of 2–3 'heads' of muscle). The papillary muscles are attached to the LV wall close to the apex and the basal ends are attached to the valve leaflets by chordae tendinae. Chordae from both papillary muscles attach to both leaflets, and are classically divided into 3 'orders', although this distinction is rarely seen well on CMR due to the thin nature of the chordae:

- **1st order chordae:** attach to leaflet tips.
- **2nd order chordae:** attach to leaflet body.
- **3rd order chordae:** run direct from ventricular wall to leaflet body (without involving a papillary muscle)

Imaging

- The three standard LV long axis views (HLA, VLA, LVOT) are good for assessing motion of the mitral valve and most segments can usually be identified on these (see Fig. 10.17).
- A short axis view through the valve is especially good at demonstrating the leaflets and segments, and can identify prolapsed segments or valve stenosis.
- For a systematic evaluation of all scallops of the mitral leaflets, a stack of parallel cine images can be obtained parallel to the LVOT view (perpendicular to the commissure), covering the entire valve (see Fig. 10.18). These should be thin (5mm) and without a gap between slices, to fully cover the valve scallops. Two additional slices at the extreme ends may be required to assess the A1/P1 and A3/P3 coaption as the commissure curves round at the ends. These slices should be perpendicular to the commissure at the ends. See Chan *et al.*, 2008, for details.

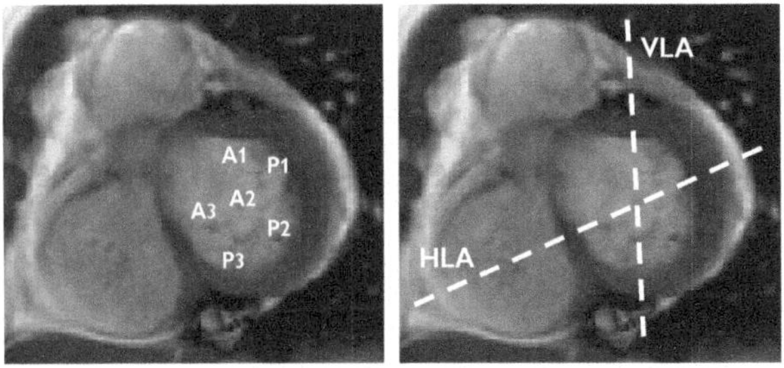

Fig. 10.16 Short axis diagram of mitral valve showing the segments (left), and approximate position of long axis planes (right).

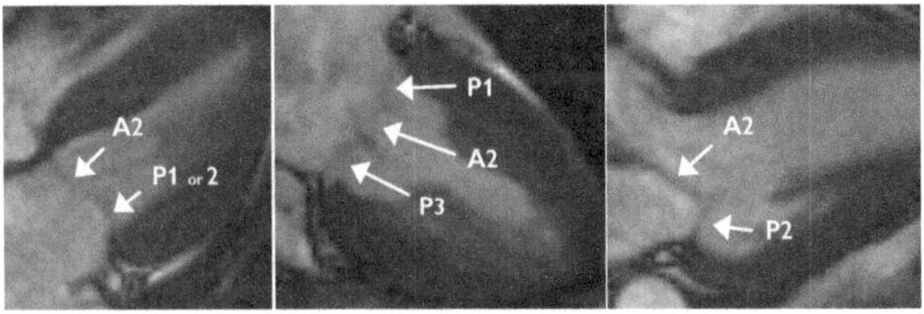

Fig. 10.17 HLA (left), VLA (middle), and LVOT (right) images showing visible segments of a normal mitral valve.

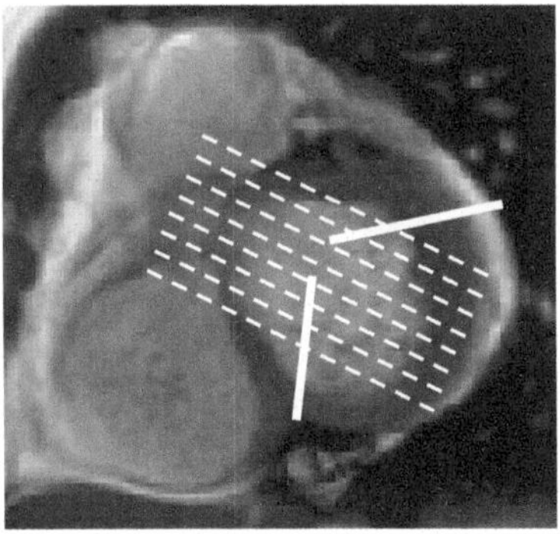

Fig. 10.18 Short axis diagram of the mitral valve, showing position of the parallel image stack to examine the individual scallops. The main stack (dashed lines) is parallel to the LVOT view, with an additional slice positioned across each end, perpendicular to the commissure (single solid lines).

Further reading

Chan et *al*. *J Cardiovasc Mag Res* 2008; **10:** 61.

Mitral regurgitation

Background

Common. May often be tolerated for years or even decades without problems. Causes include:

- Degenerative disease, often with redundant tissue (Barlow's disease).
- Prolapse.
- Infective endocarditis.
- Ruptured chordae/papillary muscles, e.g. from myocardial infarction (MI).
- Functional (due to poor LV function ± LV dilation).

Transoesophageal echocardiography provides fine detail of the valve components and function and remains the major imaging tool for most patients. CMR provides sufficient detail in many cases, however, is more tolerable than TOE for some patients, and has the distinct advantage of being able to quantify regurgitation, rather than relying on qualitative assessments.

CMR features

- **Regurgitant mitral jet:** turbulence arising from the mitral valve in systole, directed towards the LA. May be central or very eccentric. The width of the jet and jet area have a modest correlation with degree of regurgitation, but should not be relied upon and proper quantification should be undertaken.
- **± Prolapsed or flail leaflet(s):**
  - Best assessed on LVOT view (see Fig. 10.19 and 10.20).
  - Regurgitant jet usually directed away from prolapsing leaflet, e.g. if posterior prolapse, jet is directed anteriorly.
  - Regurgitation typically occurs in late systole, after prolapse has occurred.
  - Prolapse may be caused by elongated chordae or redundant leaflet tissue, and can occur in one or more scallops of a leaflet (see opposite).
  - A flail leaflet may result from a ruptured chordae/papillary muscle and is usually accompanied by severe regurgitation.
- **± Tethered leaflets:** the leaflet(s) fail to close, due to restricted movement of the chordae/papillary muscles towards the valve. Causes include:
  - Reduced LV wall contraction from poor LV function, especially following inferior MI affecting inferolateral papillary muscle. Termed 'functional regurgitation' as the valve regurgitation is secondary to poor function of the LV, rather than an intrinsic valve problem (see Fig. 10.21).
  - Shortened chordae from previous rheumatic fever.
  - Post-mitral valve repair (uncommon).
- **± Dilated LV/reduced LV function:** either secondary to significant chronic regurgitation or a cause of functional regurgitation.
- **± Dilated left atrium:** suggests chronic valve lesion and/or AF.

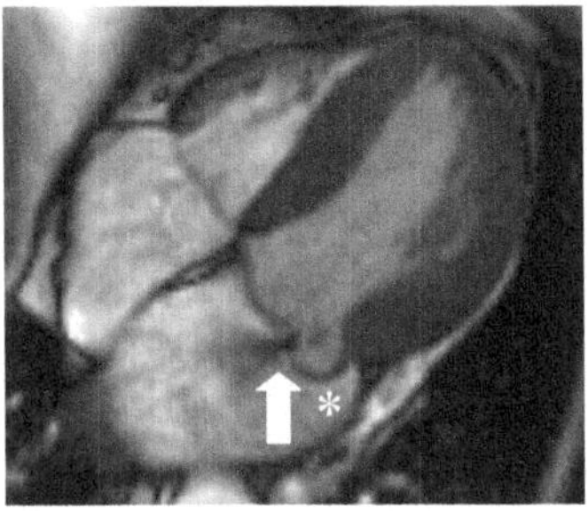

Fig. 10.19 Posterior mitral prolapse with a jet of regurgitation (arrowed). Note the bowed posterior leaflet (*) with the tip behind the mitral annulus, indicating prolapse. Systolic frame from SSFP cine in HLA plane.

Bowing, prolapse or flail?

Leaflet prolapse/bowing

Usually due to redundant leaflet tissue resulting in excessive motion of the leaflet(s) towards the LA in systole.

- '**Bowing**' is present if the leaflet body passes behind a line drawn across the mitral annulus, but the tips remain on the LV side.
- **Prolapse** is present when the leaflet tips move behind the annulus, i.e. a more severe manifestation of bowing.
- Due to the saddle shape of the annulus, this is assessed most robustly in the LVOT view (equivalent to the echocardiographic parasternal long axis view), which passes through the narrower and more atrial portion of the annulus.
- **NB:** in both cases, the leaflet tips remain 'pointing' towards the LV .

Flail leaflet

A flail leaflet nearly always results from a ruptured chordae or papillary muscle, allowing the tip of the leaflet to 'flail' backwards and point towards the left atrium. Usually results in severe regurgitation.

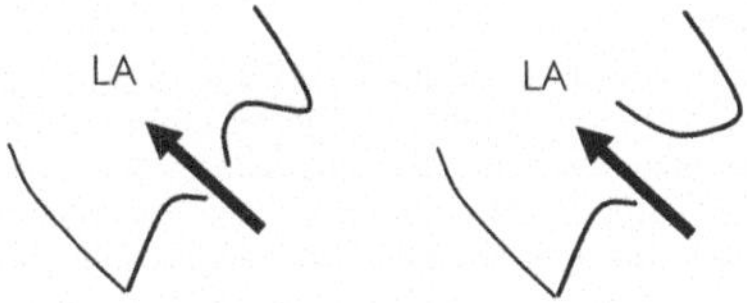

Fig. 10.20 Prolapsed leaflets (left); note the tips 'pointing' towards the LV. Flail leaflet (right) with tips 'pointing towards LA. Arrow represents mitral regurgitation.

Scanning

HLA, VLA, and LVOT long axis views

To visualize the valve anatomy and motion. Note the motion of both leaflets and any regurgitant jet.

± Short axis view of regurgitant orifice

Often well seen on one of the basal images from the LV volume stack.

± Modified long axis views

If the MR jet is not well seen, the long axis views can be modified by repositioning them through the regurgitant orifice on the short axis view.

Standard and coronal LVOT views

To position the aortic flow slice.

Through-plane flow mapping above aortic valve

To quantify forward flow through the aortic valve and facilitate quantification of the MR. Place image slice as close to the valve as possible.

Short axis stack for LV ± RV volumes

To determine effect on the LV, and allow quantification of MR.

Quantification of mitral regurgitation

This is a significant advantage of CMR and should be performed.

Standard method

The LV stroke volume must be ejected into the aorta or back through a regurgitant mitral valve (see Fig. 10.22), so subtracting aortic forward flow from LV stroke volume will quantify the mitral regurgitation. This method is robust for virtually all cardiac lesions, including aortic regurgitation (only the forward aortic flow is used in the measurement). The only exception is a ventricular septal defect. It does rely on accurate flow data, however, and uncontrolled AF may diminish the accuracy.

Mitral regurgitant volume = LV stroke volume – aortic forward flow (ml/cardiac cycle)

Regurgitant fraction = Regurgitant volume/LV stroke volume × 100% (proportion of stroke volume that flows back through mitral valve)

Alternative method

If flow imaging is unavailable/unreliable, MR can be quantified using the difference between LV and RV stroke volumes. In the absence of a shunt or another regurgitant valve, this should equal the mitral regurgitation. The reliance on other lesions being absent makes this method less robust, but it can also be used to corroborate the flow data if necessary.

Regurgitant volume (ml) = LV stroke volume – RV stroke volume

Direct mitral flow measurement

Direct measurement of the flow jet would seem attractive, but is difficult due to the mobile valve, large area of leaflet coaption, mobile nature of the jet, high (turbulent) velocities, and sometimes multiple flow jets. For these reasons, the indirect method, incorporating *aortic* flow, is used as flow measurement across the smaller aortic valve is more accurate.

Table 10.3 Assessment of severity in mitral regurgitation

	Mild	Moderate	Severe
Regurgitant fraction (%)	0–20	21–50	>50
Regurgitant volume (ml/cycle)	0–30	31–60	>60

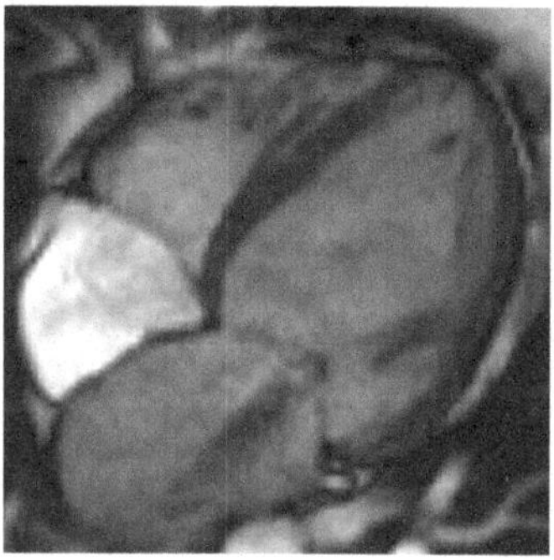

Fig. 10.21 'Functional' mitral regurgitation. Note the 'tented' leaflets held open by the reduced papillary movement towards the mitral valve, due to poor LV function. Systolic frame from SSFP cine in HLA plane.

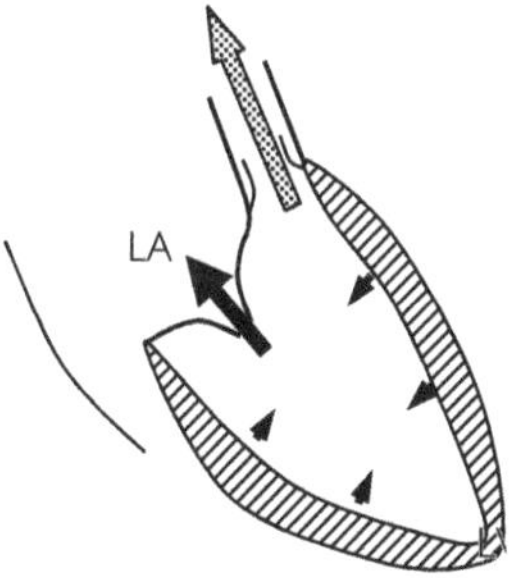

Fig. 10.22 During systole, the LV stroke volume is ejected into the aorta (grey arrow) or back through the mitral valve as regurgitation (black arrow).

Reporting should include:

- **Anatomy/function of mitral valve:** description of leaflet anatomy and motion – thickened, restricted motion, tethered, bowing, prolapse, or flail?
- **Description and quantification of regurgitation:**
  - *Description of regurgitation* – wide/narrow jet, direction, whether present throughout systole or just part of it (e.g. late systolic regurgitation in prolapse)
  - *Quantification of regurgitation* – best to use the regurgitant fraction and add descriptor of severity (see Table 10.3).
  - There are currently no accepted thresholds for intervention (i.e. valve replacement/repair) based purely on the quantity of regurgitation, and CMR quantification should be interpreted as one part of the overall clinical picture. Studies are on-going in this area.
- **Effect on LV:** mass, volumes and function.
  - If significant LV dilation/dysfunction is present, the degree of mitral regurgitation should be severe, otherwise an alternative cause of LV dilation/dysfunction should be sought
  - LV mass is usually in proportion to LV volume (roughly a 1:1 ratio, i.e. the mass in g = the volume in ml); if excessive LV mass is present, other causes of hypertrophy should be sought.

Mitral stenosis

CMR can provide useful information in the assessment of mitral stenosis, particularly direct planimetry of the valve area. However, it has lower spatial resolution for imaging the valve leaflets when compared with transoesophageal echocardiography and also lower temporal resolution than echo for diastolic flow measurement. The assessment of other aspects important for assessing the mitral valve for balloon valvuloplasty, e.g. leaflet calcification or chordal thickening, are also limited with CMR, and echocardiography may be more appropriate for this.

Causes: rheumatic valve disease, systemic lupus erythematosus, congenital (rare), degenerative (mitral annular calcification – rare).

CMR features

- **Restricted ± thickened mitral leaflets:**
  - In rheumatic mitral stenosis, fusion of the leaflets occurs at the tips, with relative sparing (initially) of the base. This causes a 'doming' of the leaflet, sometimes creating a 'hockey-stick' appearance with an angled leaflet (Fig. 10.23). The leaflets may be thickened or calcified with longstanding disease, and the whole leaflet may be poorly mobile or immobile with advanced disease. The chordae may also be thickened and/or shortened
  - In degenerative (calcific) disease, the thickening starts from the annulus and involves the leaflet base and body with relative sparing of the tips.
- **Enlarged left atrium:** best seen on HLA and VLA views. Often exacerbated by AF. Usually very large in severe stenosis.
- **± LV dysfunction:** global dysfunction can be a feature of active rheumatic carditis, but mitral stenosis in itself does not affect LV function.

Scanning

HLA, VLA, and LVOT long axis views

To visualize the valve anatomy and motion, and left atrial size. Some re-positioning of the planes may be required to see the valve opening, as the plane may pass through a fused part of the valve, which appears not to open at all!

Note the motion of both leaflets, and any thickening or regurgitation. The LVOT view is particularly good for viewing the mitral valve.

Short axis view through mitral tips

Similar to a LV short axis view, but specifically orientated to include the leaflet tips in diastole (see Fig. 10.24). Use all 3 long axis planes to position the slice. If this is placed too far towards the atrium, the valve area will be larger than the true area at the tips, and the degree of stenosis under-estimated.

Mitral diastolic flow can be measured in the same plane, but the temporal resolution is generally too low for accurate measurements.

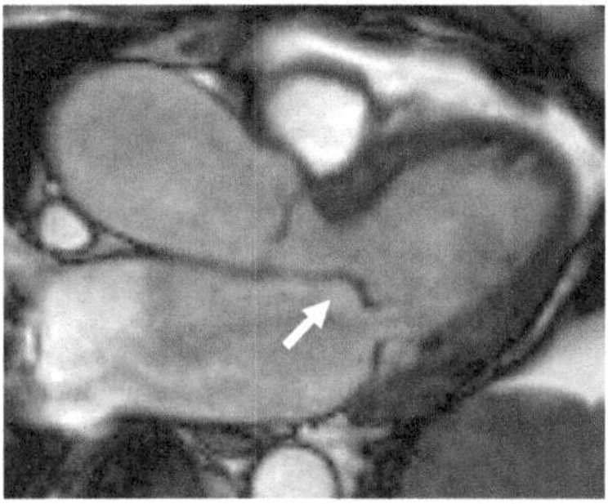

Fig. 10.23 LVOT view in diastole, demonstrating restricted opening of the mitral valve and typical angled 'hockey stick' appearance of the anterior mitral valve leaflet (arrowed).

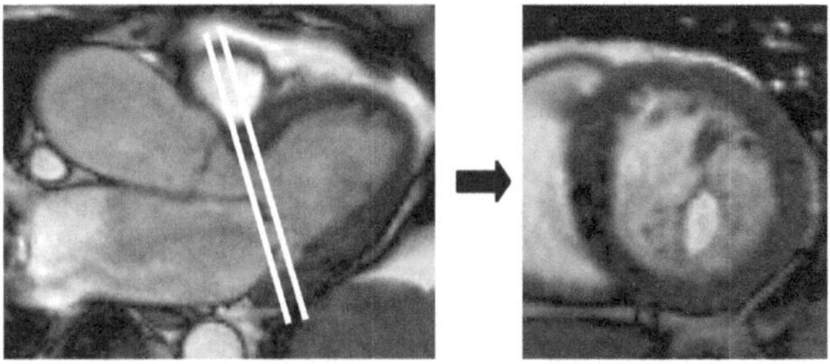

Fig. 10.24 Positioning the image slice (solid lines, left) for the through-plane image at the valve tips (right). The valve area can be measured easily.

Reporting should include:

- **Mitral valve anatomy/function and orifice area:**
  - *Description of leaflet anatomy and motion* – Is it thickened? How severely is the opening restricted? Comment on the relative motion of the base and tips to indicate likely cause, and aspects of suitability for balloon valvuloplasty.
  - Valve area from direct planimetry, with indication of severity (see Table 10.4 opposite for indication of severity).
- **Thickening/shortening of chordae?**
- **Any regurgitation present**: quantify.
- **± LV mass, volumes and function:** less important for mitral stenosis, as this doesn't specifically affect LV unless active carditis is present, but is usually part of a comprehensive CMR assessment.

Suitability for balloon valvuloplasty

CMR is not the ideal imaging modality for this – transoesophageal echocardiography provides more detail and should be performed in all cases prior to valvuloplasty. Assessing the left atrial appendage for thrombus is a crucial step pre-procedure, which also requires TOE.

CMR can, however, provide some information on the aspects needed for this decision. Important assessments are listed, with those suitable for CMR assessment marked with an asterisk (*).

- **Contraindications to balloon valvuloplasty**:
  - Thrombus in left atrial appendage
  - ≥ moderate mitral regurgitation*
  - Severe aortic or tricuspid valve disease*.
- **Predictors of long-term outcome**: valve morphology is the main determinant, and can be scored using echocardiographic criteria, the commonest of which is the Wilkins scoring system (see box 📖 p. 267). The applicability to CMR is unproven.

Differential diagnosis

- The diagnosis is usually apparent on imaging.
- Clinically, mitral stenosis may be mimicked by:
  - Atrial myxoma
  - Bulky vegetation
  - Cor tri-atriatum.

Table 10.4 Assessment of severity in mitral stenosis

	Mild	Moderate	Severe
Mitral valve area (cm^2)	>1.5	1.0–1.5	<1.0
Mean pressure gradient (mmHg; if diastolic velocity measured)[1]	<5	5–10	>10

[1] NB can be significantly affected by increased volume load (e.g. mitral regurgitation)

Wilkins scoring system for mitral valve morphology

Echocardiographic scoring system, with unproven transferability to CMR. Each feature scores between 1 and 4 points, which are added together to achieve the final score. The lower the score, the more suitable the valve for balloon valvuloplasty, though generally a score >8 suggests poor long term outcome from valvuloplasty.

* Indicates assessment with CMR is feasible

(*) indicates assessment with CMR may be possible in some cases

Leaflet mobility

- Highly mobile with restricted leaflet tips only*.
- Reduced mobility in mid-portion and base of leaflets*.
- Mostly immobile leaflets with movement only at the base*.
- Virtually no forward movement of the leaflets*.

Valve thickening

- Near normal <4–5mm (*).
- Pronounced thickening at the tips and mid-leaflet thickening (*).
- Thickening (5–8mm) throughout leaflet*.
- Severe thickening of entire leaflet (8–10mm)*.

Sub-valvar thickening

- Minimal thickening of chordae below valve.
- Thickening of up to 1/3 of chordal length (*).
- Thickening extending to distal third of chordae (*).
- Severe thickening and shortening of all chordae, extending to papillary muscles*.

Valve calcification

May be visualized as signal loss on CMR.

- A single area of increased echo brightness.
- Scattered areas of echo brightness confined to leaflet margins.
- Calcification extending to mid-portion of leaflets (*).
- Extensive calcification throughout most leaflet tissue (*).

The pulmonary valve

Normal anatomy

The pulmonary valve consists of three semi-lunar cusps – anterior, left and right, and lies just above the muscular outflow tract (infundibulum) of the RV, at the base of the pulmonary trunk. It sits adjacent to the aortic valve, but turned through 90° relative to the aortic root, due to the spiraling of the great vessels during foetal development.

Imaging

Standard RVOT view

The standard RVOT view (📖 p. 92) is the ideal plane for viewing the pulmonary valve, RV outflow tract, and proximal pulmonary trunk (see Fig. 10.25). The valve leaflets are thin and can sometimes be difficult to see, but the opening of the valve can usually be appreciated. Other features can be identified from this view, including any regurgitation, sub- or supravalvar stenosis and pulmonary artery dilation. Care should be taken to ensure the usually dynamic RVOT remains in plane throughout the cycle – the horizontal view (below) may help if problematic.

Horizontal RVOT view (see Fig. 10.26)

- This view is good for obtaining a full assessment of RVOT anatomy, particularly if any intervention may be considered, and facilitates accurate placement of an image slice across the pulmonary valve for flow or anatomical imaging.
- If pulmonary valve pathology is seen in the standard RVOT view, this view can further clarify the anatomy, including any pulmonary dilation.
- Also good for viewing the left-right motion of the RV outflow tract in systole. If the outflow tract moves out of plane on the standard RVOT view, the horizontal view can be used to modify the standard one, repositioning the image slice so that it remains within the outflow tract during the whole cardiac cycle.

Through-plane imaging

An image slice can be placed through the pulmonary valve, using the previous views for planning (see Fig. 10.26). It may be difficult to position the image with the valve remaining in plane throughout the cardiac cycle, however, as the normal RV outflow tract contracts vigorously during systole, with considerable movement towards the apex.

This view can allow assessment of individual leaflet function and overall opening of the valve, including valve area (Fig. 10.27).

Flow imaging can also be performed in this plane to quantify velocity, and pulmonary forward/regurgitant flows.

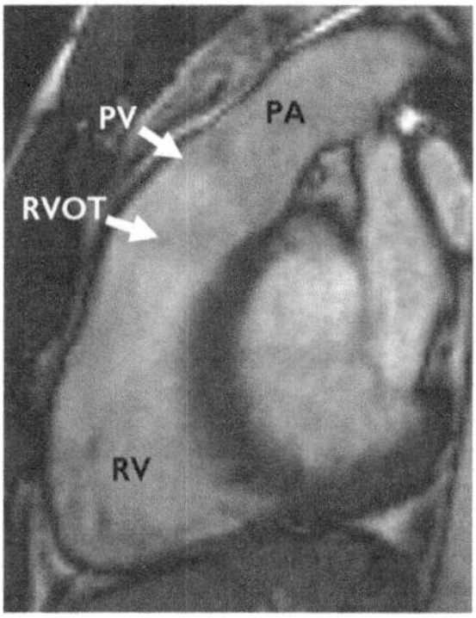

Fig. 10.25 Standard RVOT view in diastole, showing part of the mid-RV cavity, the RV outflow tract (infundibulum), the pulmonary valve (PV) – often barely seen – and the proximal pulmonary artery (PA).

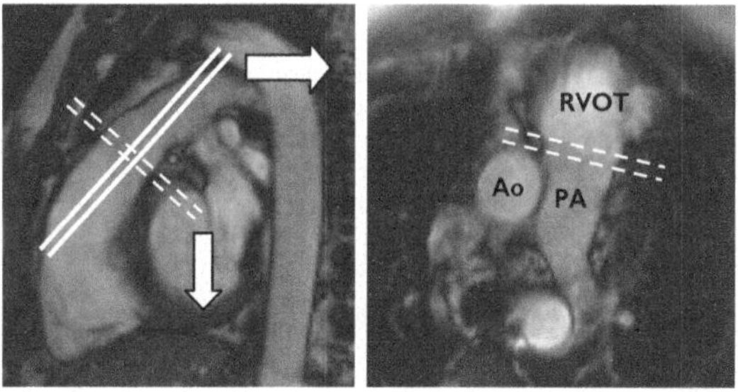

Fig. 10.26 Standard RVOT image (left) showing slice position for the horizontal RVOT image plane (solid lines) and the through-valve image (dashed lines). Horizontal RVOT view (right), showing a foreshortened RVOT, pulmonary valve, proximal pulmonary artery (PA), and dashed lines indicating the through-valve image position.

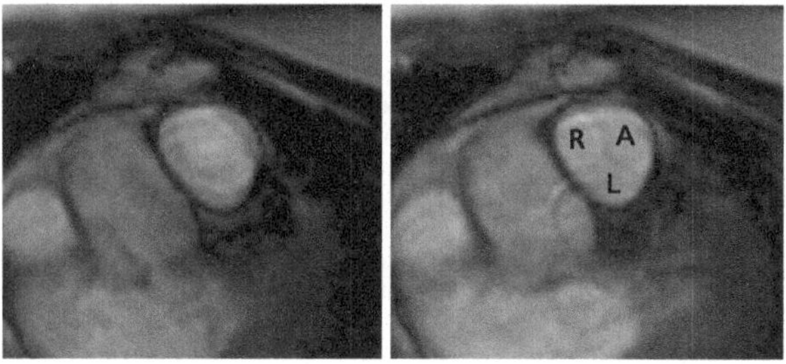

Fig. 10.27 Image through a normal pulmonary valve in systole (left) and diastole (right). Note the anterior (A), left (L) and right (R) cusps.

Pulmonary regurgitation

Background

Very mild pulmonary regurgitation is common and can be regarded as 'physiological'. Significant degrees of pulmonary regurgitation are uncommon in general, but relatively frequent following previous surgery involving enlargement of the valve or RV outflow tract, e.g. repair of Fallot's tetralogy or pulmonary valvotomy for congenital pulmonary stenosis. Rare non-congenital causes include dilation of the pulmonary artery, pulmonary hypertension, carcinoid valve disease, and endocarditis.

The RV can tolerate pulmonary regurgitation for many years, with compensatory dilation, but normal function. RV dysfunction is therefore particularly important as a sign of decompensation.

CMR is ideally suited to the assessment of pulmonary regurgitation, with clear imaging of the RVOT and pulmonary valve, accurate quantification of the regurgitation with flow mapping, and RV volume/function assessment – these are all difficult areas for echocardiography.

CMR features

- **Regurgitant pulmonary jet:** turbulence arising from the pulmonary valve in diastole, directed towards the RV. Pulmonary pressures are lower than in the aorta, so the degree of turbulence is often less and the regurgitation may be difficult to visualize (Fig. 10.28). This is particularly so if the regurgitation is very severe, when the regurgitant flow jet may be more laminar than turbulent. It is therefore often difficult to assess the degree of regurgitation by the size or appearance of the regurgitant jet, particularly on SSFP imaging in which turbulence is more difficult to visualize due to the short echo time.

▶ Quantification of the regurgitant flow is therefore very important.

- **Dilated RV ± dysfunction:** dilation indicates a significant degree of regurgitation. Dysfunction indicates RV decompensation. There is debate about whether severe dilation alone indicates decompensation.
- **± Prolapsed leaflet(s):**
  - May be caused by dilated pulmonary root, damaged leaflets from carcinoid or endocarditis, or from degenerative change in a homograft or pericardial bio-prosthetic valve
  - Use all three RVOT views to assess – through-plane flow imaging may be particularly useful for identifying the site of regurgitation.
- **± Dilated pulmonary trunk/RV outflow:** a common cause of regurgitation. Maximal diameter should be measured from a cine image placed across the PA short axis at the point of greatest dilation. Normal adult diameter <28mm for common trunk, <18mm for left or right pulmonary arteries. For smaller adults and children, the pulmonary trunk is usually the same diameter as the ascending aorta, so a large difference may indicate dilation. Causes: previous surgery, pulmonary hypertension, large left to right shunt, Marfan syndrome.

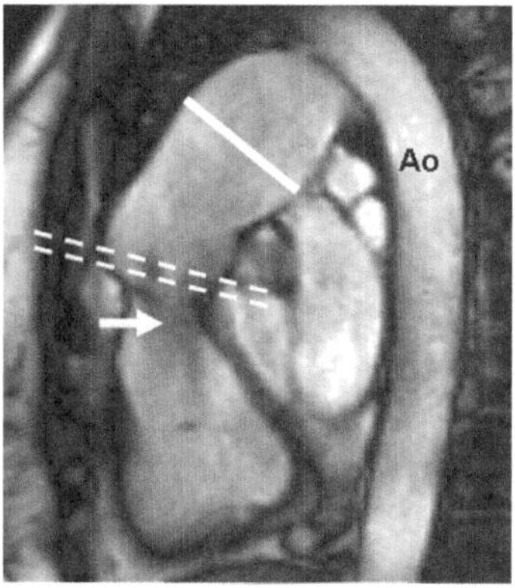

Fig. 10.28 RVOT view in diastole. Note the difficult to visualize flow jet (arrowed), and the slice position for through-plane flow imaging (parallel dashed lines). The pulmonary artery is dilated, with the single broad line indicating the slice position for a cine image at the site of greatest dilation, from which the true diameter should be measured. Ao = descending aorta.

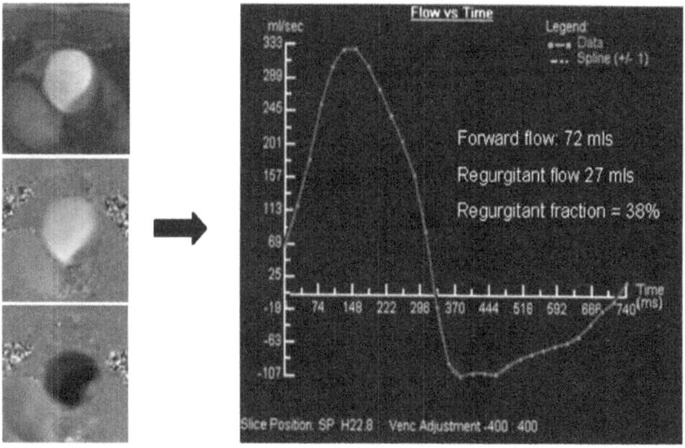

Fig. 10.29 Through-plane pulmonary flow images (left) – magnitude image (top), systolic flow (middle), and diastolic flow (bottom) showing significant regurgitation, displayed in the graph (right).

Scanning

Standard RVOT view ± horizontal RVOT view

To visualize the valve anatomy and motion, the regurgitant jet, and the anatomy of the infundibulum and proximal pulmonary trunk.

Quantify regurgitation with through-plane flow mapping

Use the through-valve view (Fig. 10.29) and place image slice just above pulmonary valve to quantify forward and regurgitant flow. Calculate pulmonary regurgitant fraction from the flow data:

Regurgitant fraction = pulmonary regurgitant volume (diastolic flow)/pulmonary forward volume (systolic flow) × 100%

If flow is unavailable, quantification may be assessed by calculating the stroke volume difference (RV – LV stroke volume) if there are no other valve leaks.

RV volumes and mass ± LV volumes

To determine effect on the RV – severe regurgitation normally results in a dilated RV (Fig. 10.30). RV function is very important, as a reduction suggests decompensation from the regurgitation. RV stroke volume should equal the pulmonary forward flow and can be used as a check.

± Further pulmonary artery imaging

Extent of any dilation; branch pulmonary artery involvement?

Reporting should include:

- **Anatomy of pulmonary valve and root:**
  - Look for any clear cause of pulmonary regurgitation (e.g. RVOT dilation, prolapsed leaflet, altered anatomy from previous surgery)
  - Pulmonary artery dimensions.
  - Any degree of pulmonary stenosis?
- **Quantification and severity of regurgitation:**
  - Best quantified as regurgitant fraction – see Table 10.5 for severity.
  - There are currently no accepted thresholds for intervention (i.e. valve replacement) based on the quantity of regurgitation, though studies are on-going. Precise assessment of the severity of regurgitation and RV dilation/dysfunction can, however, be invaluable in informing clinical decisions within the overall clinical context.
- **Effect on RV: volumes and function:**
  - Degree of RV dilation should be appropriate to the degree of pulmonary regurgitation, otherwise an alternative cause should be sought
  - Intervention based on the degree of RV dilation, or indeed RV dysfunction (in the absence of symptoms), is debated and there are no strong data to guide this.
- **Any pulmonary artery dilation/stenosis.**

Table 10.5. Assessment of severity in pulmonary regurgitation

	Mild	Moderate	Severe
Regurgitant fraction (%)	0–30	31–50	>50

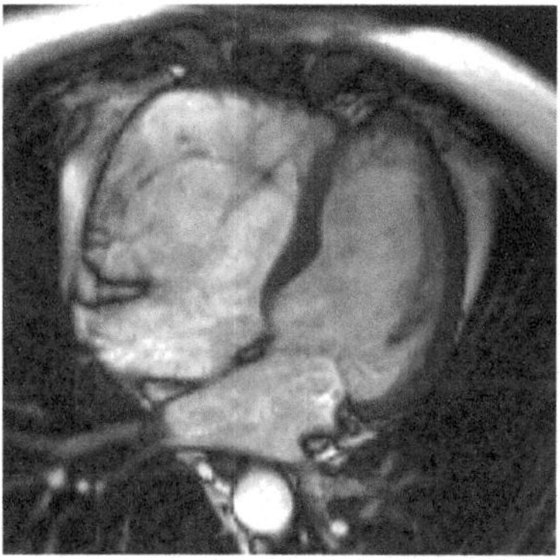

Fig. 10.30 HLA view showing dilated and trabeculated RV secondary to severe pulmonary regurgitation.

Pulmonary stenosis

Background

This can be difficult to assess with echocardiography, and CMR provides valuable information about the valve and surrounding RV outflow tract. Given the therapeutic option of a percutaneous procedure (balloon valvuloplasty or valve replacement) in severe stenosis, the outflow tract anatomy is important.

Causes

- Congenital (e.g. Fallot's tetralogy, Noonan's syndrome). Mobile leaflets with fused tips, as for congenital aortic stenosis.
- Rheumatic fever (rare).
- Carcinoid (rare).

CMR features

- **Stenotic pulmonary valve:** may be thickened, with restricted movement, or mobile with fused tips if congenital. Short axis views through the valve allow good visualization of the orifice.
- **Narrow, high velocity jet:** high signal from linear flow in the jet core, surrounded by low signal from turbulent flow (Fig. 10.31).
- **± RV hypertrophy:** if valve stenosis severe enough.
- **± Dilation of the proximal pulmonary artery.**
- **± Additional congenital abnormalities:** e.g. in Fallot's tetralogy.

Scanning

Standard RVOT + horizontal RVOT view

To visualize the anatomy and motion of the pulmonary leaflets, and identify the high-velocity turbulent jet. Modifications of the plane may be necessary to visualize the jet fully (see Fig. 10.32).

Through-plane cine image at pulmonary valve tips in systole

Position this from the RVOT views and focus on the valve tips in systole – it will be difficult to image the valve throughout the cardiac cycle. Restricted valve opening may be clearly seen, and differentiated from RVOT obstruction.

In-plane ± through-plane flow mapping

- Use the RVOT view for in-plane flow (Fig. 10.33).
- For through-plane flow, an image slice just above the valve, through the high velocity part of the jet is ideal.
- Peak velocity may be high in severe cases (up to 5m/s). Measure velocity and calculate gradient from modified Bernoulli equation.

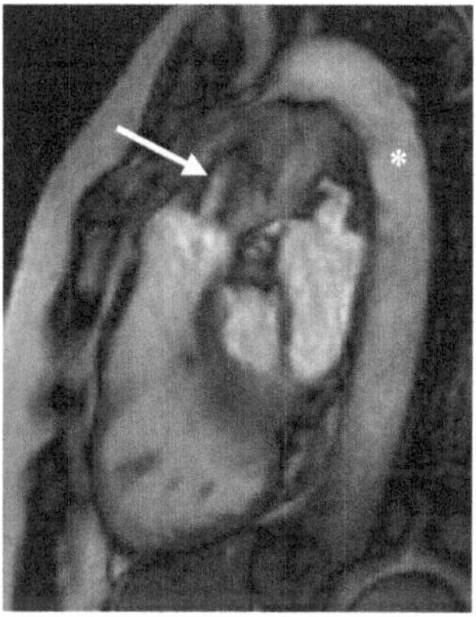

Fig. 10.31 RVOT view in systole showing high velocity jet of pulmonary stenosis (arrowed). Note the distal arch/descending aorta (*) is often seen in the RVOT view.

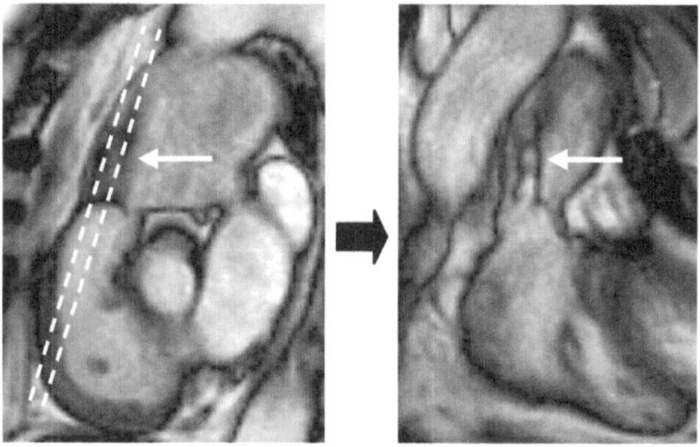

Fig. 10.32 Obtaining the best view. Standard RVOT view (left) with turbulent jet slightly out of plane (arrowed). Horizontal RVOT view (right) in the same patient clearly showing the stenotic jet (arrowed) arising from the valve tips – the leaflet bodies are relatively mobile in this case of congenital pulmonary stenosis.

Reporting should include

- **Anatomy of valve/outflow tract**
  - Description of valve function – fused tips?
  - Any abnormalities from previous surgery
  - Proximal pulmonary artery dimensions.
- **Severity of valve stenosis (Table 10.6)**
  - Valve area by direct planimetry
  - Stenotic jet velocity (and calculated gradient across the valve).
- **Effect on RV:** mass, volumes and function.
- Any associated pulmonary regurgitation, pulmonary artery dilation, or other congenital conditions.

Differential diagnosis

- Supravalvar stenosis.
- RVOT obstruction.
- Aortic stenosis (on clinical examination only – should be clear on imaging).

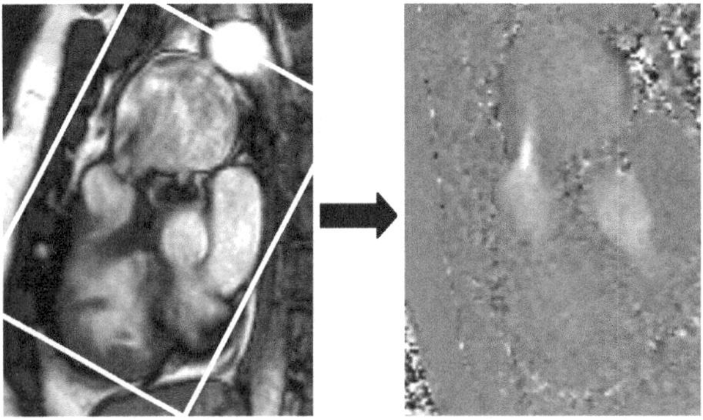

Fig. 10.33 Using the RVOT to align the in-plane flow image with the jet. Note the post-stenotic dilation of the pulmonary artery.

Table 10.6 Guide to severity of pulmonary stenosis

	Mild	Moderate	Severe
Valve area (cm^2)	>1.0	0.5–1.0	<0.5
Peak velocity (m/s)	<2.5	2.5–3.2	>3.2
Estimated gradient (mmHg)	10–25	25–40	>40

Right ventricular outflow tract obstruction

Background

Usually related to congenital disease (e.g. Fallot's tetralogy) and/or previous surgery in the RVOT. May be dynamic (i.e. little resting obstruction, but contraction of the infundibulum causes systolic obstruction).

CMR features

- **Narrowed RV infundibulum:** either in diastole and/or on systolic contraction. There is usually a turbulent flow jet visible in systole. The valve leaflets may be seen to open normally (Fig. 10.34).
- **Increased pulmonary outflow velocity:** use in-plane flow in the RVOT plane(s) to identify the site of increased velocity and differentiate this from valvar stenosis.
- **± RV hypertrophy.**

Scanning

→ See pulmonary stenosis.

► Short axis views for flow/imaging should be through the narrowest section of RVOT. May allow measurement of true minimum area and peak velocity.

Reporting should include:

- **Location and severity of obstruction:** may be qualitative description if velocity inaccurate, but short axis RVOT area is often helpful – use pulmonary stenosis for guide to severity. With dynamic obstruction, the severity may be significantly greater on exertion and the resting gradient may be misleading.
- **RV mass and function:** ?significant RV hypertrophy.

Differential diagnosis

- Pulmonary stenosis (📖 p. 274).
- Supravalvar pulmonary stenosis.

Supravalvar pulmonary stenosis

- Uncommon – usually congenital or as a result of previous surgery (e.g. pulmonary artery banding).
- May be associated with distal pulmonary artery stenosis/hypoplasia or dilation, or other congenital heart conditions (Fig. 10.35).

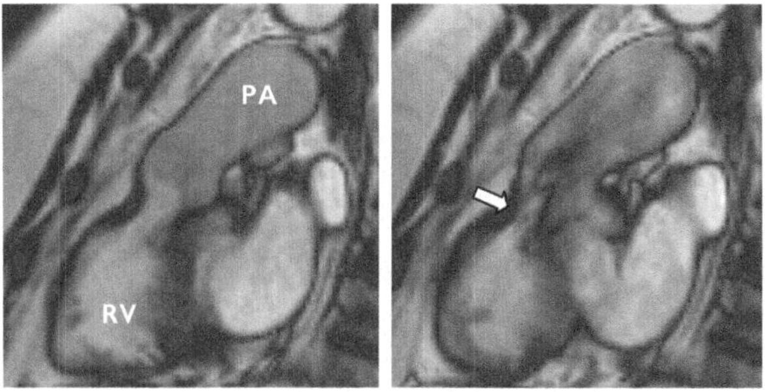

Fig. 10.34 Dynamic RVOT (infundibular) obstruction. Note the slightly narrowed RVOT in diastole (left), just below the easily discernable pulmonary sinuses. In systole (right), the infundibulum contracts, causing further narrowing, and a high velocity jet (arrowed) arising from the RVOT below the valve. RV = right ventricle; PA = pulmonary artery.

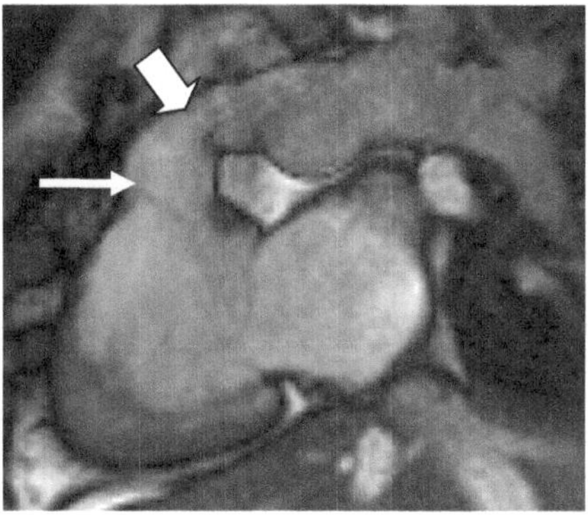

Fig. 10.35 Supravalvar stenosis (broad arrow) 2cm above the pulmonary valve (thin arrow). Note the dilated distal pulmonary artery.

The tricuspid valve

Normal anatomy

The tricuspid valve is the largest and most complex and, like the mitral valve, relies on many components to function correctly – leaflets, annulus, sub-valvar apparatus (chordae and papillary muscles), and RV wall contraction. Any may be involved in dysfunction of the valve.

Leaflets

The tricuspid valve has three leaflets (Fig. 10.36) – anterior/lateral (largest), posterior, and septal (smallest), referring to the point of insertion in the annulus/septum, although the anatomy and relative size of the leaflets is variable. The septal leaflet usually inserts in a more apical position relative to the anterior mitral valve leaflet and this 'offset' in position can be a reliable indicator of the right ventricle in complex congenital heart disease.

Papillary muscles and chordae

There are three papillary muscles in the RV, attached to the RV free wall or septum, although these can sometimes be difficult to visualize due to their smaller size and partial volume effects on CMR. Their location is more variable than for the LV, due to the variable size of the leaflets.

Chordae attach the papillary muscles to the leaflets, with chordae from each leaflet attaching to one or more papillary muscles, although the number and location of attachments is again variable.

Imaging

- The standard RV long axis views (HLA, RV 2-chamber, and RVOT views) are good for assessing the tricuspid valve (see Figs 10.37 and 10.38), as is the more specialized RV inflow-outflow view (📖 p. 94).
- A short axis view through the valve (Fig. 10.36) can demonstrate the leaflets, and identify coaption defects/regurgitant orifices or valve stenosis.

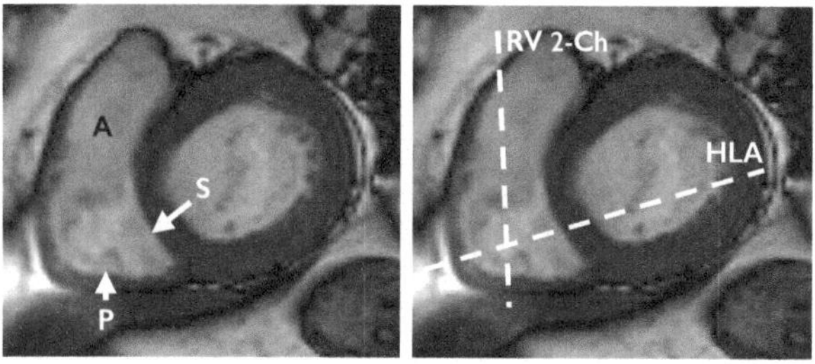

Fig. 10.36 Short axis view through tricuspid valve. Left: leaflet positions - A = anterior, S = septal, P = posterior; right: approximate position of long axis planes.

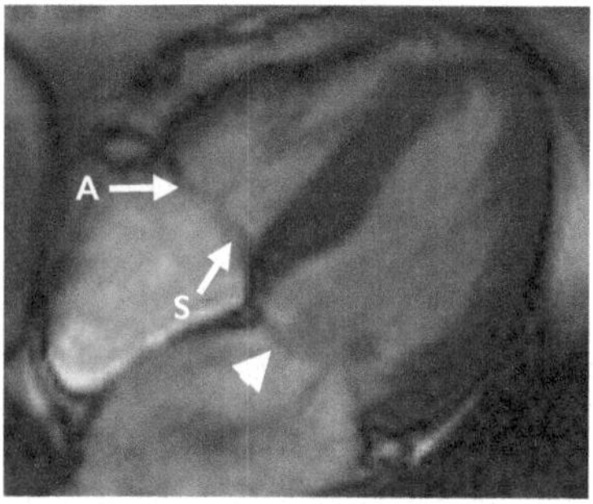

Fig. 10.37 HLA view showing a normal tricuspid valve; A = anterior leaflet; S = septal leaflet. Note the offset of the septal tricuspid leaflet relative to the anterior mitral valve leaflet (arrowhead).

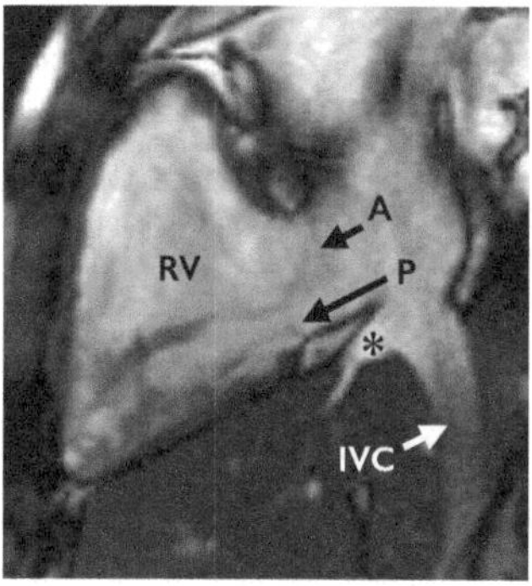

Fig. 10.38 The RV 2-chamber view shows the anterior leaflet (A), posterior leaflet (P), and the papillary muscles clearly. The hepatic vein (*) and inferior vena cava (IVC) can also be seen.

Tricuspid regurgitation

Background

CMR is good for measuring the quantity of regurgitation and RV volumes, although the regurgitant jet can be of low velocity, creating little turbulence and making visualization with CMR difficult. Mild degrees of tricuspid regurgitation (TR) are common, likely due to the irregular leaflets. The majority of pathological causes are due to RV and/or tricuspid annular dilation.

Causes

- **Dilated RV:** volume overload, cardiomyopathy (e.g. ARVC), pulmonary, or tricuspid regurgitation (can become a vicious circle!).
- **Poor RV function** ('functional' regurgitation): e.g. coronary disease, cardiomyopathy, cor pulmonale.
- **Pulmonary hypertension.**
- **Infective endocarditis** (especially IV drug users).
- **Carcinoid valve disease.**
- **Rheumatic valve disease.**
- **Ebstein's anomaly** (involves displacement of the tricuspid leaflets).
- **Uhl's anomaly.**

CMR features

- **Regurgitant tricuspid jet:** usually central; turbulence arises from the tricuspid valve in systole, directed towards the RA. The jet may be harder to visualize than mitral regurgitation, due to reduced turbulence from the lower velocity (lower pressure difference between RV and RA compared with between LV and LA), and the tendency to more laminar flow, especially with severe regurgitation (Fig. 10.39). There is normally a visible gap, however, in the leaflet coaption (Fig. 10.40). The width of the jet base has some correlation with the degree of regurgitation, but should not be relied upon and proper quantification is recommended.
- **Failure of coaption**
  - May be caused by dilated tricuspid annulus (RV/RA enlargement), shortened leaflet (e.g. Ebsteins) or large infective vegetation
  - Worsened with high pulmonary pressures
  - Best assessed on HLA and RV 2-chamber long axis views (Fig. 10.41). Can also be seen on short-axis views, in which the regurgitant orifice may be visualized (Fig. 10.40).
- **± Tethered leaflets:** leaflet(s) held open by reduced papillary muscle excursion towards the valve. Causes (all uncommon):
  - Reduced RV wall contraction (poor RV function)
  - Shortened chordae from previous rheumatic fever.
- **± Dilated RV/reduced RV function:** either secondary to significant chronic regurgitation, or a contributor to annular dilation.
- **± Dilated right atrium:** suggests chronic valve lesion ± AF.

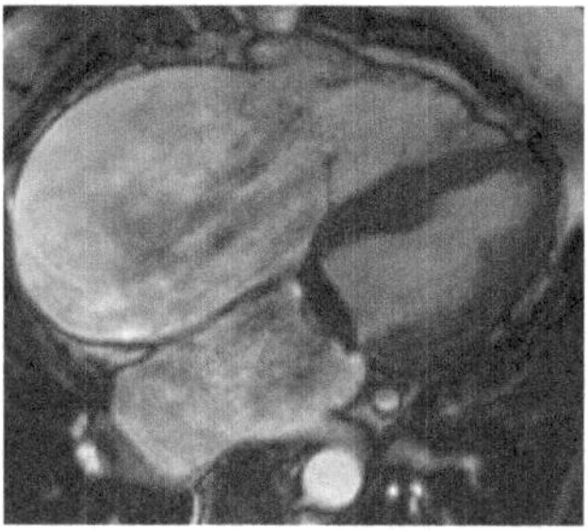

Fig. 10.39 HLA view in systole, showing minimal turbulence from severe tricuspid regurgitation into a very dilated right atrium. The edges of the tricuspid leaflets can be seen, with a notable gap between them. There is a prosthetic mitral valve (bi-leaflet tilting disc type) – this might be associated with raised pulmonary pressures (either from the valve, or the previous native valve disease), as a cause/exacerbating factor for the TR.

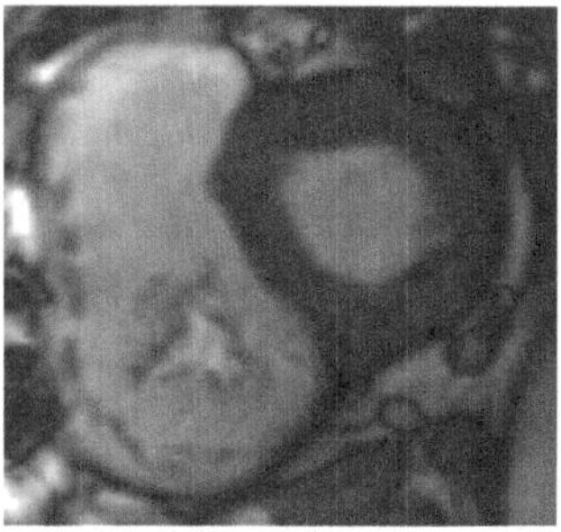

Fig. 10.40 Short axis view in systole, through the tricuspid leaflets. The failure of coaption and large defect is easily seen.

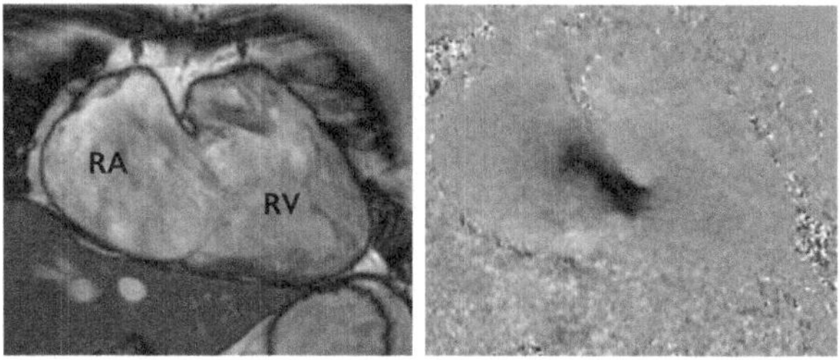

Fig. 10.41 RV 2-chamber view in systole (left) and corresponding in-plane flow image (right) showing a wide jet of tricuspid regurgitation.

Scanning

HLA and RV 2-chamber views to visualize valve anatomy and motion
Note the motion of the leaflets and any regurgitant jet. The degree of signal drop out from turbulence may be low due to the lower right-sided pressures and the floppier tricuspid valve, especially in severe TR, in which there may be a wide jet of laminar flow (see Fig. 10.41). It would be easy to underestimate the severity of TR from the SSFP images alone.

± Short axis views through the regurgitant orifice (see Fig. 10.40)
Positioned from the long axis views, aligning the image with the coaption defect. This allows good visualization of the regurgitant orifice, though no guidelines exist to assess severity. As a rough guide, an orifice diameter >7mm would indicate severe regurgitation.

± Modified long axis views through the regurgitant orifice
If the coaption defect is not well seen on standard imaging, reposition the long axis views through the regurgitant orifice on a short axis view.

± In-plane flow imaging in HLA or RV 2-chamber view
May help to visualize regurgitant flow jet more easily (see Fig. 10.41).

Standard ± horizontal RVOT views
To position the pulmonary flow slice.

Through-plane flow mapping above pulmonary valve
To quantify forward flow through the pulmonary valve and facilitate quantification of the tricuspid regurgitation.

RV ± LV volumes
To determine effect on the RV and allow quantification of the TR.

Reporting should include:

- **Anatomy/function of tricuspid valve:** description of leaflet anatomy and motion – thickened? restricted motion? tethered? abnormal position of leaflets? Comment on nature and size of coaption defect.
- **Description and quantification of regurgitation:**
  - *Description of regurgitation* – wide/narrow jet, direction, whether present throughout systole or just part of it
  - *Quantify regurgitation* – best to use the regurgitant fraction; add descriptor of severity (see box opposite and Table 10.7)
- **Effect on RV:** volumes and function ± hypertrophy.
  - If significant RV dilation/dysfunction is present, the degree of tricuspid regurgitation should be severe, otherwise an alternative cause should be sought.
  - RV volume overload (e.g. from severe TR) may be highlighted by *diastolic* septal flattening, with a return to normal LV/RV shapes in systole (Fig. 10.42).
  - RV pressure overload (e.g. from significant pulmonary hypertension) may be indicated by *systolic and diastolic* septal flattening ± RV hypertrophy if longstanding. Can either cause or exacerbate the TR.

Quantification of tricuspid regurgitation

Quantification is a major advantage of CMR and should be performed, with methods similar to mitral regurgitation (📖 p. 258).

Standard method

Use RV stroke volume and pulmonary flow. Uncontrolled AF may diminish the accuracy of the flow data:

Tricuspid regurgitant volume = RV stroke volume – pulmonary forward flow (ml/cardiac cycle)

Regurgitant fraction = Regurgitant volume/RV stroke volume × 100%

Alternative method

In the absence of a shunt or another regurgitant valve, the difference between LV and RV stroke volumes should equal the TR:

TR (ml) = RV stroke volume – LV stroke volume

Direct tricuspid flow measurement

Direct measurement of flow in the tricuspid regurgitation jet may be more reliable than for mitral regurgitation due to the less turbulent flow and the generally wider orifice, but this has not been specifically examined. It may be achieved by positioning a through-plane flow slice perpendicular to the TR jet seen on long axis imaging.

Table 10.7 Assessment of severity in tricuspid regurgitation

	Mild	Moderate	Severe
Regurgitant fraction (%)	0–30	31–50	>50
Jet width/orifice diameter (mm)	<2	2–7	>7

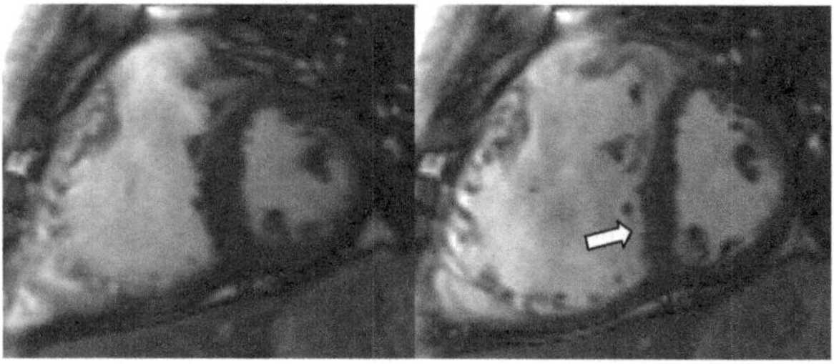

Fig. 10.42 RV volume overload due to severe tricuspid regurgitation. Note the dilated RV, with a normal LV shape in systole (left), but flattening of the septum in diastole (right, arrowed).

Tricuspid stenosis

Background

Tricuspid stenosis is very rare but when present, CMR can provide direct planimetry of the valve area.

Causes: rheumatic fever (usually with mitral stenosis), carcinoid, previous repair/replacement.

CMR features

- **Restricted ± thickened leaflets:** in rheumatic tricuspid stenosis, the leaflets may be thickened or calcified. Fusion occurs at the tips, with a relatively mobile leaflet body, causing 'doming' of the leaflet. In more advanced disease, the whole leaflet may be poorly mobile. The chordae may also be thickened and/or shortened.
- **Enlarged right atrium:** best seen on HLA and RV 2-chamber views.
- **± RV dysfunction:** tricuspid stenosis in itself does not affect RV function, but RV dysfunction may occur if active rheumatic carditis is present.

Scanning

HLA, RV 2-chamber ± inflow-outflow long axis views

- To visualize valve anatomy and motion, and right atrial size. Some re-positioning of the planes may be required to see the valve opening clearly.
- Note the motion of all 3 leaflets, and any thickening or regurgitation.

Short axis view through tips of the tricuspid valve

Similar to a LV short axis view, but positioned through the leaflet tips in diastole (see Fig. 10.43). If placed too far towards the atrium, the degree of stenosis under-estimated.

Reporting should include:

- Valve anatomy/function and orifice area
  - *Description of leaflet anatomy and motion* – thickened? How severely is opening restricted?
  - Valve area from direct planimetry, with indication of severity (see Table 10.8)
- **Thickening/shortening of chordae?**
- **Any regurgitation present:** quantify as in previous section (tricuspid regurgitation).
- **± RV volumes and function.**

Differential diagnosis

The diagnosis is usually clear from imaging, but clinical mimics include:

- Right atrial tumour.
- Large RA thrombus.
- Large vegetation.

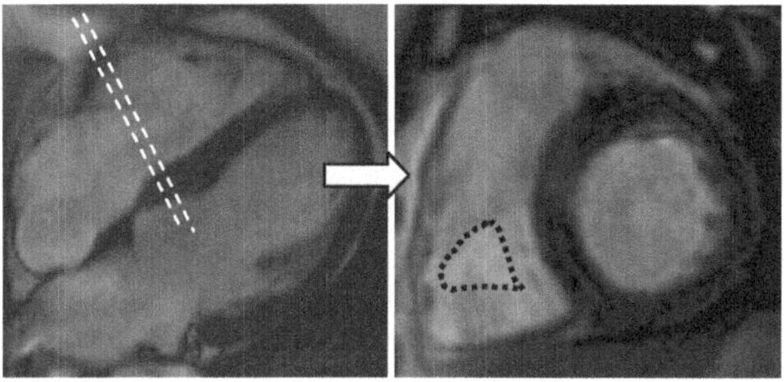

Fig. 10.43 (Left) HLA view showing position of the image slice (dashed lines) for the modified short axis image at the valve tips (right). The valve area can be measured (dotted line).

Table 10.8 Assessment of severity in tricuspid stenosis

	Mild	Moderate	Severe
Valve area (cm^2)	>7.0	1–7	<1.0

Imaging prosthetic valves

Background

Virtually all prosthetic heart valves are safe in the MR scanner at 1.5T, and can be imaged well with CMR. Most are also safe at 3T, although testing has been more limited. A fear of allowing patients with prosthetic valves into MR scanners has occurred in some centres, and many patients have been denied MR scanning unnecessarily. The few prostheses that are weakly ferro-magnetic have negligible forces exerted on the valve compared with the forces occurring with each heart beat.

The metal in the prostheses does produce an artefact, but this is generally small and only limits some aspects of scanning.

CMR features

Artefact from metallic components

May include the whole valve and small surrounding area if metallic. The largest artefact is produced by the older ball and cage valves (Fig. 10.44), but modern bi-leaflet valves have only a small artefact (Fig. 10.46). The artefact from bioprosthetic valves is variable – some contain significant metal framework, while others can produce perfect CMR images (Fig. 10.45).

Turbulent flow through valve

Virtually all prosthetic valves result in a reduced valve area relative to a normal native valve, due in part to the sewing ring, and this produces turbulence and higher than normal velocities in many cases.

± Regurgitant leak

Determine whether para-prosthetic (more likely) or transvalvar (usually bioprosthetic), and quantify leak.

Scanning

Normal views for each valve apply

- SSFP sequences can be used or sometimes FLASH sequences provide good images if SSFP artefact is too great.
- Check for well seated valve, any regurgitant leaks, their location, and a qualitative assessment of severity. The cross-sectional area of a regurgitant jet may be helpful in determining this.

Through-plane flow mapping

- To quantify any regurgitation (usual methods apply), with the image positioned just upstream of the valve.
- Can be used to assess the flow pattern and velocity, with the image slice placed just downstream of the valve. Bi-leaflet tilting disc valves have a distinctive flow pattern (Fig. 10.47).
- The image plane should avoid the area of artefact, as this will destroy any signal and give erroneous data. Aim to be as close to the valve as possible, but just beyond the area of artefact. This may miss some flow, but is better than no quantification. One advantage of prosthetic valves is that movement of the base of the heart is reduced due to post-operative (healing) fibrosis, so the valves do not move as far from the imaging plane during systole.

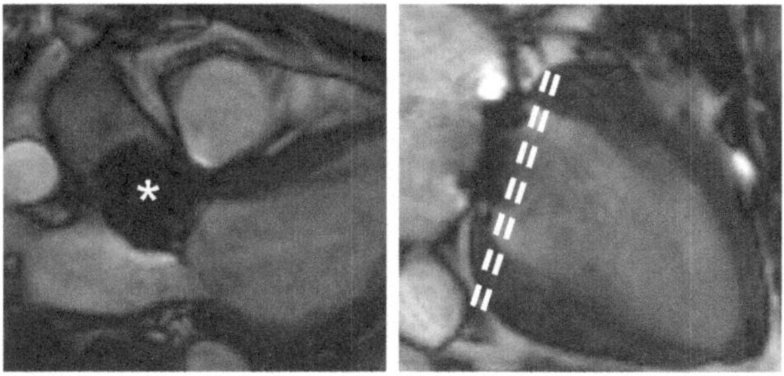

Fig. 10.44 SSFP imaging of prosthetic valves. (Left) Starr-Edwards ball and cage valve (asterisk) in aortic position (LVOT view). (Right) Bi-leaflet tilting disc valve in mitral position, with image position for through-plane forward flow assessment indicated by the parallel lines (VLA view).

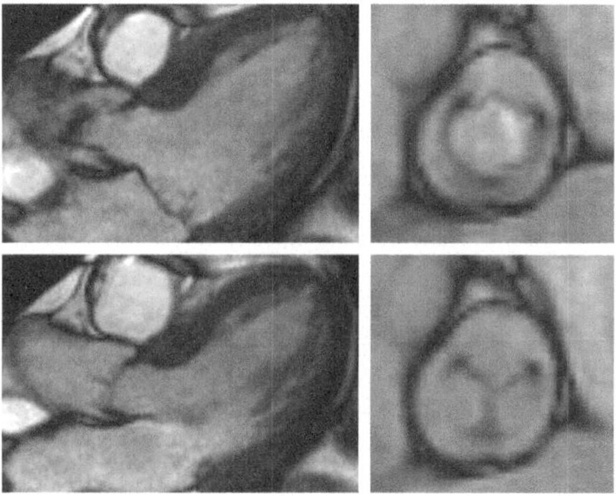

Fig. 10.45 Bioprosthetic (Carbomedics) valve in aortic position with SSFP imaging. (Left) LVOT view in systole (top) and diastole (bottom). (Right) *En-face* view through valve in systole (top and diastole (bottom).

Reporting should include:

- **Stability of the valve:** well seated or not? Any visible gaps?
- **Any regurgitation:** indicate whether paravalvar or trans-valvar, the location (clock-face positions in the short axis view can be helpful in indicating the size and position), and the degree of regurgitation.
- **Indicators of stenosis:** while leaflet motion is difficult to visualize, stenosis may be indicated by a higher than expected forward velocity for the type and size of valve, or an abnormal flow pattern (e.g. missing half of bi-leaflet flow profile).
- **Effect on the LV/RV:** as for native valve lesions. A comparison with pre-operative scans may be helpful in determining any improvement in dimensions and/or function.

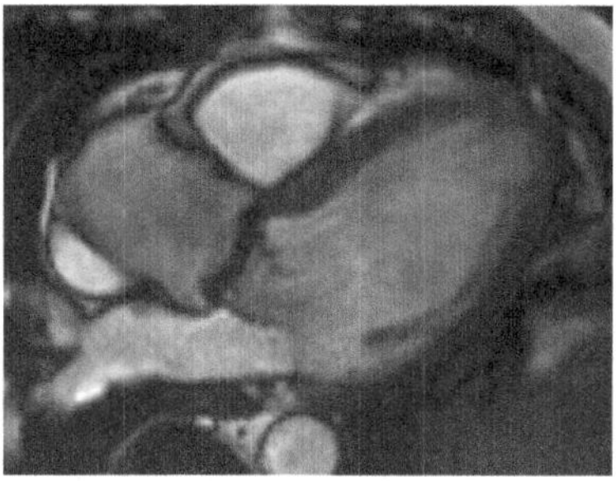

Fig. 10.46 Bi-leaflet tilting disc valve in aortic position demonstrating the minimal artefact than can occur.

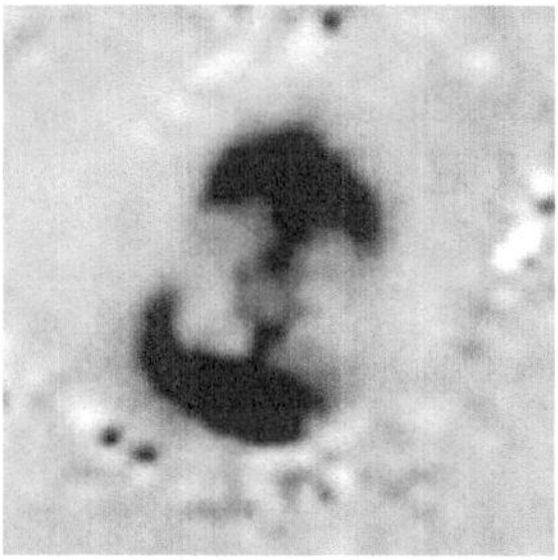

Fig. 10.47 Typical flow pattern from a bi-leaflet tilting-disc valve on through-plane flow imaging. The two discs create flow jets with crescentic shapes in cross section, joined by a smaller linear jet from the central orifice, reminiscent of a Star-Wars™ TIE-fighter viewed from the front!

Chapter 11
Pericardial disease

Imaging the pericardium

The pericardium consists of a parietal and visceral layer, usually with a small amount of fluid in between (especially in the pericardial recesses, and in children and young adults). Variable amounts of fat may be present both on the surface of the heart ('epicardial fat') and on the pericardial surface ('pericardial fat'). The thin pericardium is often not seen on CMR imaging, unless highlighted by surrounding fat, and the close proximity of fat, fluid, and fibrotic tissue within one voxel often causes a chemical shift artefact, resulting in complete absence of signal in these pixels. The pericardium may therefore appear as a thin black line.

CMR provides excellent non-invasive assessment of the pericardium, with all areas visible and good characterization of the different tissues (Table 11.1). Calcification is less well seen, however, and CT is better for assessing this.

General scanning technique

- **Standard long axis SSFP cine images (Fig. 11.1):** provide a good general impression of the pericardium and any effusion.
- **Short axis SSFP cine stack:** for comprehensive assessment of the ventricular pericardium, in addition to LV and RV functional assessment.
- **T_1- and T_2-weighted turbo spin-echo images:** in standard long axes, and any areas of interest. Image with and without fat suppression to obtain clear views of the pericardium without surrounding fat. Also good for assessment of inflammatory processes involving the pericardium and adjacent myocardium (see Fig. 11.3). Normal pericardium has a low signal on both T1-WI and T2-WI.
- **Tagged images:** T_1-weighted gradient echo 'tagged' cine images can be useful for assessing adhesion of the pericardium (2–3 long axis and 1–2 short axis images). The myocardium normally moves within (slips past) the adjacent pericardium, but can be adherent if pericardial inflammation is present (see Fig. 11.2).
- **Real-time cine imaging:** ultra-fast ('real-time') cine images in a short axis view during free breathing can be helpful for assessing constriction. Changes in RV size and interventricular septal motion during inspiration may be seen.
- **Late gadolinium imaging:** helpful for identifying any areas of peri-myocarditis.

Reporting should include:

- Thickness and signal homogeneity: the normal pericardium is thin and may not be well visualized. It should also be remembered that CMR slice thickness (5–8mm) and limited in-plane resolution (~1mm) reduce the accuracy of pericardial thickness measurements.
- Extent, composition, and localization of effusion, if present.
- Abnormal amount and distribution of fat.
- Any late gadolinium enhancement.
- For constriction: RV and RA filling, septal motion, and LV/RV volumes.

Table 11.1 CMR characteristics of the pericardium

	Normal	Effusion	Fibrous thickening	Calcification
Pericardial thickness	<4mm	Variable	Usually >4mm	Usually >4mm
T_2 and SSFP signal	Low	High (intermediate if ↑ protein)	Low	Low
T_1 signal	Low	Low (intermediate if ↑ protein)	Low	Low
Contrast enhancement	No	No	Variable	No

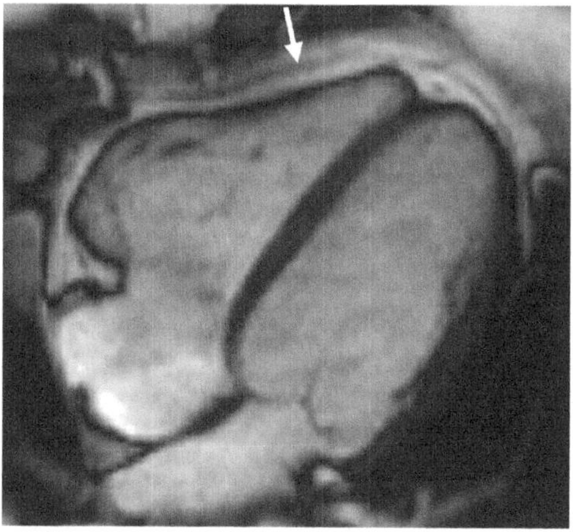

Fig. 11.1 Normal heart – HLA SSFP cine sequence in diastole. Note the thin pericardium visible between the epicardial and pericardial fat (arrowed).

Pericarditis

Commonly caused by viral infection or autoimmune conditions, although the aetiology is not always defined. It is rarely bacterial, although worldwide, tuberculosis remains one of the main causes, often leading to constriction. Uraemia is a frequent cause of pericarditis in renal patients.

CMR features

- **Pericardial thickening:** mostly present in chronic disease (rare in acute pericarditis). Not all chronic pericarditis has a thickened pericardium, but the positive predictive value is good. If calcified, the entire pericardium is often thickened.
- **Pericardial calcification:** can occur locally or globally in chronic inflammation, leading to thickening ± constriction. The pericardium has a heterogenous signal on all sequences, due to signal drop-out from the scattered calcium deposits.
- **Pericardial inflammation:** in active pericardial inflammation, increased signal on T2-WI and contrast enhancement on T_1-weighted images can be seen, with diffuse or spotty signal (Fig. 11.3).
- **Pericardial effusion:** present in many cases of pericarditis (📖 p. 298).
- **Global and regional ventricular function:** usually normal in uncomplicated pericarditis. Pericardial adhesion to the myocardium may be noted on tagged cine images (Fig. 11.2).
- **± Myocardial inflammation:** sub-epicardial myocardial inflammation (a peri-myocarditis) can be visualized as enhancement on late gadolinium imaging (Fig. 11.4). This is more commonly seen with other evidence of myocardial damage (e.g. ST segment elevation on ECG, or raised serum troponins). The usually sub-epicardial distribution should be differentiated from the sub-endocardial coronary disease pattern.

Scanning

- As for standard imaging (📖 p. 294).
- Real-time images are rarely needed for acute pericarditis.

Reporting should include:

- Pericardial thickness and any heterogeneity in signal pre/post-contrast.
- Size of any effusion in diastole and in systole.
- Areas of late enhancement, suggesting a peri-myocarditis. Report the location and transmurality.
- LV and RV volumes and mass. Comment on any regional pericardial adherence and on septal motion.

Differential diagnosis

- Myocarditis with pericardial involvement.
- Pericardial tumours (rare) – thickening is generally irregular.

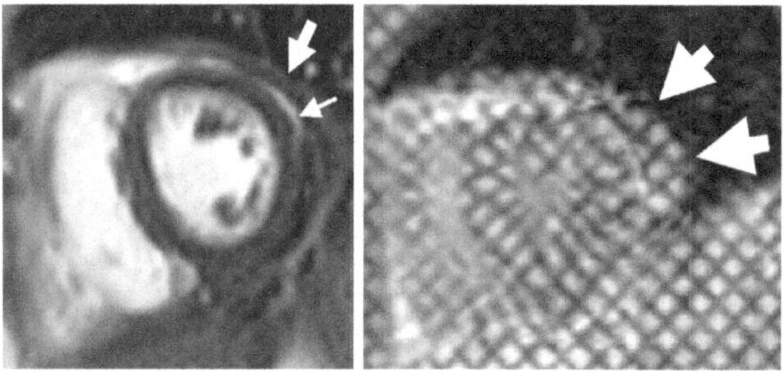

Fig. 11.2 Acute pericarditis. Short-axis SSFP cine image in diastole (left), showing thickened pericardium (thick arrow) and a small pericardial effusion (thin arrow). (Right) Tagged gradient-echo cine in systole showing lateral adhesion of the myocardium to the pericardium (arrowed).

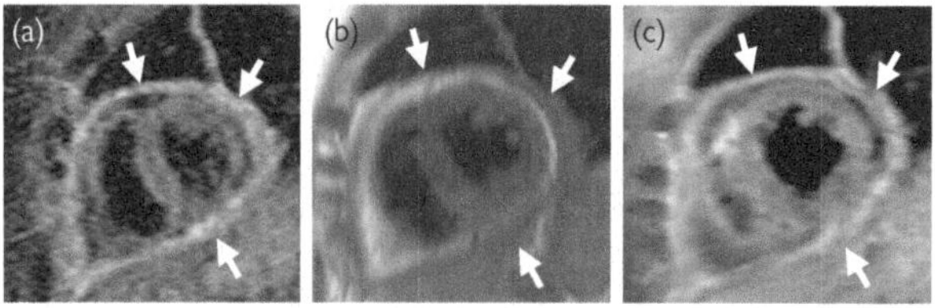

Fig. 11.3 Short axis images of a patient with acute pericarditis. The pericardium is thickened circumferentially (arrows) with features of inflammation. (A) Dark-blood fat-suppressed T_2-weighted STIR image showing increased pericardial signal. (B,C) T_1-weighted turbo spin echo images pre-contrast (B) and post-contrast, with fat-suppression (C) showing contrast enhancement.

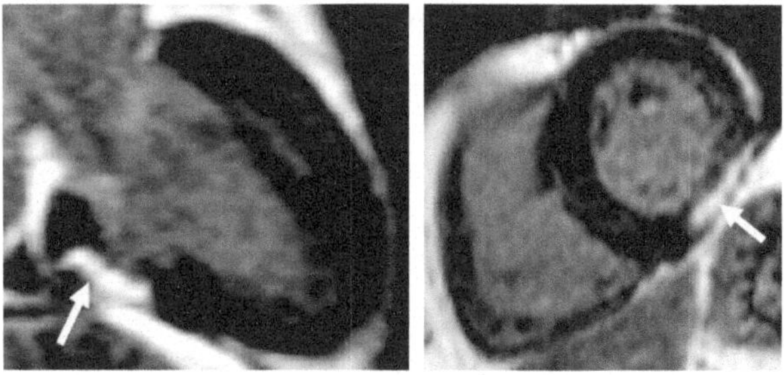

Fig. 11.4 Late gadolinium enhancement (inversion recovery) images showing peri-myocarditis. VLA image (left) and basal short axis image (right) demonstrating sub-epicardial enhancement (arrowed), indicating inflammation/necrosis.

Pericardial effusion

Causes

- Any cause of pericarditis.
- Cardiac failure (usually small effusion).
- Complication of percutaneous cardiac procedures: these often result in tamponade due to the rapid rate of fluid accumulation.
- Malignancy (usually large, and without inflammatory signs e.g. pain, friction rub, fever, diffuse ST elevation).
- Uraemia, tuberculosis (both often large).

CMR features

- **Fluid in the pericardial space:**
  - Expanded pericardial space with homogenous, low SI on T1-WI and high SI on T2-WI, STIR and SSFP cines (Fig. 11.5). Blood or protein in the effusion may lead to intermediate SI on T1- and T2-WI; a haemopericardium has high SI on T1-WI. A very low SI on phase-sensitive inversion recovery sequences with a TI of 300–400 msec is characteristic.
  - Variable size, from a few mm to very large (several cm) thick.
  - Usually circumferential distribution. Acute effusions commonly follow gravity; chronic post-inflammatory effusions can be localized.
  - Chemical shift artefact in the 'transition zone' between fluid and fat.
- **± Evidence of tamponade:** occurs when an effusion causes haemodynamic compromise, usually following rapid accumulation. Gradual increases are better tolerated (even large effusions), so the volume of pericardial fluid is not a reliable indicator of tamponade. CMR features of tamponade:
  - Diastolic collapse of the RV free wall and right atrium (right atrial collapse alone is an early sign, but may not indicate tamponade).
  - Dilated inferior vena cava with no inspiratory collapse (requires 'real-time' imaging with free breathing).
- **± Features of inflammation:** see Pericarditis, 📖 p. 296.
- **Global and regional ventricular function:**
  - Cardiac function is normal in uncomplicated effusions.
  - In tamponade, ventricular volumes are low-normal, with decreased stroke volume. Diastolic septal flattening on deep inspiration may occur.

Scanning

As for standard imaging (📖 p. 294).

Reporting should include:

- Presence of effusion and size (maximal diastolic and systolic thickness).
- Any evidence for tamponade.
- Any features of pericarditis.

Differential diagnosis

- **Pericardial fat:** high SI on T1-WI and very low SI on fat saturation images.
- **Pericardial cyst**: localized with rounded edges.
- **Pericardial tumour:** irregular mass within pericardium ± effusion.

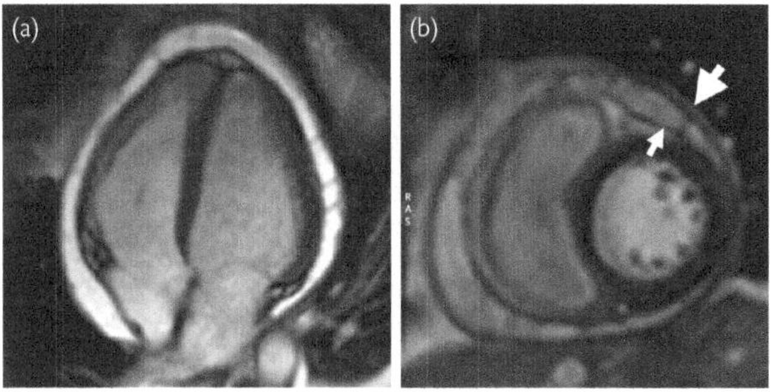

Fig. 11.5 Four-chamber view (A) and short axis (B) T_2-weighted (STIR) acquisitions in acute pericardial effusion. Note the circumferential high SI indicating transudative effusion, and low SI hyphenated structures, indicating loculation. The visceral and parietal layers of the pericardium are separated (seen best on the short axis image, arrows).

Pericardial constriction

Causes

- Most cases are idiopathic – the initial acute episode may be subclinical.
- Viral, tuberculous and pyogenic infections.
- Therapeutic irradiation.
- Post cardiac surgery.

CMR features

- **Thickened pericardium (Fig. 11.6):** usually >6mm, and may be calcified. Constriction can sometimes occur with a normal pericardial thickness. Functional assessment of possible adhesions and restricted filling patterns are the key to diagnosis.
- **± Effusion.**
- **LV and RV volumes and function:** ventricular volumes are normal-low, and atrial volumes are often increased. Typically, the first sign is ↓ systolic filling of the right atrium with almost complete emptying during diastole. Further disease progression leads to ↑ RV ejection fraction due to reduced diastolic inflow. When the systolic capacity of the right ventricle is reached, left ventricular stroke volume will also decrease.
- **Inspiratory diastolic septal flattening:** the enclosed nature of the heart impairs filling and causes equal LV and RV diastolic pressures. During inspiration, a greater volume of blood is drawn through the RV by the negative intrathoracic pressure. As compliance of the RV is limited by the constriction, diastolic pressure exceeds the LV, causing movement or 'flattening' of the septum towards the LV, which assumes a 'D' shape in the short axis view, similar to RV volume overload (📖 p. 152), but occurring particularly on inspiration (Fig. 11.7). The septum returns to its normal position during systole, when LV pressure exceeds RV pressure.
- **± Enlarged IVC with absent inspiratory collapse:** indicates high systemic venous pressures, in advanced disease.

Scanning

As for standard imaging (📖 p. 294).

Reporting should include:

- Pericardial thickness and signal heterogeneity ?evidence of calcification.
- Any associated effusion.
- Any other evidence for constriction (above).
- LV and RV volumes and mass.

It is rare to be able to make a diagnosis of constriction with certainty on CMR. In general, the features support a clinical diagnosis. Constriction normally involves a thickened pericardium, so beware making this diagnosis with a normal pericardial thickness.

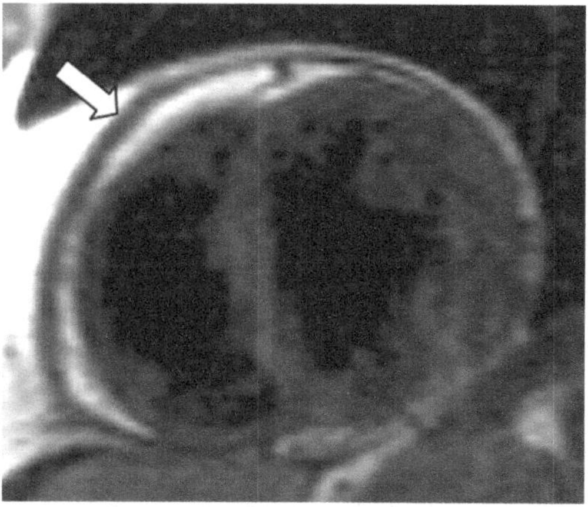

Fig. 11.6 Pericardial constriction – short axis T_1-weighted turbo spin-echo image showing thickened pericardium (arrowed).

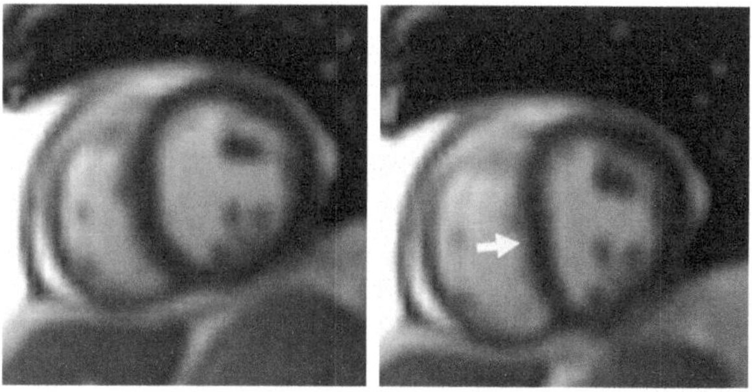

Fig. 11.7 Short axis real-time cine sequence in the same patient as above. (Left) Diastole during expiration. (Right) Diastole during inspiration, showing flattening of the septum (arrowed) and an increased RV size compared with the total cardiac diameter.

Pericardial cysts

Benign, fluid-filled structures usually found incidentally.

CMR features

- Thin-walled mass with homogenous signal intensity of the intra-cystic fluid: low-intermediate SI on T1-WI and high SI on T2-WI. They do not enhance after contrast.
- Often sited in the right cardiophrenic angle, although any location in the pericardium is possible.
- Commonly spherical or round (Fig. 11.8), but they can have unusual shapes and can invaginate into almost any part of the mediastinum.
- Characteristically have a very low signal on phase-sensitive inversion recovery sequences with an inversion time of 300–400ms.

Scanning

- As for standard scanning.
- Real time imaging and tagging are rarely required.
- First-pass perfusion or phase-sensitive inversion recovery sequence may be helpful in difficult cases.

Reporting should include:

- Location and three-dimensional size.
- Any compression of adjacent structures.
- Absence of contrast enhancement during first-pass perfusion, on T_1 post-contrast and/or on late enhancement images.

Differential diagnosis

- Pericarditis with localized effusion.
- Extra-cardiac cyst (diaphragm, liver).
- Pericardial tumour.

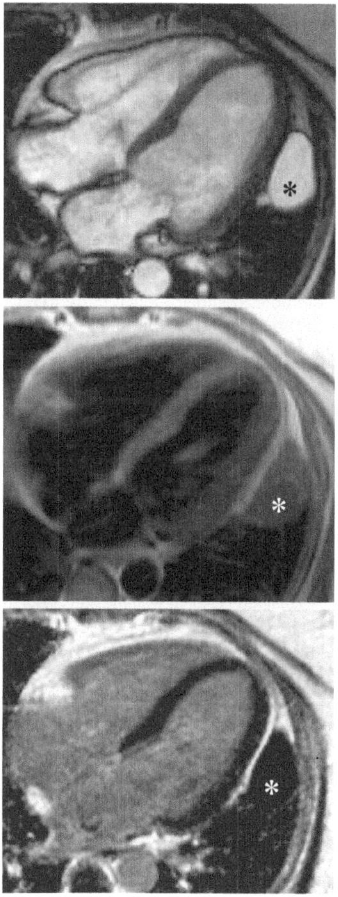

Fig. 11.8 Pericardial cyst adjacent to the lateral LV wall in the HLA view (*). (Top) SSFP sequence (high signal). (Middle) T_1-weighted turbo spin echo (intermediate signal). (Bottom) Late post-contrast phase-sensitive inversion recovery sequence (no contrast uptake and v. low SI).

Pericardial tumours

Primary pericardial tumours are rare.

Common pericardial masses

Benign

- Pericardial cyst.
- Lipoma.

Malignant

- Pericardial mesothelioma.
- Angiosarcomas.
- Lymphomas.

► Metastases to the pericardium are much more frequent than primary cardiac tumours and the pericardium is the most likely cardiac site for metastasis. The lungs or mediastinum are common primary locations.

CMR features

Benign lipomas (Fig. 11.9): localized growth of adipose tissue, usually identified by the homogenous high signal on T_1-weighted images, confirmed with fat-saturated scans. They may be difficult to differentiate from pericardial fat, although the latter is usually more diffuse around the heart.

General features of malignant tumours (see 📖 p. 222).

- Solid, localized structures (e.g. sarcoma), often with an irregular outline and hetergenous signal on many MR sequences.
- Pericardial mesotheliomas usually spread diffusely.
- Infiltration or unexplained regional wall motion abnormalities of the adjacent myocardium.
- Good blood supply on first-pass perfusion.
- Diffuse contrast enhancement on T1-WI and late imaging.
- Pericardial effusion.

Scanning

- As for standard scanning, though extra images may be required to show the extent and any infiltration of the mass.
- Contrast is often helpful - first-pass perfusion, T1-WI and late enhancement can all improve the differentiation from benign masses.
- Real time imaging and tagging are rarely required.

Reporting should include:

- Location, three-dimensional size and motion of identified masses.
- Invasion or adherence to adjacent tissues?
- Heterogenous signal, both on pre- and post-contrast imaging?
- Contrast enhancement, on first-pass perfusion and later images?
- Presence of a pericardial effusion.

Differential diagnosis

- Thickened pericardium (chronic pericarditis?) with localized effusion.
- Thrombus/fibrin in haemorrhagic pericardial effusions (e.g. post-cardiac surgery). No invasion and does not enhance with contrast.

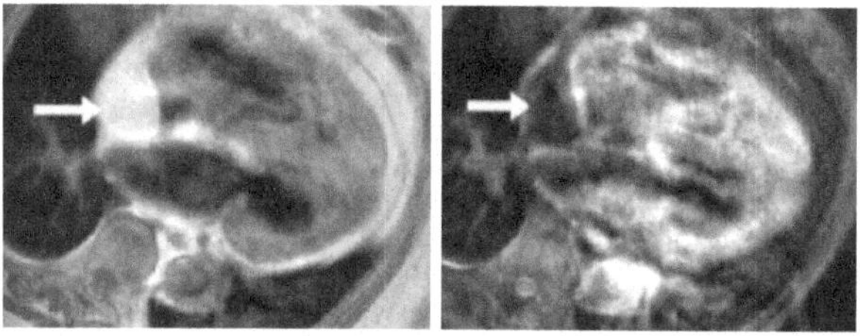

Fig. 11.9 Pericardial lipoma. Modified HLA views acquired using a T_1-weighted spin echo sequence: standard image (left); with fat suppression (right). Note the high signal from the lipoma on the standard sequence (left, arrow) and 'nulling' of the fatty tissue with the fat suppression technique (right, arrow).

Congenital absence of the pericardium

Partial and complete absence of the pericardium have been described, but are a rare finding, usually diagnosed incidentally. Patients with complete absence are usually asymptomatic, but in partial absence, herniation of the LV may lead to arrhythmias, chest pain, and atypical symptoms.

CMR features

The lack of visibility of the pericardium does not prove its congenital absence (!). Its normally thin structure is often difficult to see on CMR. Other features are, therefore, also required for the diagnosis of absent pericardium.

- **Complete absence:** the heart is displaced laterally and posteriorly (Fig. 11.10, left), and the RV is often dilated, sometimes with tricuspid regurgitation. Interposition of lung tissue between the left hemidiaphragm and the base of the heart is a typical sign on coronal anatomical slices (Fig. 11.10, right), due to the unusually posterior location of the heart. The ECG may show incomplete RBBB and a leftward axis (due to the cardiac displacement).
- **Partial absence:** indentation of the LV wall may be apparent, particularly on cine images (Fig. 11.11).

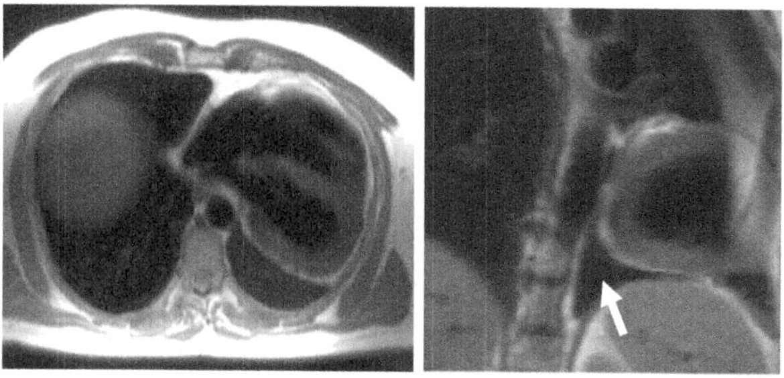

Fig. 11.10 Complete absence of the pericardium. Note the lateral and posterior displacment of the heart on the transaxial HASTE image (left) and the interposition of lung between the diaphragm and the inferior surface of the heart on coronal HASTE (right, arrowed).

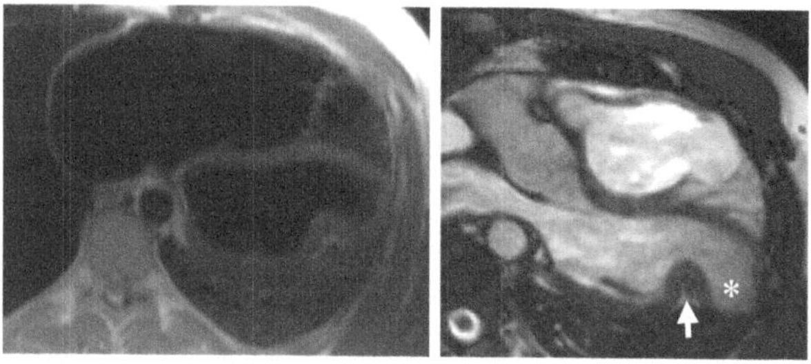

Fig. 11.11 Partial absence of the pericardium. Transaxial HASTE image (left) showing the displaced heart and dilated RV. SSFP image in the LVOT plane (right) showing indentation of the LV myocardium (arrowed) and herniation of the LV apex (*) caused by presence of the pericardium over part of the LV lateral wall.

Further reading on pericardial disease

Grizzard JD, Ang GB. Magnetic resonance imaging of pericardial disease and cardiac masses. *Magn Reson Imaging Clin N Am* 2007; **15:** 579–607.

Kim JS, Kim HH, Yoon Y. Imaging of pericardial diseases. *Clin Radiol.* 2007; 62: 626–31.

Scheuermann-Freestone M, Orchard E, Francis J *et al.* Partial congenital absence of the pericardium. *Circulation* 2007; **116:** e126–9.

Chapter 12

Congenital heart disease

Background

Advances in medicine have resulted in a steady increase in the number of patients with congenital heart disease surviving to adulthood, and thus an increase in the total number. There are currently ~150,000 adults with congenital heart disease in the United Kingdom.

CMR, in conjunction with echocardiography, angiography, and CT, plays an essential part in the management of congenital heart disease and has become the imaging modality of choice in many centres.

Advantages of CMR

- Detailed anatomy and connections, including anomalous and collateral vessels, pre- and post surgery.
- Accurate quantification of left and right ventricular volumes, mass, and function, including serial follow-up.
- Assessment of flow, including quantification of shunts.
- Assessment of valvular disease.
- Scar or fibrosis assessment with late gadolinium imaging.
- Identification of surgical or interventional complications.

What this chapter covers

This chapter provides a basic framework for imaging patients with congenital heart disease, along with specific details on the most common congenital conditions. It is not an exhaustive list of congenital diagnoses, which would be impractical in this type of guide. In addition, each patient has a different combination of lesions, so it would be impossible to cover all eventualities.

Some congenital conditions are covered in other areas of the book:

- **Coarctation of the aorta:** 🕮 p. 372.
- **Isolated valve disease:** see Chapter 10 Valve disease, 🕮 p. 235.
- **Anomalous pulmonary venous drainage:** 🕮 p. 418, 420.

General approach to congenital CMR

Preparation

Thorough preparation is essential, including:

- Knowledge of the patient's anatomy and any surgical procedures. If necessary, ask for a sketch of the patient's anatomy!
- Information required from the CMR.
- Renal function (if administering contrast).

Principles of scanning

The principles of scanning for congenital heart disease are the same as for all CMR scans, although extra anatomical images are often required and experience in congenital CMR is important. In complex cases, a sequential approach should be used, examining each aspect in turn.

Don't forget:

- Patients often have more than one lesion.
- Each patient has a unique combination of lesions and previous intervention. Being flexible is especially important for congenital CMR.

Scan protocol

The protocol usually needs tailoring to the patient, but some core components can be identified.

Standard views (for all)

- Transaxial, coronal, oblique sagittal multi-slice images – either HASTE and/or SSFP sequences for good general anatomical over view.
- HLA, VLA, LVOT, RVOT (2 views), RV 2-chamber, short-axis stack.
- If uncertain about anatomy, stack of parallel transaxial SSFP cine images from aortic arch to diaphragm (7mm thick, no gap).

Additional views (as required)

- Cine imaging of aorta, left and right pulmonary artery, atrial septum, pulmonary venous return, extra pathways.
- Velocity-encoded flow mapping - aorta, main pulmonary artery, left and right pulmonary arteries, IVC, SVC, Fontan pathway, shunts.
- Contrast-enhanced magnetic resonance angiography (CE-MRA) – very useful if surgical anatomy unknown.
- Early post-gadolinium imaging (for thrombus).
- Late enhancement imaging in HLA, VLA, LVOT, RVOT, and SA stack.
- Turbo spin-echo images.

3D datasets

Acquiring a 3D image set of the whole heart (📖 p. 405) can be particularly helpful in congenital heart disease. This can help identify anatomy and be used for planning further images.

Options for image planning

Unusual image planes are often required and several options exist for achieving these, including planning from an existing image slice, 3-point planning, using a 3D dataset to identify the image plane required and real-time interactive planning. These are reviewed on 📖 p. 96.

Starting from scratch: a sequential segmental approach to diagnosis

In many cases, patients coming for CMR scans will have at least a provisional diagnosis from other investigations and the focus for CMR will be known in advance. In some patients, however, the diagnosis will be unclear, particularly in complex cases, and in others there may be aspects of the diagnosis that have been missed. It is helpful, therefore, to have an approach for clarifying the anatomy from first principles. It pays to assume nothing and examine all the segments of the heart (atria, ventricles, great vessels) sequentially.

Determine the atrial arrangement

Atrial situs solitus

The normal arrangement, with the left atrium on the left side of the thorax, and the right atrium on the right side.

Atrial situs inversus

The mirror image, with a right atrium in the left thorax and vice versa. Normally co-exists with situs inversus (all central organs in a mirror image) – look for the normally right-sided structures (short main bronchus, liver, and IVC) and the left-sided structures (long main bronchus, stomach, spleen, and abdominal aorta). A coronal image through the bronchi or transaxial image through the upper abdomen can be helpful (Fig. 12.1).

Atrial isomerism

There are either two right-sided atria (right isomerism) or two left-sided atria (left isomerism). These usually exist with significant abdominal organ derangement. In right isomerism, the IVC and abdominal aorta lie to the right of the spine; in left isomerism the aorta and azygous vein lie to the left of the spine (the IVC is usually interrupted and continues as a posterior hemiazygous vein).

Determine the ventricular arrangement

First determine if there 1 or 2 functioning ventricles.

Biventricular

There is virtually always one of each ventricle

- **Atrioventricular concordance:** the right atrium connects to the RV and the left atrium to the LV.
- **Atrioventricular discordance:** the right atrium connects to the LV and the left atrium to the RV.
- **Ambiguous connections:** with atrial isomerism, neither concordant nor discordant ventricular connections can occur, and the ventricular arrangement is ambiguous.
- **Mitral and tricuspid valves:** in biventricular hearts, the mitral valve always exists at the LV inlet and the tricuspid valve at the RV inlet.

Identifying atria

The most reliable method of identification is to image the atrial appendages, as anatomical connections to the atria are variable. Multiple transaxial, sagittal, or coronal views can help with the identification:

- **Left atrium:** small, claw-shaped appendage with a narrow orifice.
- **Right atrium:** large triangular appendage with a broad orifice.

Identifying ventricles

Wall thickness is not a good identifier as the ventricles may be subject to abnormal loading conditions.

Right ventricle

- More heavily trabeculated, with a moderator band traversing the apical portion of the ventricle between the free wall and septum.
- Septal attachment of the atrioventricular valve (the tricuspid valve) is more apical than for the LV.
- Possesses a muscular infundibulum (outflow tract).
- Has a tricuspid valve (in biventricular hearts).

Left ventricle

- Smoother walled.
- No moderator band.
- Mitral valve (in biventricular hearts).

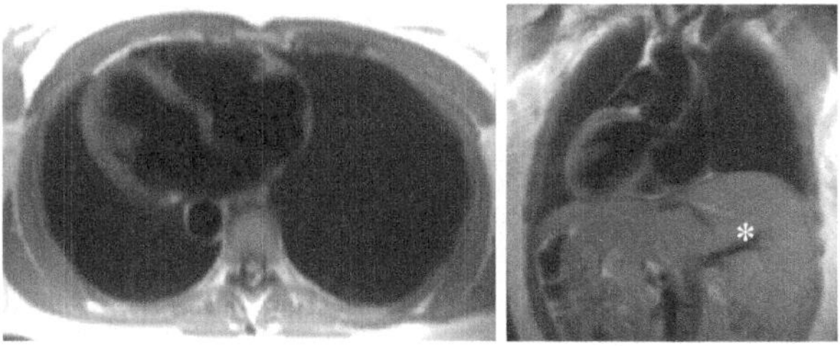

Fig. 12.1 Total situs inversus. Transaxial HASTE image (left) and coronal image (right). Note the heart positioned on the right side of the chest, with the apex towards the right lateral wall, and the right-sided aorta. The liver is on the left side (*).

Uni-ventricular

- **Dominant left ventricle (rudimentary RV).**
- **Dominant right ventricle (rudimentary LV).**
- **Solitary ventricle:** in a uni-ventricular heart, 3 main atrioventricular valve configurations are possible.
  - *Absent right AV valve* – right atrium has no ventricular connection
  - *Absent left AV valve* – left atrium has no ventricular connection
  - *Double inlet* – both atria connect to the main ventricle.

Determine arrangement of the great vessels

Identify whether the ventricles are connected to the correct great vessel – the LV to the aorta and the RV to the pulmonary artery. Rarely, a common arterial trunk occurs (Truncus arteriosus, 📖 p. 344).

The aorta and pulmonary artery are identified by their branching pattern (the pulmonary artery bifurcates early; the aorta ascends in the thorax to give rise to the head and neck vessels), and the coronary arteries (which arise from the aortic sinuses).

Determine the cardiac position

The heart may lie mainly in the left thorax, centrally, or in the right thorax, independent of the apex position or other abnormalities.

Dextrocardia

The apex points towards the right lateral chest wall, usually existing with the heart lying in the right side of the thorax (Fig. 12.1). Cardiac anatomy may otherwise be normal, with little functional consequence.

Check for other lesions

Examine all aspects of the connections in turn:

- Systemic and pulmonary venous return – all correctly connected?
- Atrial size and any shunt (ASD).
- Atrioventricular (mitral/tricuspid) valve function.
- Ventricular function (LV and RV).
- VSD?
- Outflow tracts: dynamic/valvar/sub- or supravalvar stenosis?
- Great vessels: position, size, abnormalities, e.g. coarctation.

Atrial septal defect

A common congenital defect, often associated with other congenital cardiac anomalies (~30%). Left to right shunting occurs at the atrial level, causing increased pulmonary flow. This can result in pulmonary hypertension if severe enough and Eisenmenger's syndrome in severe cases. For this reason, ASD's are usually closed if large enough to cause RV dilation (generally >1.0cm in size or 1/3 of the length of the septum). The development of percutaneous closure devices for secundum ASD's has lowered the threshold for closure, although there is no clear consensus on which ones to close. It has resulted in CMR becoming a valuable tool for assessing patients for percutaneous closure, as the precise anatomy is important, and in particular whether there is a sufficient rim of atrial septum on which to lodge the device. The posterior location of the atria make this difficult with echocardiography.

Types of atrial septal defect

Secundum

The commonest type. Situated in the region of the fossa ovalis (Fig. 12.2), although may extend beyond the fossa. Variable in size. Usually a single defect is present, but multiple ASD's are not uncommon.

Primum

Anterior to the fossa ovalis, adjacent to the ventricular septum. Usually part of a combined atrioventricular septal defect, (📖 p. 326), but can exist in isolation (partial AVSD). Usually associated with an abnormal tri-leaflet ('cleft') mitral valve.

Sinus venosus

Adjacent to the mouth of the superior or inferior vena cavae (Fig. 12.3), and may be associated with an anomalous pulmonary vein. Superior sinus venosus defects are more common and often associated with anomalous drainage of the right upper pulmonary vein to the SVC.

Coronary sinus

Rare. The defect is in the wall of the coronary sinus, at the opening into the right atrium, allowing communication with the left atrium. In its severest form, the whole superior roof of the coronary sinus is absent (an 'unroofed' coronary sinus), with significant shunting.

CMR features

- **Defect in the atrial septum:** variable in size and position.
- **Dilated RA and RV:** due to volume overload if significant left to right shunting is present.
- **Increased pulmonary flow:** the pulmonary to aortic flow ratio (Qp/Qs) can be calculated – a ratio >2 indicates a large shunt.
- **± Anomalous pulmonary venous drainage:** if sinus venosus defect.

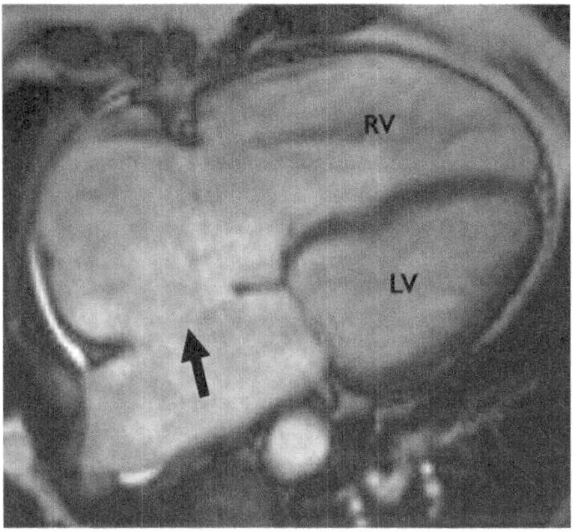

Fig. 12.2 HLA cine showing a large ASD (arrowed), dilated right atrium and ventricle.

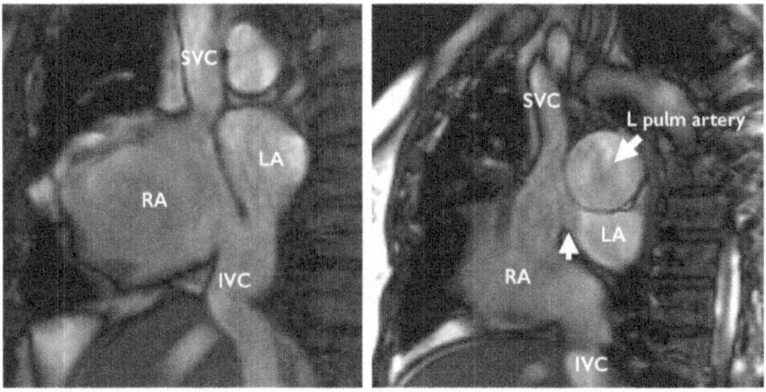

Fig. 12.3 Inferior sinus venosus ASD (left) and superior sinus venosus ASD (right), both on modified atrial short axis views.

Scanning

HLA cine

Gives a good impression of the RV size and can identify the defect.

Ventricular short axis cine stack

For RV and LV volume quantification. Can measure the shunt this way and also indicates the effect on the RV.

Atrial short axis stack

Continue the image stack from the ventricles into the atrium, but without a gap. This provides a comprehensive assessment of the atrial septum.

Perpendicular views through the ASD

- A modified HLA view through the ASD (seen on the atrial SA view). Gives a good impression of the anterior and posterior septal rims (Figs 12.5, 12.6). If difficult to position through the ASD, use the *en-face* view to guide planning.
- An oblique coronal view, perpendicular to the ASD in the (modified) HLA view (Figs 12.5, 12.6). Visualizes the superior and inferior rims. This view can be further modified to pass through the IVC (by rotating the plane to include the IVC seen on a transverse HASTE image). This visualizes the junction with the IVC, where little rim may be present.

En-face view of the atrial septum

This is a view along the atrial septum, accurately demonstrating the ASD location (see Fig. 12.4). It is positioned by placing the image plane along the atrial septum in the (modified) HLA view and also in the oblique coronal view. The septum is not perfectly flat, so some compromise is required, but good views can usually be obtained. A spoiled gradient echo cine (e.g. FLASH) is usually better than SSFP cines.

Pulmonary and aortic flow

Through-plane flow just above the pulmonary and aortic valves (📖 p. 235) can quantify the degree of shunting (Qp/Qs ratio).

± Flow through the ASD

If a good *en-face* view is obtained, flow can be measured through the ASD itself by using this image position for through-plane flow imaging.

± Pulmonary venous angiography

If anomalous pulmonary venous drainage suspected. Pulmonary veins may also be identified on SSFP multislice transaxial images.

Reporting should include:

- Site, size and number of defects ?sinus venosus type
- Degree of shunt - calculate Qp/Qs from aortic and pulmonary flow
- Dilation of RV (if present)
- Suitability for percutaneous closure. Potentially suitable ASD's are secundum type with a sufficient (0.5–1.0cm) rim surrounding most of the defect. Proximity to the aortic root is not usually a problem, but absence of a significant inferior rim usually reflects an unsuitable ASD (Fig. 12.6).
- Confirmation of normal pulmonary vein locations, or anomalous pulmonary venous drainage.

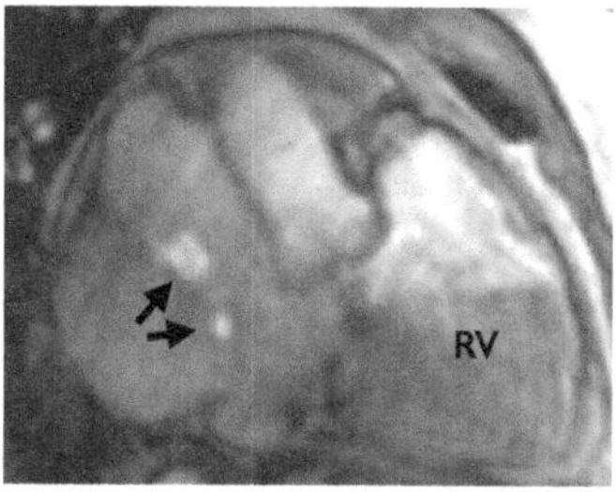

Fig. 12.4 En-face view showing two small secundum ASD's (arrowed).

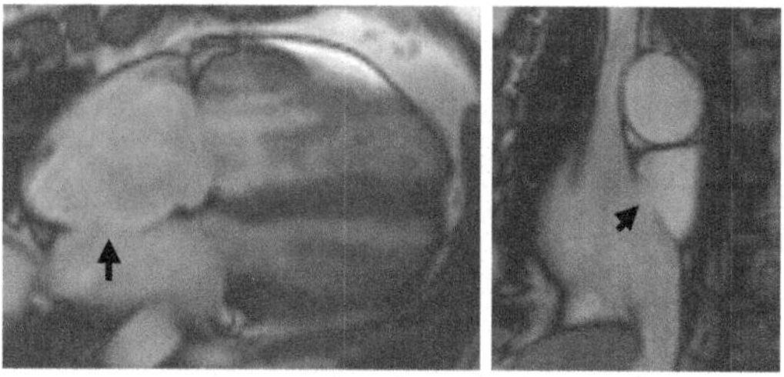

Fig. 12.5 This patient was previously told that her ASD was too large to close percutaneously. The HLA view (left) and the atrial short axis view (right) show the ASD (arrowed) to be large, but with reasonable peripheral rims of septal tissue and the patient subsequently had a successful percutaneous ASD closure.

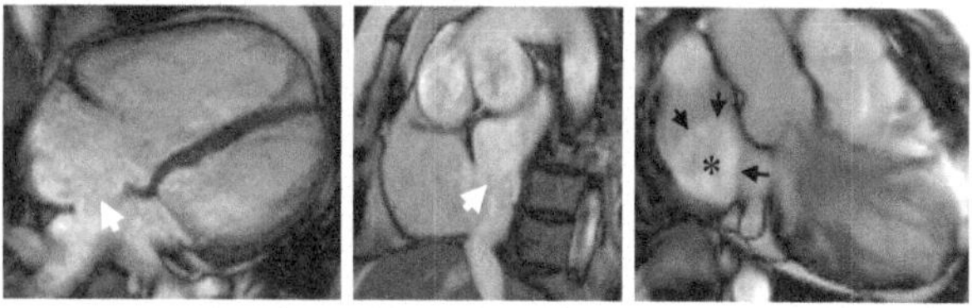

Fig. 12.6 Large ASD, initially thought to be suitable for percutaneous closure on echocardiography, which the HLA view (left) suggests. The atrial short axis view, however, shows an inadequate inferior rim (middle) and the *en-face* ASD view (right) shows the ASD (*) with clear rims of tissue superiorly and anteriorly (black arrows), but no significant inferior rim.

Eisenmenger syndrome

A condition resulting from uncorrected left-to-right shunting, with progressive pulmonary hypertension eventually exceeding systemic pressure, and leading to reversal of the shunt and cyanosis. Mostly caused by uncorrected large ASD, VSD, and AVSD's.

Atrial septal aneurysm

The atrial septum is aneurysmal if it is thin/membraneous, with at least 15mm of side-to-side (left to right) movement during the cardiac cycle (Fig. 12.7). In itself, this is not clinically relevant, but can be associated with a patent foramen ovale (PFO), and may increase the risk of a right to left shunt through a PFO. Best imaged on an HLA cine ± an atrial short axis cine.

Patent foramen ovale

The foramen ovale closes shortly after birth following the increase in left atrial pressure, and in most cases fuses closed in time. In ~25% of the population, however, it fails to fuse and remains a flap of tissue with the potential to open if pressure in the right atrium exceeds that in the left atrium. The vast majority of people with a PFO are asymptomatic, but it has the potential to facilitate a right to left shunt (as opposed to the left to right shunt of an ASD), due to its flap-like nature. This could cause a paradoxical embolus, e.g. from thrombo-embolus in the systemic venous circulation. There is also debate about the role of PFO's in causing migraine. Percutaneous PFO closure is now possible, and is considered in some patients with cryptogenic stroke or migraine with aura.

CMR is not sensitive for identifying PFOs, due to their small size, and contrast echocardiography is the usual imaging method of choice.

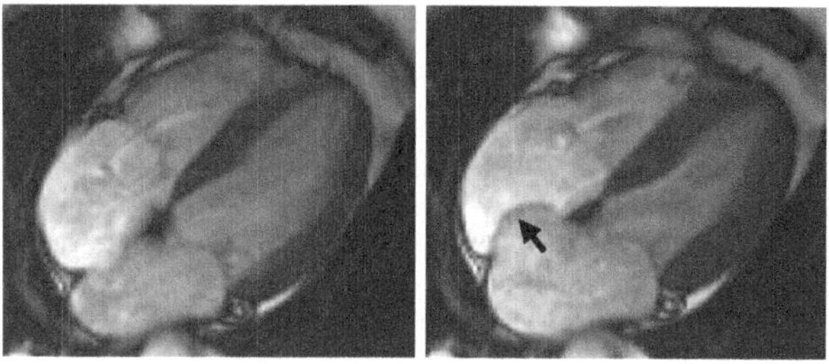

Fig. 12.7 Atrial septal aneurysm. Note the membraneous atrial septum with significant movement from diastole (left) to systole (right, arrowed). The septum is intact and RV size is normal.

Ventricular septal defect

Defect in the ventricular septum, causing a left to right shunt dependent on the size of defect and pulmonary vascular resistance (see box Restrictive and non-restrictive VSD, 📖 p. 325). Large defects often require closure to prevent pulmonary hypertension.

Types (Fig. 12.8)

- **Peri-membraneous (~80%):** located within the membraneous portion of the ventricular septum.
- **Muscular (~15%):** located in the muscular septum, and can be multiple.
- **Sub-arterial (~5%):** located just under the aortic/pulmonary valves. May damage the aortic cusps, due to a Venturi suction effect. Even mild degrees of aortic regurgitation are thus of concern, and may indicate the need for VSD closure.

CMR features

- **Defect in the ventricular septum:** if small, may be difficult to see with CMR.
- **Dilated LV ± RV:** if haemodynamically significant shunt. As the majority of shunting occurs during systole, the LV ejects the blood across the VSD into the pulmonary circulation, and is subject to the majority of the volume loading.
- **± Increased pulmonary flow:** if haemodynamically significant. A pulmonary to aortic flow ratio (Qp/Qs) >2 indicates a large shunt.

Scanning

HLA and LVOT cines

Can often identify the defect from these views. Look for turbulent flow into the RV/RVOT (see Fig. 12.9).

Ventricular short axis cine stack

To identify the VSD and for RV and LV volume quantification. Indicates the effect on the LV.

Specific views through the VSD

A modified HLA or LVOT view, positioned through the VSD seen on the SA stack, often provides good visualization of the shunt.

Pulmonary and aortic flow

Through-plane flow just above the pulmonary and aortic valves to quantify the degree of shunting (Qp/Qs ratio), and any aortic regurgitation.

Reporting should include:

- Size, location, and type of defect (location and restriction to flow).
- Degree of shunt: calculate Qp/Qs from aortic and pulmonary flow.
- Any aortic regurgitation (and quantity).
- Dilation of LV ± RV (if present).

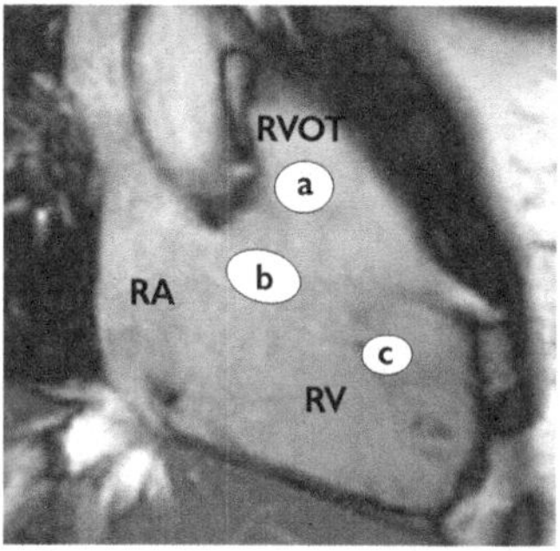

Fig. 12.8 Location of the various types of VSD, viewed from the RV. (a) Sub-arterial; (b) membraneous; (c) muscular.

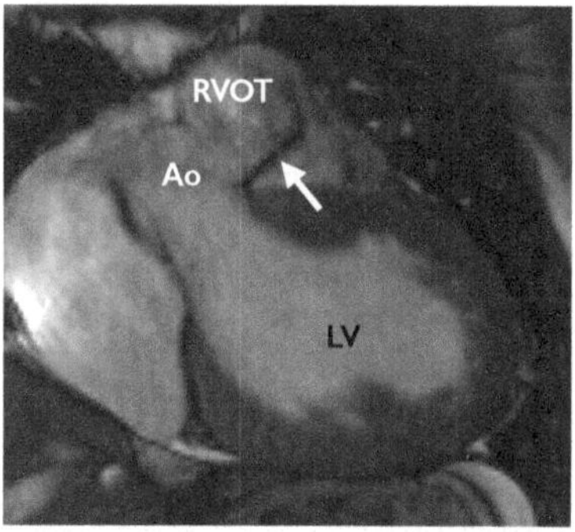

Fig. 12.9 Small sub-arterial VSD in a modified LVOT view. The narrow jet can be seen (arrow), although the defect itself is poorly visualized. Ao = aortic sinuses.

Restrictive and non-restrictive VSD

- **Restrictive:** 'restrict' flow across the defect. They are thus small (<1/3 of the aortic root diameter), with a pressure gradient between left and right ventricles. RV pressures and pulmonary resistance are normal.
- **Moderately restrictive:** ~½ the size of the aortic root, with moderate-severe shunting. ↑ RV pressures, but not to systemic levels. Pulmonary resistance can be raised, and the LV can be dilated.
- **Non-restrictive:** large, with equal LV and RV pressures. The pulmonary circulation is subject to systemic pressure and significantly increased flow, leading to increased pulmonary resistance. This reduces the left-to-right shunt and ultimately results in reversal of the shunt (causing right-to-left flow) – Eisenenger syndrome (📖 p. 321).

Atrioventricular septal defect

This defect occurs at the junction between atria and ventricles, and results from inadequate fusion of the endocardial cushions. A common atrioventricular valve with 5 leaflets serves both side of the heart, with two bridging leaflets straddling the septum. Significant left to right shunting can develop, but depends on the pulmonary vascular resistance. Most (70–80%) AVSD's occur in patients with Down syndrome (trisomy 21). There are two main types:

- **Complete AVSD:** both atrial and ventricular septal defects, with the bridging leaflets usually floating between the atrial and ventricular septum.
- **Partial AVSD (septum primum ASD):** a membrane of tissue connects the ventricular septum to the bridging leaflets, resulting in a shunt at atrial level only.

Post-repair, a degree of atrioventricular valve regurgitation may remain, particularly with the left atrioventricular ('mitral') valve (Fig. 12.10).

CMR features

- **Septal defect at the atrial ± ventricular level.**
- **A 5-leaflet common atrioventricular valve:** the 5 leaflets can often be appreciated on a short axis view, and are not truly tricuspid or mitral. There is a lack of offset of the valves, as the two bridging leaflets straddle the septum, in the same plane.
- **Atrioventricular valve regurgitation:** both from the RV ('tricuspid') and the LV ('mitral') valves, of varying degree.
- **LV / RV dilation:** dependent on the degree of shunting and valve regurgitation.
- **± LV or RV outflow tract abnormalities (e.g. stenosis).**

Scanning

- **HLA cine:** often demonstrates the AVSD.
- **Short axis ventricular stack:** for LV and RV volumes, and basal slices can also demonstrate the septal defect and atrioventricular valve leaflets.
- **Aortic and pulmonary flow:** to quantify shunting.
- Further images to demonstrate the ASD or VSD as appropriate.
- LV/RV outflow imaging as required.

Reporting should include:

- Size of defect.
- Degree of shunting (Qp/Qs ratio).
- Severity of regurgitation.
- Degree of leaflet bridging.
- LV and RV volumes.
- Any other defects.

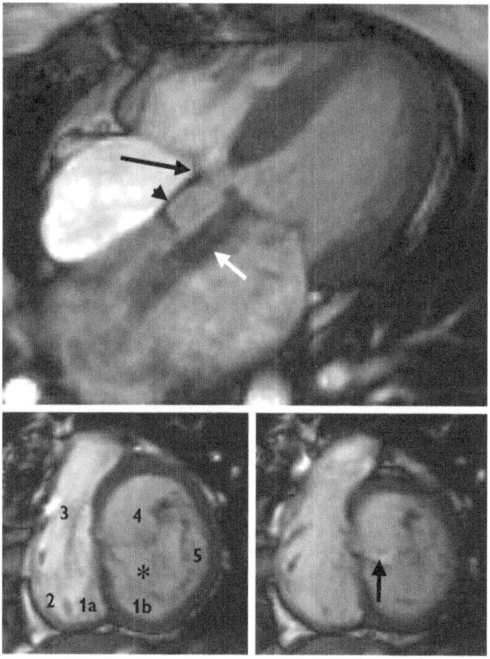

Fig. 12.10 Repaired atrioventricular septal defect. SSFP HLA view in systole (top). Note the lack of offset of the two atrioventricular valves (long black arrow), the patch in the atrial septum (black arrowhead) and the residual 'mitral' regurgitation (white arrow). (Bottom) Short axis SSFP views in diastole (left) and systole (right). The five valve leaflets can be appreciated in diastole (numbered), with the inferior bridging leaflet (1) split between the two AV orifices, but minimal bridging of the superior bridging leaflet (4). The gap between these two leaflets on the LV side can be seen in diastole (*) and systole (arrowed); this is sometimes erroneously referred to as a 'cleft'. In this patient, failure of coaption causes the 'mitral' regurgitation. There is no true mitral valve, as it has three leaflets, and is better referred to as the left atrioventricular valve.

Ebstein anomaly

Background

Dysplasia of the tricuspid valve, with apical displacement, particularly of the septal and posterior leaflets. The anterior leaflet is often large and abnormally attached to the RV free wall. Tricuspid regurgitation commonly results, causing RV dilation, and dysfunction in severe cases. There is a wide range of severity, however, and patients may be asymptomatic.

CMR features

- **Apical displacement of the tricuspid leaflets:** the septal ± posterior leaflets insert within the ventricle, resulting in 'atrialization' of the RV (a normal septal leaflet attaches 0.5–1.0cm more apical than the anterior mitral leaflet). The degree of displacement is variable, but can be severe, resulting in a very small true RV chamber (see Fig. 12.11).
- **Tricuspid regurgitation:** can be severe. Results from failure of coaption of the malformed valve.
- **Dilated RV:** secondary to the tricuspid regurgitation.
- **Other associated defects:** RVOT abnormalities, ASD, VSD, tetralogy of Fallot.

Scanning

LV and RV long axis views

HLA, VLA, RV 2-chamber for visualization of the tricuspid valve leaflets. RVOT views to check anatomy and plan pulmonary flow images.

Short axis cine stack

For RV ± LV volume measurement. A transaxial cine stack can be used instead if only RV volumes are required. This may facilitate easier visualization of the tricuspid valve position.

▶ Volumetric assessment can be difficult, as the abnormal position of the tricuspid valve is hard to judge from the short axis view. If available, processing software that incorporates RV long axis planes in the analysis should be used. These allow identification of the tricuspid valve plane to automatically exclude short axis images on the atrial side of the valve.

Pulmonary valve flow

Through-plane flow just above the tricuspid valve, for quantification of the regurgitation (📖 p. 270)

Reporting should include:

- Location and anatomy of the tricuspid valve leaflets: degree of 'atrialization' of the RV.
- Quantity and severity of tricuspid regurgitation.
- RV volume and function: quote 'true' RV volumes (i.e. on the ventricular side of the tricuspid valve).
- Any other defects.

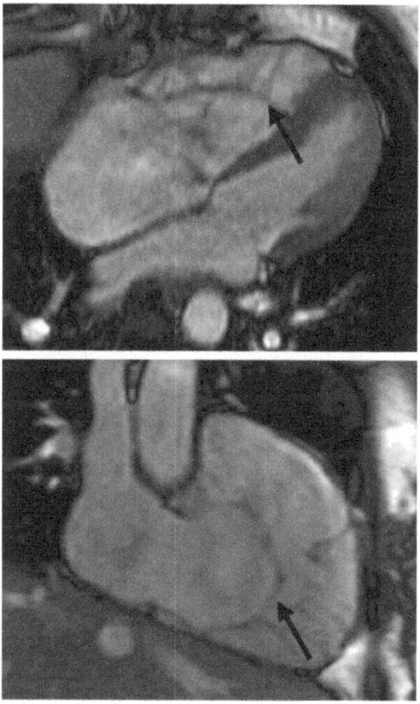

Fig. 12.11 Ebstein anomaly. HLA view (top), RV 2-chamber view (bottom) demonstrating the apical insertion of the tricuspid leaflet (arrowed).

Tetralogy of Fallot

Background

The commonest cyanotic congenital cardiac lesion, with a tetrad of features – ventricular septal defect (VSD), sub-pulmonary stenosis, aortic 'over-ride' of the interventricular septum, and 2° RV hypertrophy (see Fig. 12.12). The primary embryological abnormality is an anterocephalad deviation of the outlet ventricular septum. There is a spectrum of severity and some overlap with other congenital defects:

- Severe pulmonary hypoplasia (overlap with pulmonary atresia).
- Minimal RVOT obstruction, large VSD, and significant aortic over-ride (overlap with double-outlet RV).

Significant right to left shunting occurs, facilitated by the over-riding aorta, and causing cyanosis. Most patients are repaired as a child, with closure of the VSD and widening of the RV outflow tract, sometimes with a patch to facilitate enlargement. Significant pulmonary regurgitation can occur if a transannular patch is required (across the pulmonary annulus) and modern surgical approaches attempt to preserve pulmonary valve function. Many adult patients will have had a palliative shunt (often Blalock-Taussig 📖 p. 352) as a first procedure to improve pulmonary flow, with complete repair performed at a later date.

Associated anomalies

- Right sided aortic arch (📖 p. 380)
- Left SVC (📖 p. 412)
- Anomalous coronary arteries (📖 p. 406)
- ASD/VSD/AVSD (📖 p. 318; 📖 p. 324; 📖 p. 326).
- Aortopulmonary collaterals (if severe pulmonary stenosis).

CMR features (unoperated)

- **RV outflow tract obstruction:** hypoplasia of the infundibulum, often with a small and abnormal pulmonary valve (usually contributing to the obstruction).
- **± Pulmonary artery hypoplasia:** both the main and branch pulmonary arteries may be stenosed.
- **Ventricular septal defect:** usually large and membraneous, with significant right to left shunting.
- **Aortic 'over-ride' of the ventricular septum:** the aorta is positioned over the centre of the septum, straddling both ventricles. There is a very variable degree of over-ride, with 5–95% of the aorta positioned above the RV.
- **RV hypertrophy:** 2° to RVOT obstruction and systemic LV pressures from the large VSD.

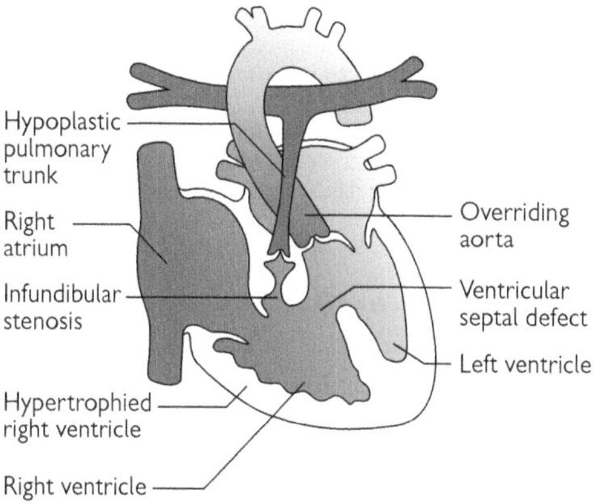

Fig. 12.12 Features of Fallot's tetralogy. Reproduced from Myerson S, Choudhury R, and Mitchell A (2009) *Emergencies in Cardiology* 2nd edn, Oxford University Press.

CMR features (post-repair)

- **Abnormal RV outflow tract:** often dilated and non-contractile (sometimes aneurysmal), due to the patch enlargement (Fig. 12.13). Occasionally, residual obstruction.
- **Pulmonary regurgitation:** severe pulmonary regurgitation may result from the surgery. Sometimes well tolerated, but can result in RV dilation/dysfunction. May be difficult to see on SSFP cines, as minimal turbulence may be present.
- **Dilated RV ± dysfunction:** secondary to severe pulmonary regurgitation.
- **Residual pulmonary arterial hypoplasia.**

Scanning

LV long axis views

HLA, VLA, and LVOT.

Modified HLA or LVOT view

Angled to pass through the VSD – can show the aortic over-ride and relationship with the VSD well.

RVOT views, RV 2-chamber view.

Ensure the RV outflow and pulmonary valve are well visualized. Any stenosis or dilation? Measure dimensions of the RVOT and proximal pulmonary artery in at least 2 views (this helps determine suitability for any percutaneous intervention).

Pulmonary and aortic flow

Through-plane flow mapping just above the valves. For quantification of pulmonary or aortic regurgitation. Consider flow mapping across both left and right pulmonary arteries if asymmetric stenosis is present.

Short axis cine stack

For LV and RV volume measurements. Look for RV hypertrophy (unoperated group) or dilation (post-surgery).

Branch pulmonary arteries

See Fig. 12.4. Look for hypoplasia or stenosis at site of previous anastomosis.

± Contrast (late gadolinium enhancement)

RV scar may be detected and has some correlation with outcome.

Reporting should include:

- **State of RVOT:** general anatomy, severity of stenosis, degree of pulmonary regurgitation.
- **Pulmonary artery anatomy:** dilated proximal trunk? Branch stenosis?
- **Size of VSD and degree of aortic over-ride.** if post-repair, whether any residual VSD is present.
- **RV and LV volumes and function:** compare with previous scans.
- Any ventricular scar, if present.
- Aortic dilatation or aortic regurgitation.
- Any other associated abnormality.

(a)
(b)

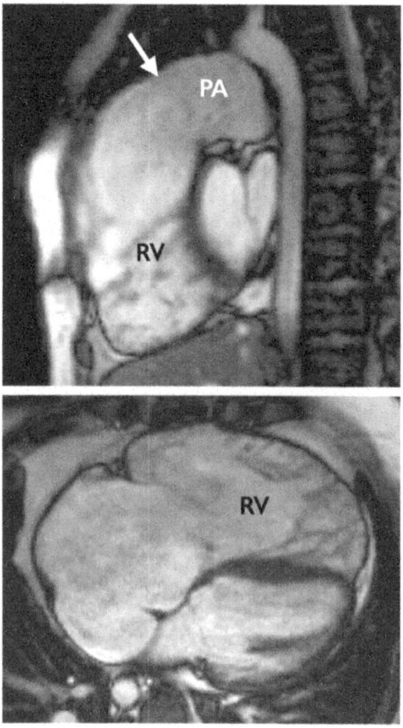

Fig. 12.13 Post-repair RVOT view (above), showing a dilated outflow with a transannular patch. The site of the (regurgitant) pulmonary valve is indicated by the arrow. (Below) Dilated RV secondary to the severe pulmonary regurgitation. (a) reproduced from Thorne S and Clift P (2009) *Adult Congenital Heart Disease*, Oxford University Press.

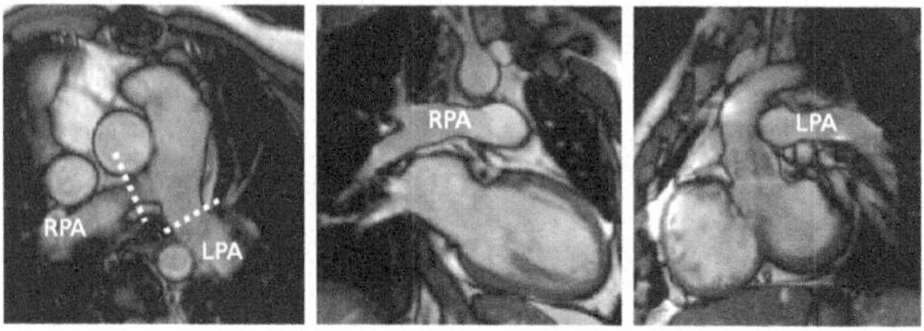

Fig. 12.14 (Left) Transverse image of the pulmonary bifurcation, with a mild stenosis of the proximal right pulmonary artery (RPA). The dotted lines represent the image planes for through-plane flow mapping of the pulmonary arteries. (Middle and right) Oblique coronal/sagittal views through the long axes of the branch arteries, positioned from the transverse view. Middle and right images reproduced from Thorne S and Clift P (2009) *Adult Congenital Heart Disease*, Oxford University Press.

Double outlet right ventricle

This represents a range of anatomical defects in which >50% of both great vessels arise from the RV and a large, usually sub-arterial, VSD is present (Fig. 12.15). The spectrum ranges from a Fallot-type anatomy, with pulmonary outflow stenosis, to a uni-ventricular heart physiology, with one rudimentary ventricle, and may include transposition of the great arteries. The degree of shunting depends on the anatomy, pulmonary pressures and degree of 'streaming' of outflow tract flows. Complex surgical repair techniques are required.

CMR features

- **Large VSD:** usually sub-aortic or sub-pulmonary and non-restrictive.
- **RV outflow to both great arteries:** the anatomical arrangements vary.
- Other features include:
  - RVOT stenosis (Fallot-type anatomy)
  - Transposition of the great arteries (📖 p. 336)
  - Small/rudimentary left ventricle.

Scanning

This is very dependent on the anatomy involved, but usually involves:

Transaxial stack (HASTE or SSFP)

For general anatomical arrangements. Can include a transaxial cine stack.

LV and RV long axis cines

For assessing the arrangement of the ventricles and relative size.

RV and LV outflow tract cines

Often demonstrate the VSD and arterial positions well.

Short axis cine stack

For LV and RV volumetric, and functional assessment.

Aortic and pulmonary flow

Through-plane flow mapping above the aortic and pulmonary valves to determine the degree of shunting.

Other imaging

As required by the associated features.

Reporting should include:

- Nature of the anatomical connections and relationship of the VSD to the great arteries.
- Any outflow tract stenosis.
- Degree of shunting and direction.
- LV and RV size and function (may effectively act as one ventricle).
- Any other features.

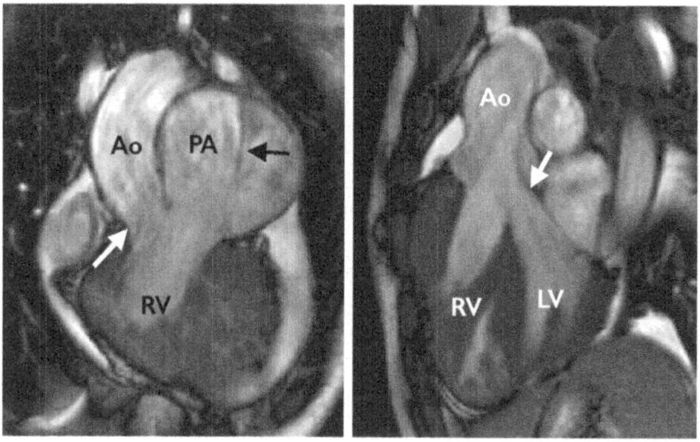

Fig. 12.15 Double outlet RV. Oblique RVOT view (left) showing the RV emptying into the aorta (Ao) through the VSD (white arrow), in addition to the normal connection to the pulmonary artery (PA). The pulmonary artery is dilated with a dissection (black arrow). LVOT view (right) showing the rightward displacement of the aorta, and the VSD (white arrow).

Transposition of the great arteries

The great vessels arise from the wrong ventricle – the aorta from the RV and the pulmonary artery from the LV. Thus, systemic blood cannot pass to the lungs for oxygenation (Fig. 12.16). Neonates are dependent on a patent ductus arteriosus and thus need intervention in the first few days of life before this closes. A balloon atrial septostomy is commonly performed first to create an ASD, followed by a more definitive operation. Unoperated patients do not exist as adults!

Associated conditions: VSD, LVOT obstruction, aortic coarctation.

Surgical options

Atrial switch operation

The most common operation amongst current adults, but has been replaced since the 1980s by the arterial switch operation. Atrial blood flow is redirected with a baffle so the LV receives systemic venous blood (and pumps to the lungs); while the RV receives pulmonary venous blood (and pumps into the aorta). The disadvantage is that the RV remains the systemic ventricle, and is prone to late failure. There are 2 variants:

- **Senning operation:** this uses the right atrial wall and atrial septal tissue to create the baffle.
- **Mustard operation:** uses extrinsic pericardium or synthetic material to create the baffle.

Arterial switch operation (Jatene procedure)

The aorta and pulmonary artery are separated from the ventricles, and reattached in the anatomically correct position, with re-implantation of the coronary arteries. The operation is more technically challenging than the atrial switch, but results in a systemic left ventricle. In the longer term, outflow tract stenosis can occur. The Lecompte manoeuvre is a variant in which the pulmonary artery is brought more anterior to the aorta, with the branch pulmonary arteries often straddling the aorta (Fig. 12.20).

Rastelli operation

For TGA with a large sub-aortic VSD and pulmonary stenosis. A baffle is placed in the RV to channel blood from the LV through the VSD to the aorta. The pulmonary trunk is ligated and a separate RV to pulmonary artery conduit is created (usually valved). The LV becomes the systemic ventricle, but longer-term problems involve outflow tract obstruction, which can occur in either pathway, and subsequent operations are usually required.

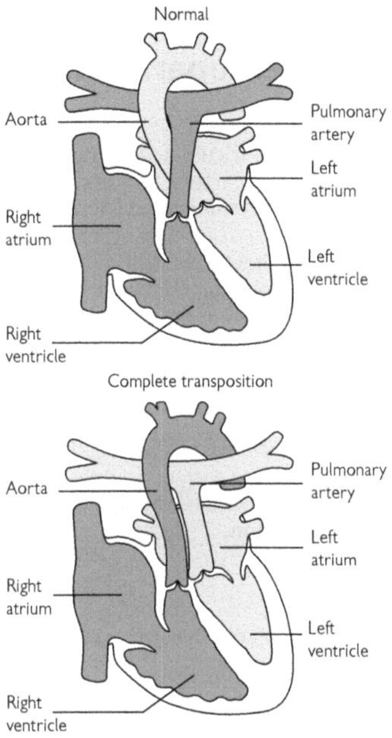

Fig. 12.16 Features of transposition of the great arteries. Reproduced from Myerson S, Choudhury R, and Mitchell A (2009). *Emergencies in Cardiology*, 2nd edn, Oxford University Press.

Transposition of the great arteries post-atrial switch operation

CMR features

- **Discordant ventricles:** ventriculo-arterial discordance (LV connected to pulmonary artery; RV connected to aorta).
- **Hypertrophied ±dilated ±dysfunctional RV:** 2° to systemic pressure loading ± tricuspid regurgitation. RV dysfunction is common and is the main source of concern in these patients (Fig. 12.17).
- **Atrial baffle:** directing systemic blood towards the LV (and into the pulmonary circulation) and pulmonary venous return to the RV (and into the aorta) (see Fig. 12.18). Baffle obstruction or leak can occur at any point along the path.
- **Tricuspid regurgitation:** related to the systemic RV pressures and altered septal geometry.
- **Parallel great vessels:** a hallmark of TGA (Fig. 12.19). The aorta and pulmonary artery lie parallel to each other, rather than at 90°. The aorta is usually more anterior and to the right of the pulmonary artery.
- **± Residual LVOT obstruction.**

Scanning

LV and RV long axis views

For general assessment of function. The atrial baffle may be seen, particularly on the HLA and VLA views.

LV and RV outflow tract views

To assess any obstruction.

Specific imaging of the atrial baffle

Several images may be required for adequate visualization. Each pathway should be examined along the whole route for stenosis or leaks:

- The pulmonary venous route can usually be visualized with a modified HLA view passing through the pulmonary venous 'corridor' (Fig. 12.17).
- The systemic venous pathway can usually be visualized in an oblique sagittal view passing through SVC, IVC and the mitral valve (Fig. 12.18). Separate views may be required for each limb.

Short axis cine stack

For LV and RV functional assessment.

Aortic and pulmonary flow

To assess any baffle leak (shunt), or valve regurgitation.

Reporting should include:

- Systemic RV and sub-pulmonary LV volumes and function.
- Status of systemic and pulmonary venous pathways – obstruction/leak?
- Any LVOT or RVOT obstruction.
- Degree of tricuspid regurgitation.

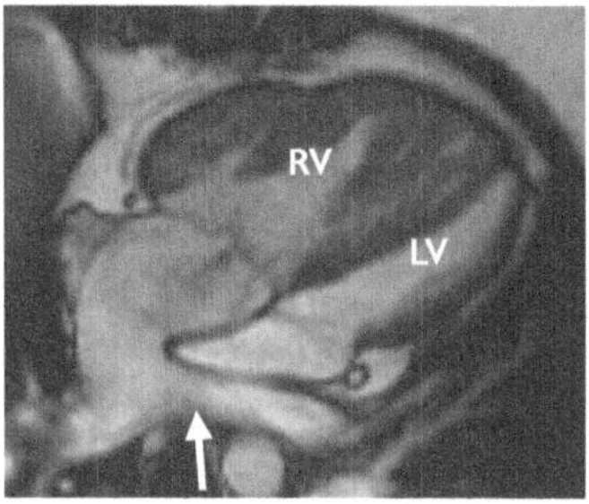

Fig. 12.17 Modified HLA view showing pulmonary venous pathway (arrowed) in a patient post-Mustard operation. Note the severely hypertrophied systemic RV and thin-walled, compressed sub-pulmonary LV.

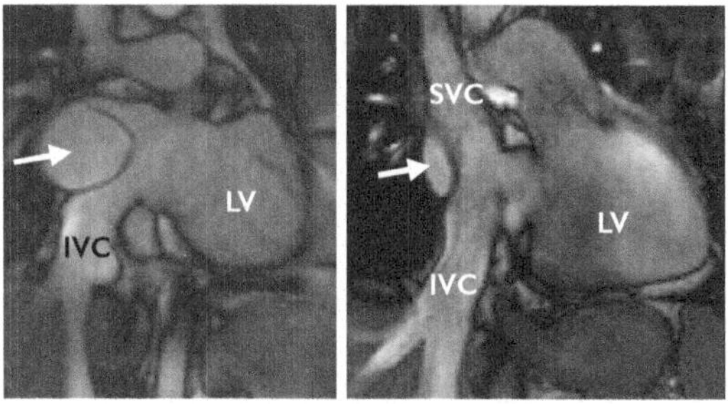

Fig. 12.18 Modified oblique sagittal views showing the variation in systemic venous pathways in two patients post-atrial switch procedures. The pulmonary venous channel can be seen in cross section (arrowed). Image on the right reproduced from Thorne S and Clift P (2009) *Adult Congenital Heart Disease*, Oxford University Press.

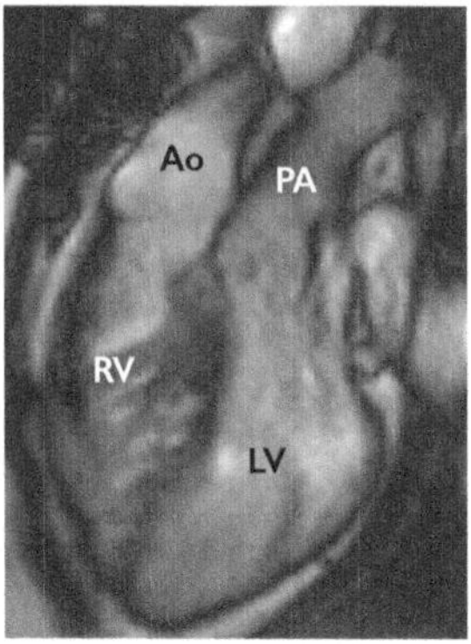

Fig. 12.19 Parallel great vessels in a patient with TGA.

Transposition of the great arteries post-arterial switch/Rastelli

CMR features

- **Normally connected LV and RV:** ventricular function is often normal, but residual dysfunction is possible in either ventricle, related to previous pressure loading or outflow tract stenosis.
- **LV or RV outflow tract obstruction:** the re-fashioned outflow tracts are often somewhat angulated and are prone to obstruction. Re-operations are often required, particularly post-Rastelli operation.
- **± Aortic regurgitation:** the (neo)aortic valve can become regurgitant following the arterial switch procedure.
- **Parallel great vessels:** as for the atrial switch operation, the aorta and pulmonary artery remain parallel to each other, rather than at 90°. This is a hallmark of TGA. The aorta is usually more anterior and to the right of the pulmonary artery.
- **± Coronary artery disease:** the coronary arteries can be obstructed in up to 20% of patients, related to the surgical repair. Viability assessment with late gadolinium imaging can aid the assessment of any LV/RV dysfunction.

Scanning

LV and RV long axis views

For general assessment of function.

LV and RV outflow tract views

To assess obstruction. May require modified views to fully assess the extended outflow tract after the Rastelli operation.

Short axis cine stack

For LV and RV functional assessment.

Aortic and pulmonary flow

To assess any outflow tract/valvar stenosis or regurgitation.

± late gadolinium enhancement

If coronary disease suspected (particularly if ventricular function is impaired).

Reporting should include:

- Biventricular volumes and function.
- Assessment of LV and RV outflow tracts for obstruction (particularly the RV conduit in the Rastelli operation).
- Assessment of ascending aorta and pulmonary arteries for stenosis.
- Any aortic regurgitation.
- Any evidence for infarction if ventricular dysfunction is present.

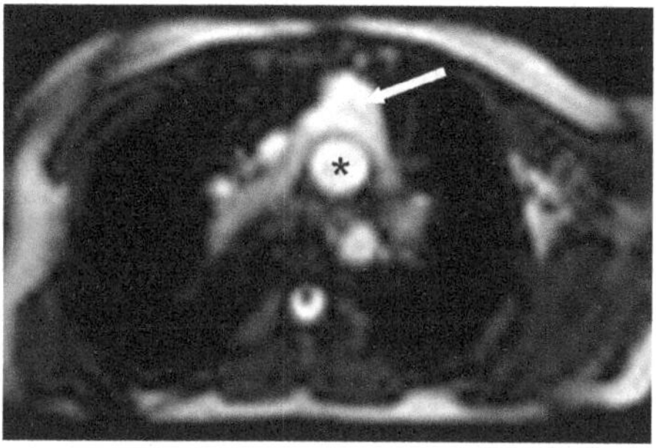

Fig. 12.20 Arterial switch with Lecompte manoeuvre in a young patient (hence the poor image quality). Transaxial SSFP image showing the pulmonary arteries (arrowed) straddling the aorta (*). Reproduced from Thorne S and Clift P (2009) *Adult Congenital Heart Disease*, Oxford University Press.

Congenitally corrected transposition of the great arteries

In congenitally corrected transposition of the great arteries (ccTGA), the ventricles are 'inverted' (positions swapped), with the RA connected to the LV and the LA connected to the RV. In addition, there is ventriculo-arterial discordance, with the RV connected to the aorta and the LV connected to the pulmonary artery. This is sometimes called 'double discordance'. Patients are not cyanotic as blood flows to the appropriate circulation - systemic venous return enters the LV, which ejects into the pulmonary artery. Pulmonary venous return enters the RV which fills the aorta. The circulation is therefore 'physiologically corrected' but the RV supports the systemic circulation, which creates long term problems with RV dysfunction. Patients can occasionally remain undiagnosed into adult life, though surgery is common if discovered in childhood, to repair the pulmonary outflow obstruction or tricuspid regurgitation. Full 'correction' is sometimes performed, which involves both an atrial and arterial switch procedure. This is a complex operation, but avoids the long-term risk of RV dysfunction.

Associated cardiac defects are common, with the most likely being:

- VSD.
- Pulmonary/subpulmonary stenosis.
- Tricuspid regurgitation (± Ebsteins).
- Dextrocardia.

CMR features: the unoperated patient

- **Discordant ventricles:** both atrioventricular and ventricular-arterial discordance, atrial situs is usually normal.
- **RV hypertrophy ± dysfunction:** RV dysfunction is common in the longer term, 2° to chronic systemic pressures.
- **± Tricuspid regurgitation:** related to systemic pressures ± a dysplastic valve.
- **Parallel great vessels:** as for the atrial switch operation, the aorta and pulmonary artery remain parallel to each other. The aorta is usually more anterior and to the right of the pulmonary artery.

The operated patient

Patients may have been operated for their associated lesions (e.g. VSD closure, conduit formation from LV to pulmonary artery, tricuspid valve repair). CMR features are those relevant to these.

Scanning

- ***LV and RV long axis views*** Confirms double discordance, and provides a general assessment of ventricular and valvalar function.
- ***LV and RV outflow tract views*** To confirm connection to great vessels and assess any obstruction.
- ***Short axis cine stack*** For LV and RV functional assessment.
- ***Aortic and pulmonary flow*** For outflow tract stenosis or regurgitation.

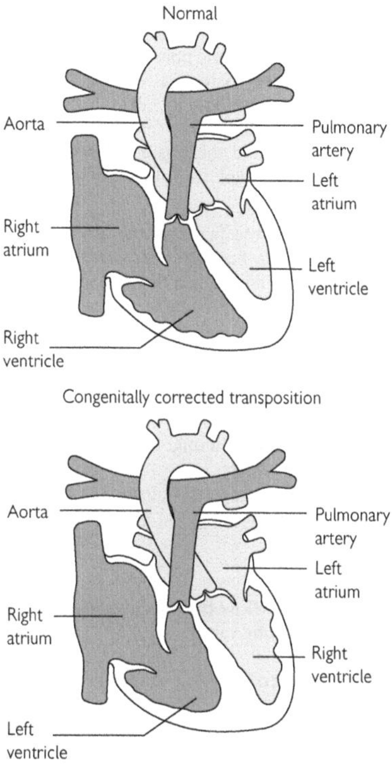

Fig. 12.21 Features of congenitally corrected transposition of the great arteries. Reproduced from Myerson S, Choudhury R, and Mitchell A (2009) *Emergencies in Cardiology*, 2nd edn, Oxford University Press.

Truncus arteriosus

Rare condition in which the aorta and pulmonary artery arise from a common trunk, although there are anatomical variants. A single truncal valve is present, which may be quadricuspid in ~20% of cases and regurgitation is common. Other aortic abnormalities can occur, including interrupted aortic arch and coarctation, and there is an association with DiGeorge syndrome. A large VSD underlies the common trunk, which straddles (over-rides) the septum.

Patients undergo surgery in the first months of life to create separate outflow tracts, usually with a homograft prosthetic valve and synthetic conduit from the RV to the pulmonary artery. Re-operations are the norm, to replace the conduit, which can become narrowed, and/or to replace the truncal valve which can develop severe regurgitation. Most patients presenting for CMR are post-surgery. The main longer-term problem is stenosis of the outflow tracts.

CMR features: without corrective surgery

- **Combined aortic/pulmonary trunk:** the pulmonary artery usually arises from the posterior aspect.
- **Large sub-arterial VSD:** the common trunk sits astride the septum.
- **Other associated lesions:** interrupted aortic arch, aortic coarctation, right aortic arch, ASD.

CMR features: post-corrective surgery

- **Abnormal LV and RV outflow tracts:** these may include a conduit and usually involve prosthetic valves.
- **± Aortic root dilation.**
- **± LV/RV dysfunction:** secondary to previous surgery and/or coronary artery abnormalities.
- **± Residual VSD.**
- **± Branch pulmonary artery stenosis.**

Scanning

- LV and RV long axis cines.
- LV and RV outflow tract views – may need to be modified to visualize the whole tract.
- Aortic and pulmonary through-plane flow to assess valve function.
- Short axis cine stack for LV and RV functional assessment.
- Aortic views – include the whole thoracic aorta.

Reporting should include:

- LV and RV function.
- Status of the outflow tracts and prosthetic valves.
- Aortic anatomy ± root dilation.
- Other residual defects.

Pulmonary atresia with ventricular septal defect

The pulmonary outflow tract is absent and RV blood flow passes through the large VSD to the aorta (Fig. 12.22). Pulmonary blood supply is from major aorto-pulmonary collateral arteries (MAPCA's) and/or a persistent ductus arteriosus, and pulmonary artery abnormalities are common. There is some overlap with Fallot's tetralogy.

Patients with well formed pulmonary arteries may undergo repair, with an RV to pulmonary artery conduit; the VSD may also be closed. Those with more severely hypoplastic pulmonary arteries may undergo palliative surgery with a shunt to increase pulmonary blood flow (e.g. Blalock-Taussig or Waterston; Fig. 12.23).

CMR features: post-repair

- **RV to PA conduit:** may include a prosthetic valve. The conduit can become stenosed.
- **Pulmonary artery hypoplasia/stenosis.**
- **Major aorto-pulmonary collateral arteries (MAPCA's):** often arise from the aortic arch, but can originate from the branch vessels. Very variable in size and number.
- **± RV dysfunction and/or hypertrophy.**
- **± Tricuspid regurgitation:** may be due to RV dysfunction.
- **± LV dysfunction:** due to longstanding volume overload from MAPCA's.
- **± Aortic root dilation ±regurgitation.**

CMR features: unoperated or palliated patients

- **Small hypertrophied RV.**
- **VSD.**
- **± LV dysfunction:** due to longstanding volume overload from MAPCA's.
- **Pulmonary artery hypoplasia/stenosis.**
- **± Systemic-pulmonary shunt.**
- **Major aorto-pulmonary collateral arteries (MAPCA's):** as above.

Scanning

- Long axis views of the LV and RV.
- Short axis stack for LV and RV function.
- LV and RV outflow tract views.
- Aortic ± pulmonary through-plane flow.
- Pulmonary artery views.
- MR angiography timed to the aorta to visualize the MAPCA's – take great care to avoid venous emboli in cyanotic patients (these can embolize to the systemic circulation).

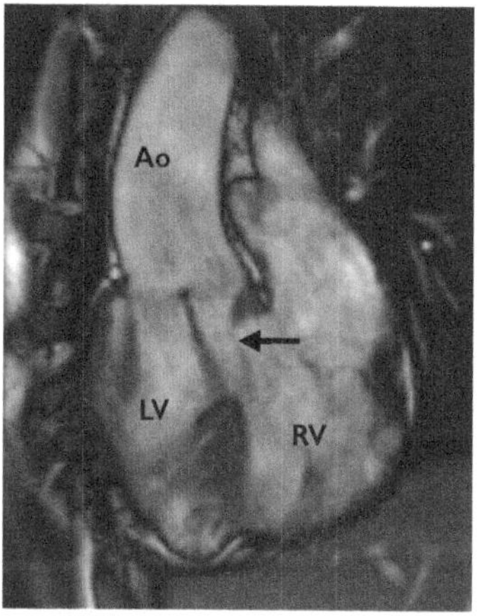

Fig. 12.22 Pulmonary atresia with VSD. There is a large VSD (arrowed) and no effective RV outflow tract, with both ventricles essentially functioning as a single ventricle ejecting into the enlarged aorta (Ao).

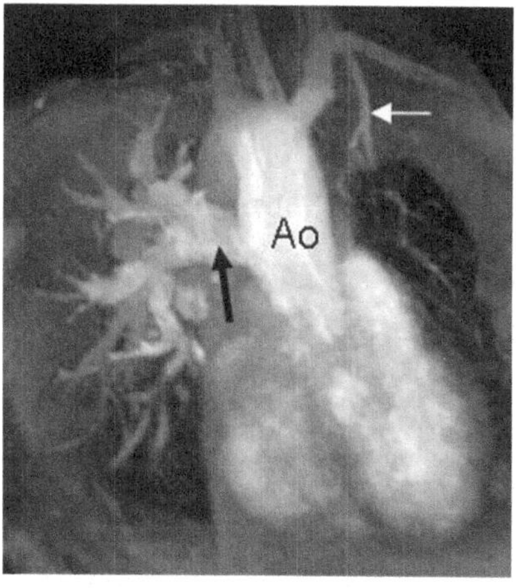

Fig. 12.23 MR angiogram (MIP) of the patient shown in Fig. 12.22, showing a large Waterston shunt from the aorta to the right pulmonary artery (black arrow), with reasonable right lung perfusion. There is little left lung perfusion, with the largest aorto-pulmonary collateral seen here. (white arrow).

The single ventricle

This comprises a spectrum of uni-ventricular hearts, including tricuspid atresia and double inlet ventricles, in which there is a single functioning ventricle, sometimes with a rudimentary second ventricle. See 📖 p. 314 for anatomical assessment. There is a wide spectrum of anatomy and previous surgical procedures, and all available anatomical information and details of surgical procedures should be obtained prior to CMR scanning.

CMR scanning

No specific protocol can be defined due to the wide range in anatomy, but imaging should focus on:

- Defining the anatomy (especially if not previously known).
- Ventricular function: if a rudimentary chamber contributes to the ventricular function, it should be included in the volumetric analysis. However, the rudimentary ventricle may have a negative effect on the stroke volume, enlarging during systole of the dominant ventricle.
- Evidence of significant valvular regurgitation.
- Evidence of pulmonary artery, pulmonary vein, or Fontan pathway stenosis or obstruction.
- Differential pulmonary artery, IVC, and SVC blood flow by phase encoded velocity mapping.
- Evidence of thrombus formation: slow flow may give the impression of a thrombus, but contrast and early gadolinium images should be acquired if there is any concern (Early gadolinium enhancement 📖 p. 112)

► Care should be taken with contrast injections for all cyanotic patients, as systemic emboli may result – use a filter.

The Fontan circulation

The original Fontan operation was for patients with uni-ventricular hearts (tricuspid atresia initially) and created a connection from the systemic venous circulation to the pulmonary arteries, by-passing the right ventricle and separating the two circulations (Fig. 12.24). There are several variations in anatomy, including:

- Lateral tunnel within the right atrium, connecting SVC and IVC, and also connected to the pulmonary artery.
- Extracardiac pathway from the IVC to the pulmonary artery.
- Glenn anastomosis (SVC to right PA) + conduit between the right atrium and pulmonary artery (modification of the original Fontan).

CMR imaging should be focused on the systemic venous pathways, which need to be imaged along their length to exclude significant obstruction and ventricular function.

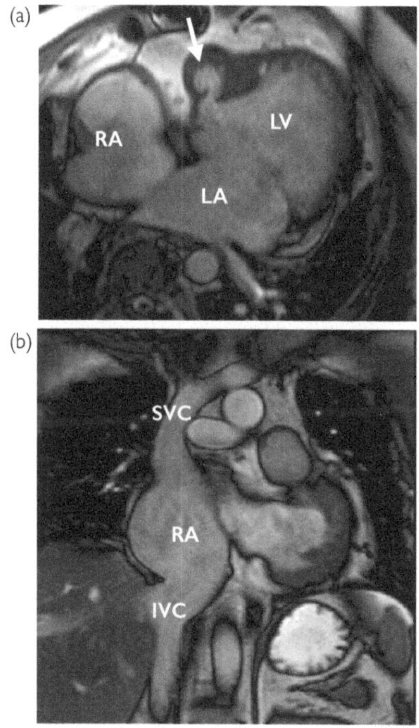

Fig. 12.24 Uni-ventricular heart with a dominant left ventricle and rudimentary right ventricle (arrowed, top on HLA view). The SVC and IVC enter the dilated right atrium (bottom), which connects to the pulmonary artery via a conduit (out of plane), forming a Fontan circulation. Reproduced from Thorne S and Clift P (2009) *Adult Congenital Heart Disease*, Oxford University Press.

Surgical shunts and conduits

These are used in a number of palliative and reparative surgical procedures for congenital heart disease, often to improve the pulmonary circulation. These include:

- Systemic to pulmonary artery shunts, e.g.
  - Blalock-Taussig (subclavian artery to pulmonary artery). See 📖 p. 352.
  - Waterston (ascending aorta to right pulmonary artery). See 📖 p. 354.
- Cavopulmonary anastomosis (e.g. Glenn shunt).
- Right ventricle to pulmonary artery conduits.

The shunts should be assessed for stenosis, occlusion, aneurysms, or thrombus. Contrast-enhanced MR angiography can visualize the course of the shunt and assess patency.

Glossary of surgical procedures

Arterial switch operation or Jatene procedure Operation for TGA patients. Involves switching the great arteries to bring the aorta to the former pulmonary artery position and the pulmonary artery to the former aortic position. The coronary arteries have to be transposed from the aortic root to the former pulmonary artery root (neo aorta). Ultimately, the left ventricle will perfuse the aorta and the right ventricle will perfuse the pulmonary artery. See 📖 p. 336.

Bentall operation Replacement of the ascending aorta and aortic valve, with a composite graft (conduit) and valve, and re-implantation of the coronary arteries into the conduit.

Brock procedure Palliative procedure for ToF patients. Closed resection of right ventricular musculature from the outflow tract using a biopsy like instrument and dilatation (valvotomy) of the pulmonary valve.

Blalock-Taussig shunt (classic) Subclavian artery to ipsilateral pulmonary artery anastomosis (direct end-to-side junction).

Blalock-Taussig shunt (modified) Same shunt using a prosthetic graft.

Damus Kaye Stansel operation For patients with single ventricles, transposition of the great arteries and a restrictive VSD causing 'subaortic' stenosis. The operation connects the aorta and pulmonary artery in a side-to-side fashion to provide unrestricted blood flow from the systemic ventricle to the aorta.

Fontan operation Palliative operation for patients with 'single' ventricle physiology (📖 p. 348). Diversion of the systemic venous return to the lung without interposition of a subpulmonary ventricle. Leads to volume unloading of the 'single' ventricle and, ideally, to normalization of the arterial oxygen saturation.

Multiple variations of the procedure exists regarding the type of connection between the systemic veins and the pulmonary arteries (Fig. 12.25):

- **Classic Fontan:** connection between right atrium and pulmonary artery.
- **Extracardiac Fontan:** inferior vena cava connected to pulmonary artery via an extracardiac conduit combined with a Glenn shunt.
- **Bjoerk or RA-RV Fontan:** valved conduit between the right atrium and the right ventricle.
- **Total cavopulmonary connection (TCPC):** inferior vena cava connected to pulmonary artery via an intra atrial tunnel (also called lateral tunnel), combined with a Glenn shunt to the SVC.

Glenn shunt SVC to pulmonary artery anastomosis

- **Classical Glenn shunt:** anastomosis of the superior vena cava to the distal right pulmonary artery with ligation of the SVC below the anastomosis and division of the proximal right pulmonary artery from the pulmonary bifurcation.
- **Bi-directional Glenn shunt:** anastomosis of the superior vena cava to the undivided pulmonary artery.

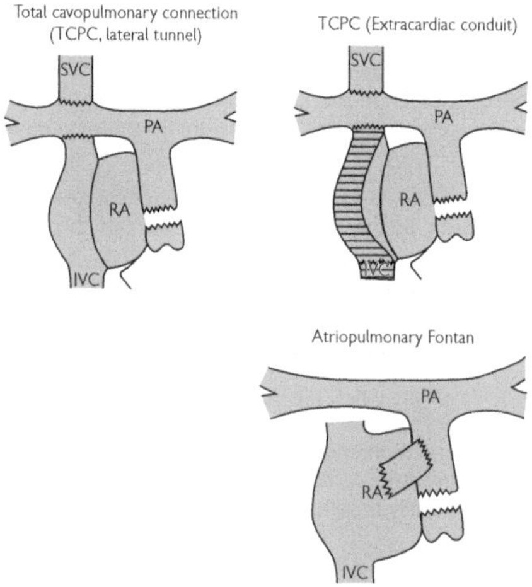

Fig. 12.25 Types of Fontan operation. Reproduced from Myerson S, Choudhury R and Mitchell A (2009) *Emergencies in Cardiology*, 2nd edn, Oxford Unviersity Press.

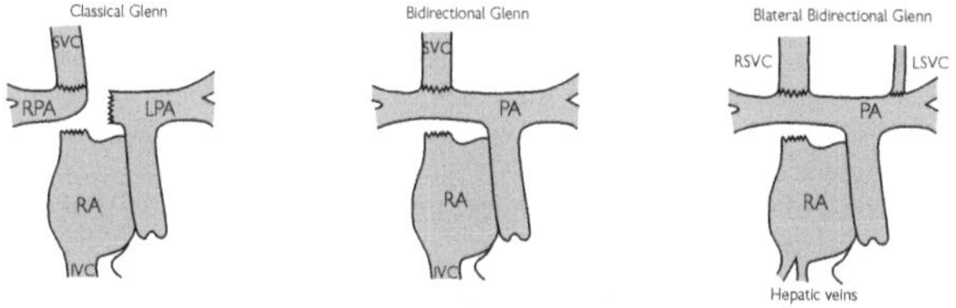

Fig. 12.26 Types of Glenn shunt. Reproduced from Myerson S, Choudhury R, and Mitchell A (2009). *Emergencies in Cardiology*, 2nd edn, Oxford University Press.

Konno operation Complex repair and reconstruction of the LV outflow tract for patients with tunnel-like subvalvar left ventricular outflow tract obstruction. The operation involves enlargement of the outflow tract by inserting a patch in the interventricular septum and aortic valve replacement, as well as enlargement of the aortic annulus and the ascending aorta.

Lecompte manoeuvre Manoeuvre that brings the pulmonary artery in a position anterior to the ascending aorta (part of the arterial switch operation).

Mustard operation Atrial switch operation for patients with TGA. Redirection of the venous blood to the contralateral ventricle using pericardial or synthetic patches. See 🕮 p. 336.

Norwood operation Initial palliative procedure for the treatment of hypoplastic left heart syndrome with aortic atresia and hypoplasia of the ascending aorta. Operation involves the reconstruction of 'neo-ascending' aorta using the pulmonary valve and trunk, and the creation of an aorto-pulmonary shunt (usually modified BT shunt).

Pott's anastomosis shunt Descending aorta to left pulmonary artery anastomosis.

Rastelli operation For patients with TGA, VSD, and pulmonary stenosis. Involves closure of the VSD in a way that the patch forms the left ventricular outflow tract to the aorta. The right ventricle is connected to the main pulmonary artery using a valved conduit.

Ross operation Aortic valve replacement involving transplantation of the patient's pulmonary valve into the aortic position (pulmonary autograft) and replacement of the pulmonary valve using a homograft valve. Major advantages are:

- Potential of the 'neo-aortic' valve (former pulmonary valve) to grow.
- No need for anticoagulation.

Senning operation Atrial switch operation for patients with TGA. Redirection of the venous blood to the contralateral ventricle using the atrial wall and the septum. See 🕮 p. 336.

Waterston shunt Ascending aorta to right pulmonary artery anastomosis.

Chapter 13

Aortic disease

Imaging the aorta

Introduction

CMR brings many advantages to aortic imaging, including the free choice of imaging planes, flow measurement and 3D angiography, in addition to excellent anatomical imaging. These make imaging the aorta straightforward, but there are still important aspects to be aware of to obtain the best pictures, gain the best from CMR, and avoid the pitfalls that catch the unwary.

Other aortic imaging techniques – transoesophageal echocardiography and computed tomography (CT) – also have their strengths, particularly in the acute setting, when the MR environment may not be the best place for a patient. The combination of features that CMR provides, however, suggest that it has become the 'Gold standard' for aortic imaging.

General tips

Make good use of cine imaging

Although most sequences start with a standard 'static' sequence (e.g. HASTE), the aorta is a mobile organ! SSFP cine imaging is excellent for visualizing the aorta throughout the cardiac cycle, avoiding blurring, and identifying narrowed sections. The high contrast between blood and aortic wall allows good visualization of the wall and any dissection flaps.

Be creative in your choice of image plane

Although the aorta can be imaged satisfactorily in standard transverse and sagittal planes, much better images can often be obtained in non-standard planes, which demonstrate pathology more clearly and quantify the severity accurately.

Don't always try to image the whole aorta in one plane

While many aortic arches can be imaged within a single plane, significant features are often present in more difficult and tortuous aortas, and aiming to get too much in one image may miss or underestimate important pathology. Sometimes it pays to image just the relevant section to demonstrate the important features well.

Standard imaging technique

Transverse image stack through thorax

Usually with a single-shot fast spin echo (e.g. HASTE) sequence. This gives a general guide to the aortic anatomy and allows positioning of subsequent images.

± Coronal image stack

Can be useful, but often the oblique sagittal images are more helpful.

Oblique sagittal image stack

- Usually provides a good representation of the thoracic aorta.
- 5–7 parallel images piloted from the transverse image stack, through the longitudinal plane of the aorta. A HASTE sequence is appropriate (no gap between slices). Position the image slices parallel to a line between the central axis of both ascending and descending limbs (see Fig. 13.1), ideally with the ascending and descending aorta in the same slice.

The longitudinal plane (the 'candy-stick' view)

Cine sequences (e.g. SSFP) are ideal. Aim to display as much of the ascending arch and descending aorta as possible in a single slice (Fig. 13.2). You may be fortunate enough to acquire this in one of the oblique sagittal images above. If not, choose one of the following:

Modify an oblique sagittal slice closest to the desired image.

Often, the ascending and descending limbs of the aorta will be in view, but not the apex of the arch. If this image position is projected onto a coronal view through the arch, it may be rotated to pass through the apex of the arch, while remaining in the ascending and descending limbs.

Identify the image plane from 3 points (if software allows this)

Use the transverse or coronal image stacks to choose the 3 points:

- Mid-ascending aorta (usually at the level of the pulmonary artery).
- The apex of the arch.
- The mid-descending aorta.

If necessary, repeat to obtain a better image, using the transaxial or sagittal images to re-pilot or modify the plane.

- Provides excellent representation of the course of the aorta, relative diameters, and tortuosity without the mental re-construction required for an image stack. The aortic sinuses are often out of plane however.
- Less good for measurement of diameter as the plane may miss the true central axis of the aorta.
- Transaxial images of the aorta (i.e. perpendicular to the long axis of the aorta) can be positioned perpendicular to this view, however, which provide accurate measurement of the true diameter.

► It may not be possible to image the whole aorta in a single plane, particularly if tortuous. In this case, aim to acquire several long axis images covering the thoracic aorta.

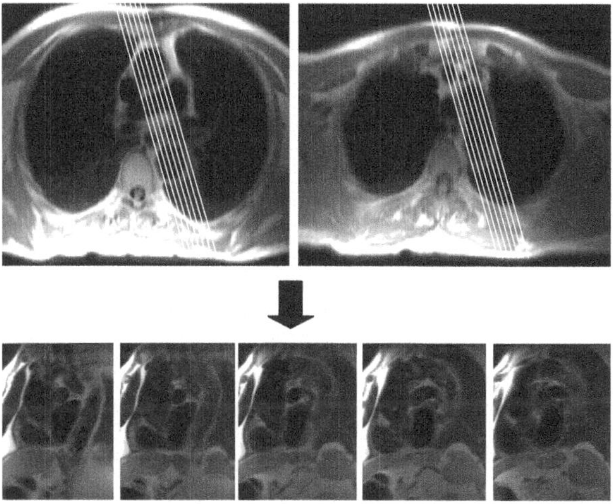

Fig. 13.1 Transverse views through the ascending and descending aorta (left), and aortic arch (right), showing the image position for the oblique sagittal series (bottom).

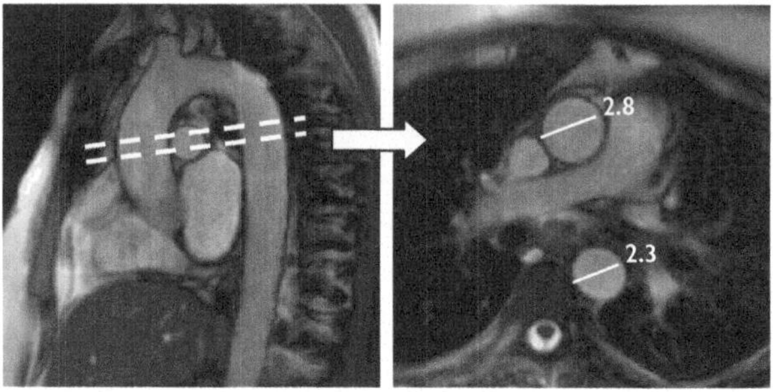

Fig. 13.2 Long axis through the thoracic aorta – the 'candy-stick' view (left). The aortic sinuses lie slightly out of plane. The parallel lines indicate good positions for obtaining transaxial views of the aorta, from which to measure the true short axis diameter (right).

± Transaxial (short-axis) aortic images

Positioned perpendicular to the longitudinal view. These provide accurate images from which to measure aortic diameter.

± Oblique coronal images of the descending aorta

Separate imaging of the descending aorta is sometimes required if this is tortuous or the lower thoracic aorta is particularly relevant (Fig. 13.4). This should also be cine imaging, and can be either mostly sagittal or coronal, depending on the orientation of the aorta at this point. To position the slice, either modify an appropriate coronal/sagittal HASTE image or pilot from 3 points as above.

Aortic root

The aortic root is a common site for disease and should not be omitted when assessing the aorta. The coronal LVOT view (Fig. 13.3) is particularly useful for demonstrating the sinuses and proximal ascending aorta. This view may not always show the whole ascending aorta, however, and a second image is often needed to demonstrate this. This should be planned either as an oblique sagittal view (using the transverse HASTE images as a reference) or created using the 3-point technique. In both cases, the plane should be planned passing through/using the following 3 points:

- Aortic sinuses.
- Mid-ascending aorta.
- Apex of the arch.

Note, this view is similar to the 'candy stick' view, but the focus is on the root and ascending aorta, and not the distal arch/descending aorta.

± MR angiography

When imaging of the arch and major branch vessels is difficult, MR angiography of the aorta can be helpful. Complex anatomy is easily visualized, and dilation/stenosis can be appreciated well, for example, in Takayasu's arteritis (Fig. 13.5). 3D reconstruction software and surface rendering are ideal for providing the best images.

Aortic wall imaging

If imaging of the aortic wall is important, both SSFP and turbo spin echo images are helpful, either in longitudinal or transaxial planes (relative to the aorta). On SSFP imaging, flowing blood is high signal (bright), in contrast to the low signal (dark grey) of the aortic wall, which helps to delineate the two. On turbo spin-echo imaging, the contrast between the black flowing blood and mid-grey aortic wall is helpful. On both images, thrombus (either luminal or intramural) is usually mid-dark grey. Atheroma is usually the same signal intensity as the aortic wall, but large plaques with a high lipid content may have a central core of high signal from the lipid visible on turbo spin echo images.

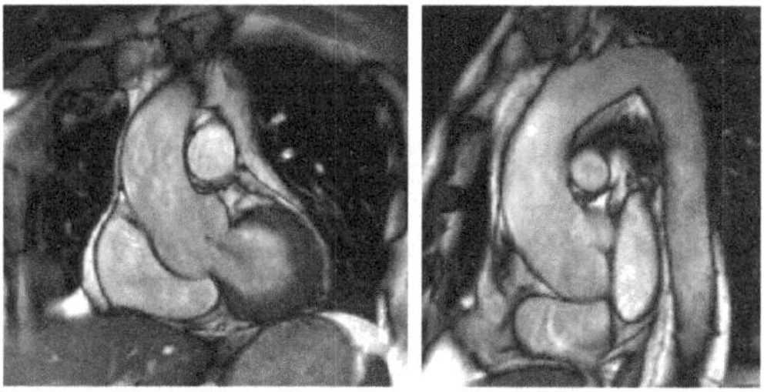

Fig. 13.3 SSFP images in the coronal LVOT view (left) clearly showing the anatomy of the aortic root. A small jet of aortic regurgitation is also seen. Oblique sagittal view (right), visualizing the whole ascending aorta and arch.

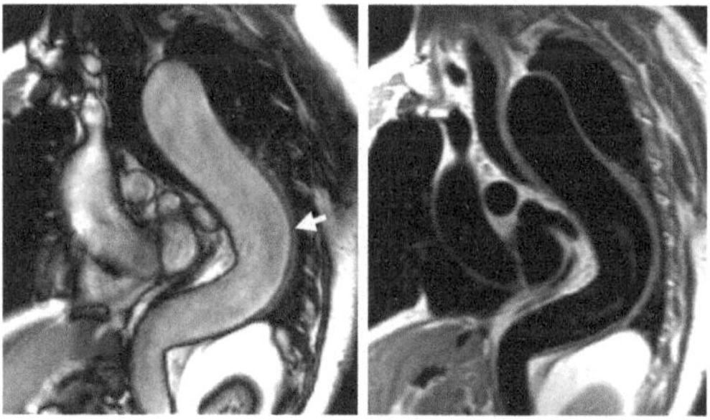

Fig. 13.4 Oblique coronal image of the descending aorta. Note the tortuous course and thickened lateral wall suggestive of atheroma or intramural haematoma (arrowed). Still image from SSFP cine sequence (left); turbo spin echo sequence (right).

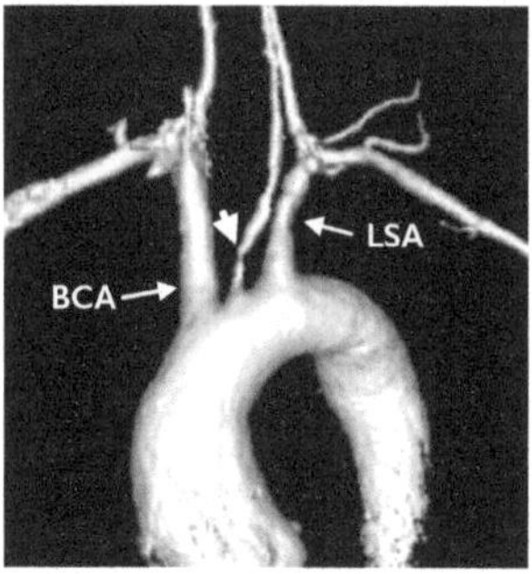

Fig. 13.5 MR angiogram of the aortic arch in a patient with Takayasu's arteritis. Note the irregular outline to the left common carotid (arrowhead) and left subclavian (LSA) arteries and the significant stenosis of the proximal left common carotid. BCA = brachiocephalic artery.

Aortic dilatation

Background

CMR is ideal for imaging dilated aortas, with good visualization of the anatomy and true diameter, and 3D angiography has a role in visualizing the anatomy in more complex cases. These aspects are important for deciding on the need for and the planning of any intervention (surgical or percutaneous).

Causes: hypertension, atheroma, bicuspid aortic valve*, aortic stenosis*, Marfan syndrome (* = usually ascending aorta only).

CMR features

- **Enlarged aortic dimensions:** may be one small section, multiple sections, or the whole thoracic aorta (Fig. 13.6). In patients with Marfan syndrome, the aortic sinuses are typically most severely involved and may be the only dilated segment.
- **Irregular wall:** suggests atheroma.
- **Thickened wall:** suggests atheroma and/or intramural haematoma.
- **± Abnormal aortic valve:** both bicuspid and stenotic aortic valves have an association with dilation of the mid-ascending aorta. The mechanisms are debated, but it is believed an intrinsic aortopathy may accompany bicuspid valves, while altered flow ± pressure patterns may be involved for both lesions. A bicuspid valve may of course also be stenotic! Dilated aortic roots can cause aortic regurgitation, due to reduced leaflet coaption, and this should also be looked for.

Scanning

Longitudinal planes

As described in previous section. To visualize the whole thoracic aorta, including aortic root.

Aortic short axis views

Accurate measurement of aortic diameter requires a short axis view, planned perpendicular to the aortic longitudinal axis as indicated in Fig. 13.7. This takes full advantage of the capabilities of CMR and avoids:

- Underestimation, common in long axis views as these may not pass through the central axis of the aorta.
- Overestimation from parallax error (see Fig. 13.8) in views transverse to the whole body.

Imaging is usually required at several points.

± MR angiography

If complex anatomy requires a better 3D assessment (see Fig. 13.11).

± Aortic flow measurement

If aortic regurgitation present.

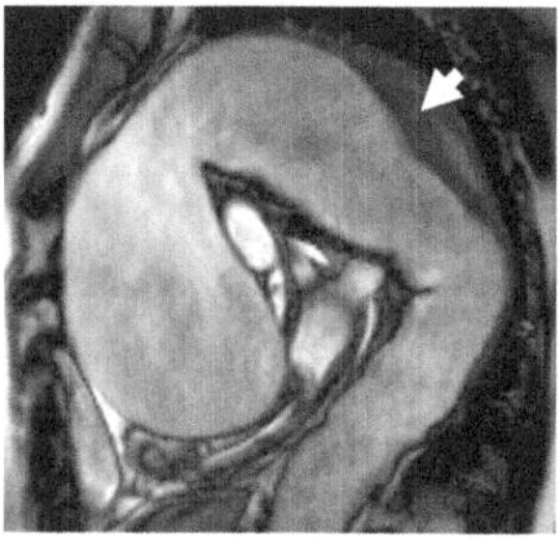

Fig. 13.6 Longitudinal aortic view showing the benefits of CMR in portraying complex anatomy of the thoracic aorta. The ascending aorta is dilated, which tapers to a normal diameter before enlarging again in the arch and descending aorta. There is a thrombosed dissection or intra-mural haematoma present in the distal arch (arrow).

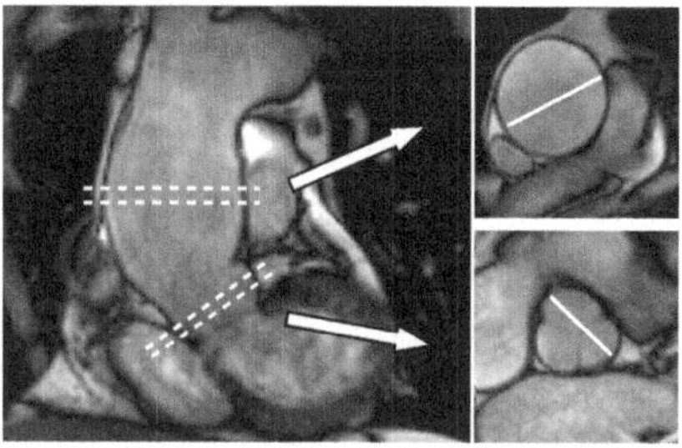

Fig. 13.7 Dilated ascending aorta in ascending aortic view (left), showing positions for short axis images (right). Note the slightly irregular outline to the aortic wall, suggestive of atheroma as the cause.

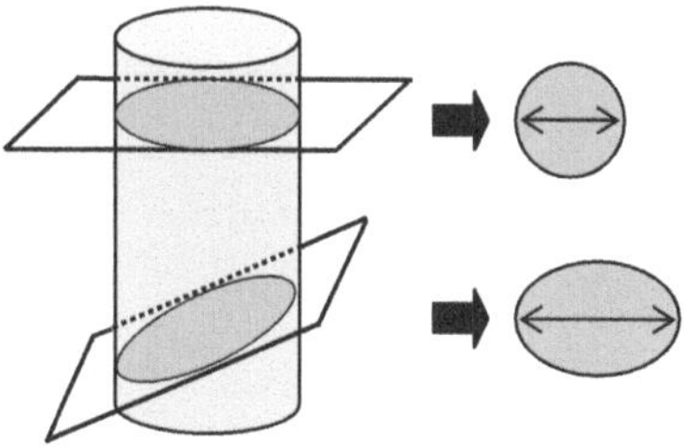

Fig. 13.8 Parallax error. The top half shows the correct short axis position perpendicular to the long axis of a representative aorta, with corresponding circular short axis image. The bottom half shows an incorrectly positioned image slice at an angle to the aorta, with a resultant ellipse shape of the aorta in the 'short axis' view, and potential overestimation of the true diameter (arrows).

Reporting should include:

Description of site and degree of dilatation

Also describe where the aorta returns to normal diameter – e.g. 'the ascending aorta is dilated but tapers to a normal sized arch and descending aorta'. Look for features of specific conditions, e.g. dilated sinuses/root in Marfan syndrome or coarctation with post-stenotic dilation (Fig. 13.10).

Maximum diameter of dilated segment(s)

Best measured from the aortic short axis views to ensure true diameter. Normal ranges exist for the adult aortic root, indexed to body surface area (see Fig. 13.9). Another technique, particularly for smaller adults or children, is to compare the ascending to the descending aorta – the ascending aorta should be less than twice the diameter of the descending. For other sections, a diameter >4.0cm is generally considered to be dilated.

Any associated pathology

E.g. atheroma, intramural haematoma/dissection, bicuspid, or stenosed aortic valve.

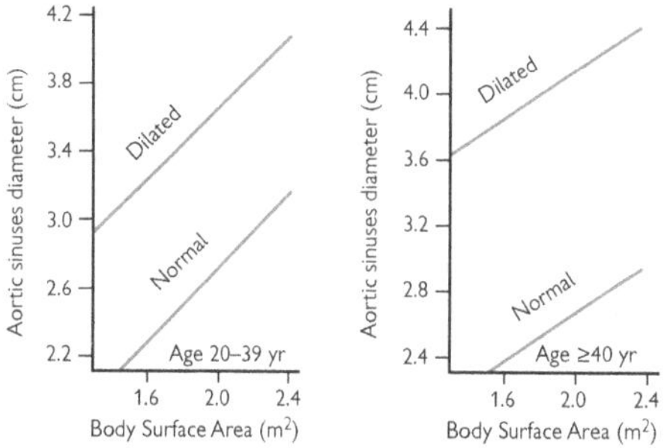

Fig. 13.9 Normogram showing aortic diameters indexed to body surface area. Reproduced with permission from the British Society of Echocardiography.

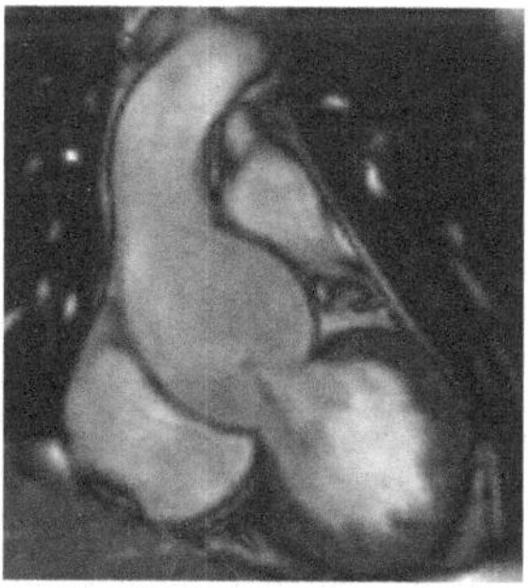

Fig. 13.10 Typical dilated sinuses of a Marfan aorta.

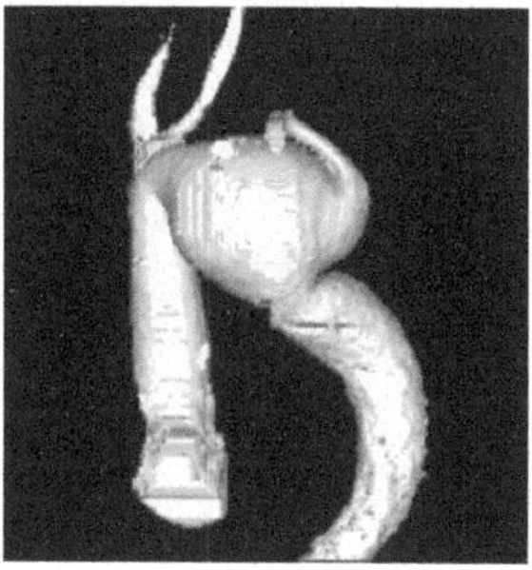

Fig. 13.11 MR angiogram with 3-D reconstruction and surface rendering of a complex dilated aortic arch. The proximal arch is hypoplastic, the distal section has a likely coarctation, while the middle arch is dilated, with the left subclavian artery arising from the dilated section. This complex anatomy can be difficult to view with 2-D image slices, even with CMR.

Scanning

SSFP cine sequences are ideal

Longitudinal plane(s) of the aorta

Give a good representation of the dissection flap and extent (Fig. 13.13). If a dissection isn't seen on the images and the suspicion of dissection is high, the image plane may be parallel to the flap – modify the image plane to be perpendicular to any flap, using a short axis image if necessary (Figs 13.14, 13.15).

LVOT views

To assess the aortic root and integrity of the aortic valve.

Short axis images

Images transverse to the body or the aorta can often show a dissection flap clearly.

Standard cardiac views

Look for any features of high risk in acute dissection – pericardial effusion ± tamponade, poor LV function?

Through-plane flow mapping

This can be useful for identifying the true lumen (highest flow) in difficult cases or for measuring the degree of any aortic regurgitation present.

▶ For follow-up studies, care should be taken to image in the same positions as previous scans to ensure an accurate comparison.

Reporting should include:

- Presence, origin, and extent of dissection.
- Evidence of continued flow and/or thrombus in the false lumen.
- Involvement of any major branch vessels.
- Dimensions of aorta (including false lumen).
- Any involvement of the aortic valve or heart (e.g. pericardial effusion/ tamponade).
- Comparison to previous imaging (especially CMR).

Differential diagnosis

Intra-mural haematoma (Fig. 13.4, 📖 p. 361)

Usually a more restricted area of aorta is involved, with a smaller, more uniformly thickened aortic wall/false lumen. However, a dissection with a completely thrombosed false lumen may be impossible to differentiate from an intramural haematoma.

Transverse sinus of the pericardium

The pericardium has complex reflections onto the heart, and the visceral pericardium in the transverse sinus extends down the aortic root, reflecting back up the right atrium. To the unwary, this potential gap can appear similar to a dissection (Fig. 13.16).

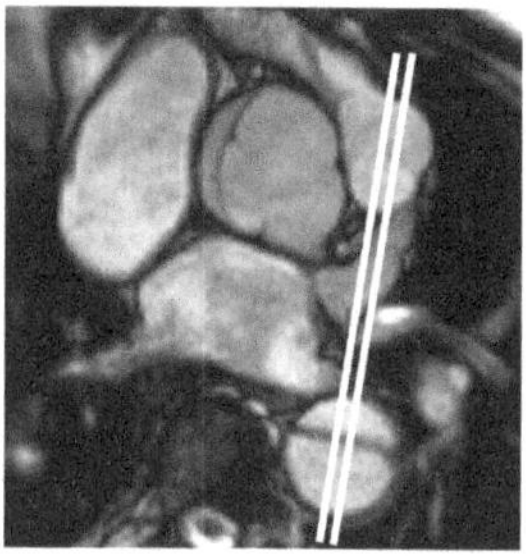

Fig. 13.14 Indication of the ideal plane for demonstrating the dissection flap in the descending aorta in longitudinal section – perpendicular to the flap itself. Note the dissection is also present in the aortic sinuses, indicating a type A dissection.

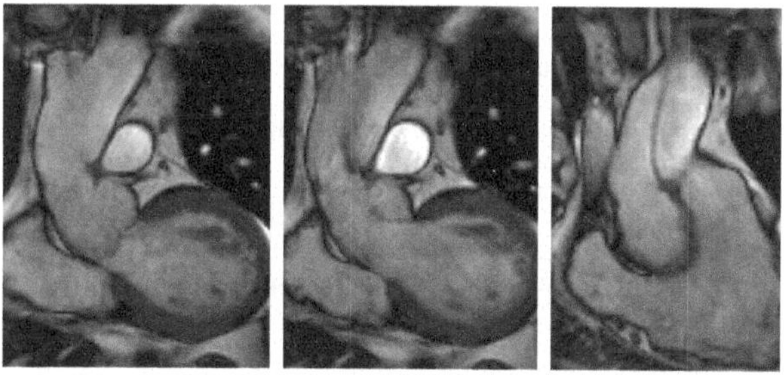

Fig. 13.15 Demonstration of the importance of finding the correct plane. The diastolic SSFP image in the LVOT plane (left) does not demonstrate a dissection. The systolic frame of the cine (middle) shows turbulence in the ascending aorta, suggesting a dissection, but this is not well visualized. The image on the right is a modified position, more sagittal, and clearly demonstrates the dissection flap. In this case, the flap is above an interposition graft repair for the type A dissection.

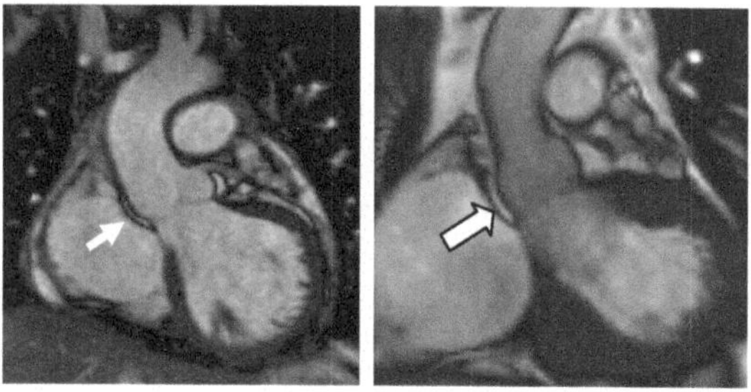

Fig. 13.16 LVOT views showing the gap created by the transverse sinus as it descends between aorta and right atrium (arrows). The impression of a 'flap' is exacerbated by the chemical shift artefact on SSFP imaging creating a 'black' edge to the aortic wall.

Post type A dissection repair

Background

Acute type A dissection carries a high mortality, due primarily to cardiac complications from dissection in the aortic root – compromised coronary flow, acute severe aortic regurgitation from dehiscence of the valve, and cardiac tamponade. Emergency cardiac surgery is thus recommended and, as patients often require imaging of the aortic root in the future, it is important to understand the CMR appearances following surgery.

CMR features

There are different surgical approaches, dependent on individual patient circumstances and the surgical skills available:

- **Interpositional graft:** a short tubular interpositional graft in the mid-ascending aorta, usually just above the sinotubular junction. This is the most common operation as it is quick to perform and requires less specialist surgical expertise. Appearances on CMR can be subtle, but there is usually an irregularity in the aortic wall at both ends of the graft, and a sharper angle to the curve in the ascending aorta (see Fig. 13.17).
- **Combined aortic valve and root replacement:** provides more robust protection against complications. CMR appearances of the valve are similar to other metallic valves. The graft portion may be less identifiable, but is straighter than a normal root, lacks sinuses, and there is usually a break in continuity at the distal end (see Fig. 13.18).
- **Aortic root replacement with valve re-suspension:** the aortic root is replaced down to the valve, which is resuspended in the proximal portion of the graft. This can provide an excellent long-term result, but the operation is longer and more complex. CMR appearances of the valve will be normal, and the graft appearances are as above.
- **Residual dissection flap:** the dissection flap distal to the graft usually remains. The false lumen has the potential to expand in the future and should be monitored.

Scanning

As for aortic dissection. Look for expansion of the aortic arch and descending aorta from the residual dissection.

Reporting should include:

- Describe the anatomy of the aortic root, arch, and descending aorta.
- Any residual dissection – location, extent.
- Any dilation of the unoperated sections of the aorta.
- Integrity of the aortic valve – well seated? regurgitation? obstruction?
- Any changes from previous scans.

Differential diagnosis

Residual dissection and surrounding atheroma can cause irregularities in the aortic wall, which resemble the junction between a graft and aorta.

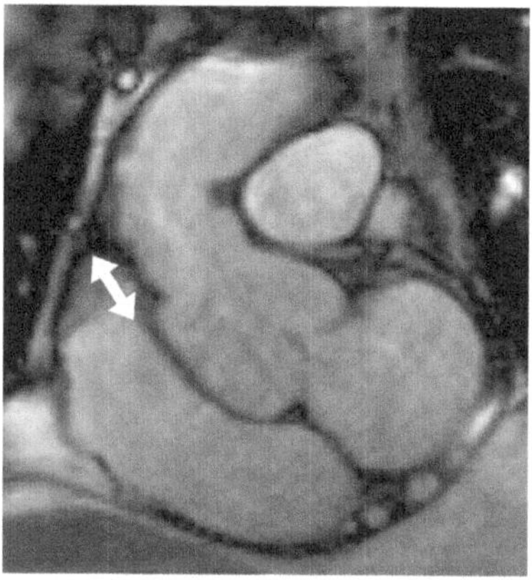

Fig. 13.17 Coronal LVOT view following an interpositional graft for acute type A dissection. The position of the short graft (arrow) can be appreciated by the change in aortic wall continuity at either end and the sharp angulation of the aorta at the distal end. Note the irregular aortic wall distal to the graft due to atheroma or thrombus in a small residual false lumen.

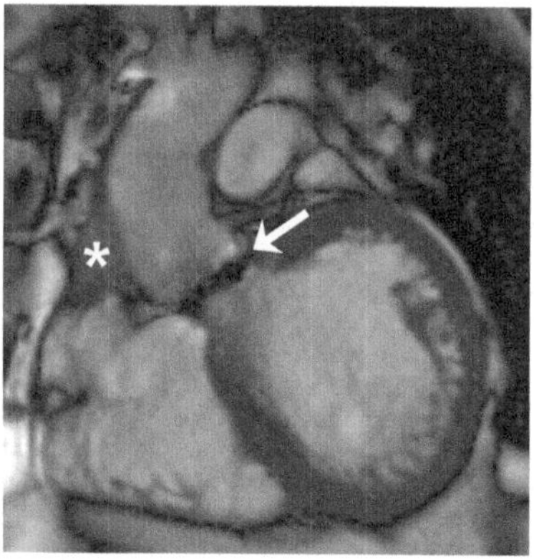

Fig. 13.18 Coronal LVOT view following combined aortic valve and root replacement. The metallic prosthetic aortic valve is easily seen (arrow), but the graft is less discernable, with only a slight angulation in the distal ascending aorta providing a clue to its presence. This scan was performed a week following surgery and some residual thrombus surrounding the root can be seen (*).

Aortic coarctation

Background

Coarctation is a narrowing of the aorta just distal to the left subclavian artery, where the ligamentum arteriosum is attached. Rarely, coarctation can occur in the abdominal aorta. There is a wide spectrum of severity, from mild kinking/narrowing (Fig. 13.19) to complete coarctation (total obstruction), and it may co-exist with the cervical arch syndrome (📖 p. 380).

The pathophysiology is debated, and may be due to alteration of intra-uterine aortic flow patterns or post-natal constriction as the ductus arteriosus fibroses (with excess fibroductal tissue). It may also be part of a more generalized aortopathy, with a genetic/developmental origin.

Over 50% of patients with coarctation have a bicuspid aortic valve. There is a pre-disposition to arterial stiffness and dilation, which may be due to the generalized aortopathy mentioned above, and this persists after coarctation repair and can lead to hypertension.

CMR features

- **Narrowed proximal descending aorta:** virtually always just distal to the left subclavian artery, the origin of which may also be involved with narrowing of the ostium. There may be mild post-stenotic dilation of the aorta.
- **Tortuous/kinked distal arch:**
  - Development of the surrounding aorta *in utero* may also be abnormal and a tortuous distal arch is common. This has some overlap with a cervical arch, which can co-exist
  - If considerable tortuosity or kinking is present without significant narrowing, a '*pseudo coarctation*' is said to be present. It is not associated with a significant pressure gradient and has no proven clinical consequences, although may be associated with an underlying aortopathy similar to coarctation.
- **Increased turbulence ± high velocity jet:** a narrowed turbulent jet is present in systole unless the coarctation is very mild (see Fig. 13.20). This may be flattened against the greater curve of the distal arch/descending aorta, or with a tortuous aorta may be angulated away from the midline. Persistence of the turbulent flow into diastole (a 'diastolic tail') suggests a more severe coarctation
- **± Dilated ascending aorta:** usually related to the severity of coarctation and the resultant proximal hypertension, but may also be exacerbated by the underlying aortopathy.
- **± Dilated head and neck vessels, and collateral circulation:** if severe coarctation is present, large collateral vessels develop from branches of the head and neck vessels to supply the lower body (see Fig. 13.21).
- **± Bicuspid aortic valve:** occurs in >50% of patients with coarctation. Should be imaged to confirm nature of valve and identify any significant obstruction/regurgitation (see 📖 p. 244).

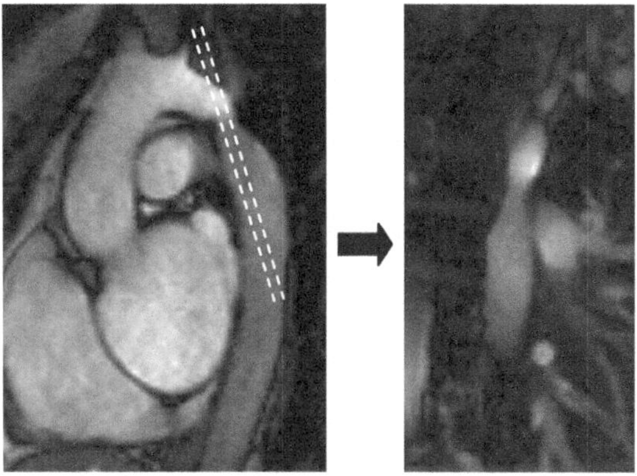

Fig. 13.19 Longitudinal aortic view of a mild coarctation (left), demonstrating the position for the orthogonal image slice (right) to fully appreciate the anatomy.

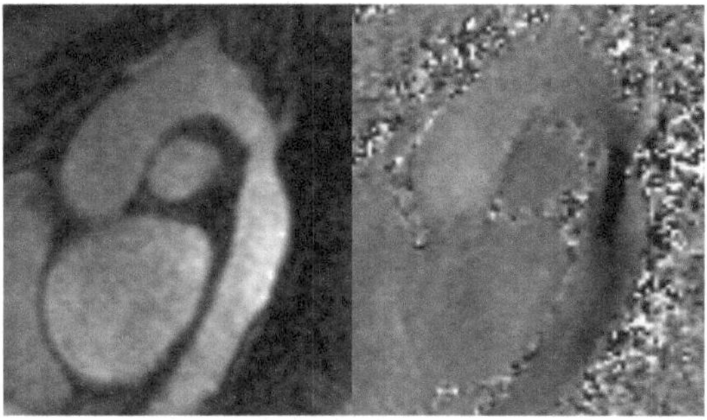

Fig. 13.20 In-plane flow mapping in the above patient, slightly rotated to align the direction of flow measurement with the likely jet (magnitude image, left). The flow image (right) shows the higher velocity jet arising from the coarctation.

Scanning

Transverse and oblique sagittal HASTE image stacks

These provide a good basis for further image planning and may sometimes provide the required information.

Longitudinal aortic view through the coarctation (SSFP cine)

This is the most useful to obtain, but often tricky – the coarctation is commonly surrounded by a tortuous section of aorta and it can be hard to visualize in a single plane. Multiple attempts may be required, starting with one plane, imaging through the coarctation to obtain an oblique coronal view (see Fig. 13.19), and imaging back through this to obtain a modified longitudinal plane through the coarctation. The aim should be to image only the coarctation section - including the rest of the aorta in the same image is not necessary and often impossible.

The turbulent jet can usually be seen in this view. In severe/complete coarctation obtaining a satisfactory image may not be possible, however, due to partial volume effects from the thick image slice.

Dilated head and neck vessels, and large collaterals can sometimes be seen on this image.

Oblique coronal view perpendicular to the longitudinal aortic view

Planned as in Fig. 13.19. This is useful for appreciating the full 3D anatomy as the coarctation may be worse in one plane.

± Short axis view through the coarctation

If mild–moderate, the true diameter of the coarctation may be imaged.

Velocity/flow mapping

To measure the velocity across the coarctation, in a similar fashion to stenotic valves. In-plane flow is helpful and can provide the peak velocity in mild-moderate cases – one of the longitudinal planes acquired above is usually best, rotated to align the flow direction with the expected flow through the coarctation (Fig. 13.20). Through-plane flow is better for more severe cases, with the image plane placed just distal to the coarctation. As for valves, flow mapping has a tendency to underestimate peak velocity.

In severe coarctation, there may be such a small or turbulent jet that accurate flow measurement is impossible. The severity of coarctation in these cases is usually clear from anatomical or cine images, and there is often persistence of forward flow into diastole (a diastolic 'flow tail'), which can be seen on flow or cine images.

Aortic valve imaging ± the ascending aorta

Ideally, the aortic valve should be imaged if not already characterized.

MR angiography of the aorta

Can be useful, especially if the coarctation is severe or the anatomy difficult (Fig. 13.21). Some advocate its use in all cases. Surface rendered images are helpful, but some detail is lost in these, and maximum intensity projection (MIP) images are better for visualizing very small channels.

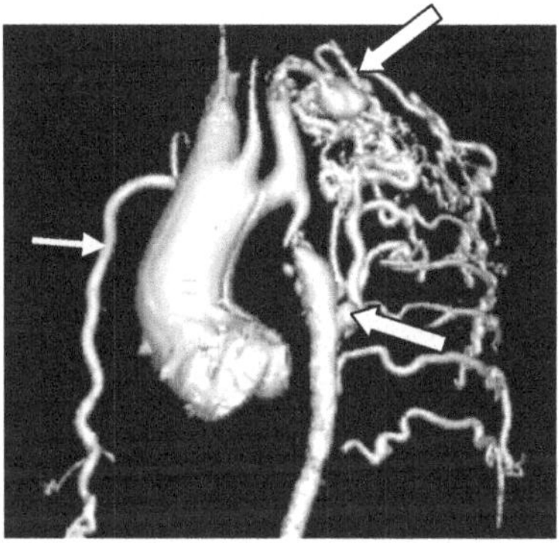

Fig. 13.21 Surface rendered MR angiogram of a complete coarctation. Note the dilated ascending aorta, the small descending aorta and the large collateral circulation with a dilated right internal mammary artery (short arrow). Intercostal artery aneurysms can also be seen (long arrows).

Reporting should include:

- **Description of coarctation and surrounding aorta:** include minimum diameter of the coarctation and the aorta above/below (this may be difficult if the mid arch is hypoplastic or there is post-stenotic dilation, but aim to measure a normal looking section). Include the severity (see Table 13.1).
- **Consequences:** dilated ascending aorta, head and neck vessels, and any collaterals (best seen on the angiogram). Note any intercostal artery aneurysms if seen.
- **Nature of aortic valve:** bi/tricuspid, whether narrowed etc.

Differential diagnosis

- Hypoplastic aortic arch – the mid arch is small in diameter but usually not severely narrowed. Can co-exist with coarctation.
- Cervical aortic arch (📖 p. 380)
- 'Pseudocoarctation' – significantly tortuous (and often narrowed) aorta but without severe narrowing.
- Interrupted aortic arch – more severe and complex abnormality, involving a failure of the mid-section of the aorta to form.

Guide to severity of coarctation

Table 13.1 Guide to severity of coarctation

	Mild	Moderate	Severe
Minimum diameter (proportion of reference aortic diameter)	>2/3	1/3-2/3	<1/3 or <5 mm diameter
Peak velocity (m/s)	< 3.0	3.0-4.0	>4.0
Estimated gradient (mmHg)	< 36	36-64	>64

NB This is only a rough indication and does not have a rigorous evidence base. An indication of mild/moderate/severe is helpful however when reporting.

Coarctation post-surgery/intervention

Surgery is usually performed in childhood, and residual or 're-coarctation' may occur if the surrounding aorta grows, but the repaired segment does not. In adults, angioplasty and stenting of the coarctation is an option, but the stent precludes any subsequent intra-stent MR imaging.

► Beware the artefact from metal surgical clips when imaging. This can cause the aorta to appear narrowed at the site of coarctation (see Fig. 13.23).

Types of repair

End-to-end anastomosis

The narrowed segment is removed and the two ends pulled together. Often results in a satisfactory result if the coarctation segment is short, particularly as the joined sections will grow with the child. The aorta appears mostly normal, but may have a narrowed section at the join.

Interpositional graft

An option if the resected segment is too long to join the remaining ends of the aorta together. Less common as this doesn't grow with the child.

Subclavian flap

The left subclavian artery is tied off and the proximal section used as a flap to widen the narrowed aorta. The left arm receives its blood supply from collaterals. CMR appearances similar to above, although the left subclavian artery will, of course, be absent.

Patch angioplasty

An elliptical patch is used to enlarge the aorta at the site of coarctation. Rarely used now due to a high incidence of late aneurysm formation, particularly with synthetic patches.

Aortic bypass graft

Bypassing the coarctation and inserting in the descending aorta beyond the coarctation. Can be from the subclavian artery (Fig. 13.22), the proximal descending aorta/arch or, occasionally, from the ascending aorta.

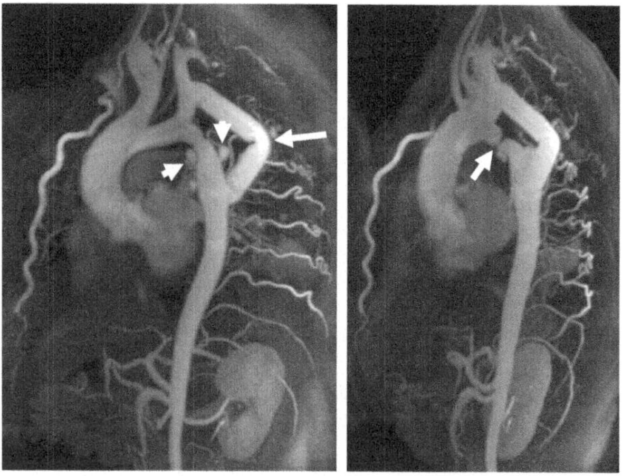

Fig. 13.22 Post-coarctation repair with a subclavian bypass graft (MIP images from 3D MR contrast angiography). The graft can be seen connecting the left subclavian artery to the descending aorta and has a slight kink (left, long arrow). There are also two small intercostal artery aneurysms close to the aortic origin, just distal to the coarctation (arrowheads). The severity of the coarctation is not well appreciated in the left image, due to the orientation, but a slightly rotated view (right) clearly demonstrates the tight stenosis (arrow) and also highlights the importance of image orientation in assessing tight coarctations. Note the hypoplastic aortic arch, and the dilated collateral circulation (head and neck vessels, intercostal and mammary arteries).

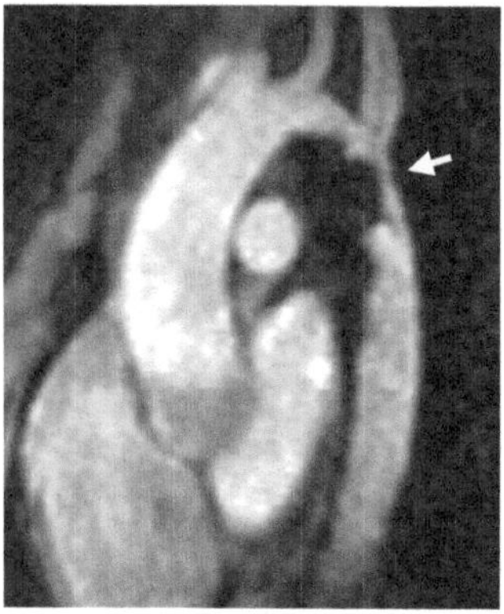

Fig. 13.23 Gradient echo sequence showing an apparently narrowed aorta following coarctation repair (arrow). Multiple metal surgical clips are present on the lesser curve at the coarctation site, causing the loss of signal and the apparent narrowing. Aortic catheterization did not demonstrate any significant stenosis or gradient.

Congenital variants

Cervical aortic arch

A congenital variant in which the aortic arch courses higher than normal and in part lies behind the left clavicle. It is an important finding to report, particularly if central venous cannulation is considered. The arch is often tortuous and/or hypoplastic, and a coarctation may be present.

Imaging can be difficult, but oblique sagittal HASTE images can identify the position of the arch relative to the clavicle, and MR angiography can be helpful (see Fig. 13.24).

It is believed to occur as a result of a failure in formation of the fourth left branchial arch (which normally forms the aorta). The aorta is formed from the third left branchial arch instead, which lies higher in the thorax.

Right-sided aortic arch

The aorta lies to the right of the spine in the chest, although may return to the left side in the abdomen. The ascending aorta is straighter than normal and the branching of the head and neck vessel may differ. Clinical consequences are nil unless there are additional lesions.

Transverse ± coronal HASTE imaging usually provides the diagnosis (Fig. 13.25), but this can be complimented by oblique sagittal imaging and/or MR angiography.

It is believed to occur due to atresia of the left dorsal aorta and left fourth branchial arch *in utero*, with the aorta formed from the corresponding right sided vessels.

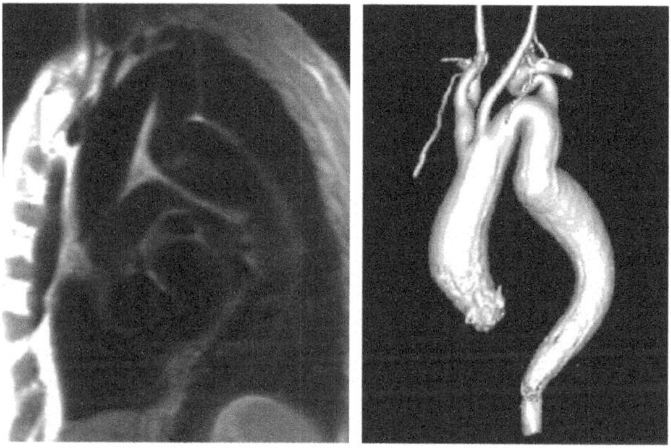

Fig. 13.24 Cervical aortic arch. Oblique sagittal HASTE image (left) and 3D rendered MR angiogram (right). Note the high position of the arch and the tortuous course. The origins of the head and neck vessels can be seen easily on the angiogram.

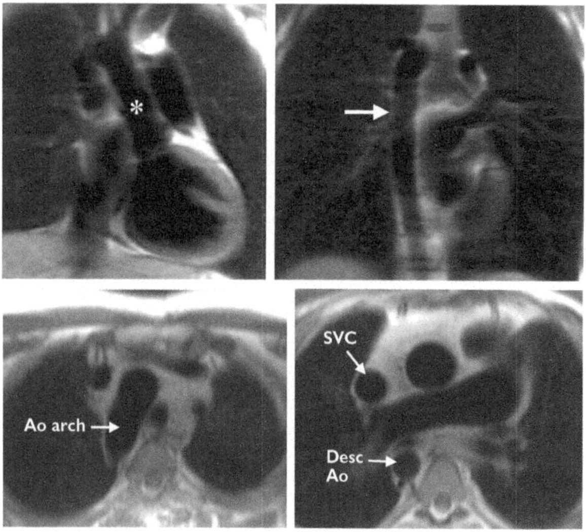

Fig. 13.25 Right-sided aortic arch. Coronal HASTE images (top) demonstrating the straight ascending aorta directed towards the right side (*) and the descending aorta to the right of the spine (arrow). Transverse HASTE images in another patient (bottom) showing the aortic arch (Ao arch) on the right side (bottom left) and the descending aorta (Desc Ao) lying to the right of the mid-line (bottom right). SVC = superior vena cava.

Chapter 14

Peripheral arteries

Introduction

Digital subtraction (x-ray) angiography (DSA) has been the gold standard for the diagnosis of carotid disease for many years. There are risks associated with the technique however (e.g. cerebral ischaemia/stroke, the invasive nature of the technique) and limitations due to variation in projection of the 2-dimensional images and interobserver variability. These led to the development of non-invasive imaging, particularly magnetic resonance angiography (MRA), which has become a common method of investigation. It offers both 2D and 3D imaging techniques for an accurate assessment of carotid, vertebral, and subclavian artery disease, with and without the use of gadolinium contrast. These vessels can be examined in a single scanning protocol with high image quality.

Non-contrast techniques

Non-contrast-enhanced techniques include time-of-flight (ToF) and phase-contrast (PC) methods. While the former can be used for the precise display of the carotid artery lumen anatomy, the latter is mainly used to obtain hemodynamic information, e.g. flow velocity. Both techniques rely on their inherent flow sensitivity and are thus not only time-consuming, but also prone to pitfalls associated with slow flow, turbulence, or patient motion during data acquisition.

Contrast-enhanced methods

Contrast-enhanced (CE) 3D MRA, on the other hand, is an ideal method for robust and time-efficient assessment of arterial lumen morphology. The high vascular signal due to T1-shortening of the blood pool by gadolinium and the insensitivity to flow artefacts are significant advantages, and imaging can be acquired in virtually any plane for optimal display of carotid, vertebral, and subclavian artery stenoses. Recently, higher field strength and parallel acquisition methods have enabled sub-millimetre spatial resolution in all three dimensions. Hence, changes of the lumen including eccentric stenosis can be detected and accurately assessed.

Further reading

Leiner T, Nizenhuis RJ, Maki JH *et al.* Use of a three-station phased array coil to improve peripheral contrast-enhanced magnetic resonance angiography. *J Magn Reson Imaging* 2004; **20:** 417–25.

Meaney JF. Magnetic resonance angiography of the peripheral arteries: current status. *Eur Radiol* 2003; **13:** 836–52.

Nael K, Michaely HJ, Villablanca P *et al.* Time-resolved contrast enhanced magnetic resonance angiography of the head and neck at 3.0 tesla: initial results. *Invest Radiol* 2006; **41:** 116–24.

Schoenberg SO, Rieger J, Nittka M *et al.* Renal MR angiography: current debates and developments in imaging of renal artery stenosis. *Semin Ultrasound CT MR* 2003; **24:** 255–67.

Steffens JC, Schafer FK, Oberscheid B *et al.* Bolus-chasing contrast-enhanced 3D MRA of the lower extremity. Comparison with intraarterial DSA. *Acta Radiol* 2003; **44:** 185–92.

Yang CW, Carr JC, Futterer SF *et al.* Contrast-enhanced MR angiography of the carotid and vertebrobasilar circulations. *Am J Neuroradiol* 2005; **26:** 2095–101.

Scanning and reporting: general aspects

A contrast-enhanced 3D angiographic dataset is usually acquired of the relevant region. Images can be acquired pre- and post-contrast with subsequent image subtraction for greater contrast-to-noise ratio. Patients therefore require an intravenous cannula in a large vein.

- See p. 116 for general acquisition techniques and p. 142 for post-processing.
- Recommended gadolinium does 0.1mmol/kg body weight.
- A typical injection rate for both the contrast bolus and the saline flush (20–30ml) is 2ml/s.
- **Image parameters:** TR and TE should be as short as possible (typically TR < 5–7ms; TE < 2–3ms). *Flip angle*: 30–45°, field of view 40–50cm, and a matrix of ideally 512 voxels, although 256 can be used for the larger vessels.
- Precise timing of imaging to the contrast bolus arrival in the relevant vessels is important for optimal imaging and to avoid signal contamination from venous contrast.

Post-processing

It is important to remember that although post-processing techniques are good for 3D visualization of vessel anatomy, degradation of the image quality can occur during processing, either obscuring or exaggerating pathology, particularly surface rendering techniques. The most robust way to detect pathological changes is still a careful evaluation of the unprocessed image data in all three major planes (coronal, sagittal, and transverse), though maximum intensity projection (MIP) viewing is usually robust.

Reporting: general

An MRA report should cover all of the following, if present:

- Anatomic variants.
- Tortuosity.
- Atherosclerotic changes.
- Inflammatory disorders (e.g. Takayasu arteritis).
- Stenosis severity.
- Occlusion.
- Aneurysm.
- Penetrating ulcer.

Head and neck vessels

Background

Carotid disease

Carotid disease, most frequently at the bifurcation, is the leading cause of cerebral ischaemia and stroke. Symptomatic patients with carotid stenosis >70% of the vessel lumen benefit from carotid endarterectomy, hence accurate measures of stenosis severity are important.

Subclavian and vertebral arteries

Clinically relevant atherosclerotic disease is rare. The left subclavian artery is more frequently involved than the right and, importantly, stenotic disease tends to include the origins of the vertebral arteries.

Significant proximal subclavian stenoses often cause retrograde flow in the ipsilateral vertebral artery, especially during exercise, resulting in 'subclavian steal' syndrome. Phase-contrast velocity measurements or time-resolved 3D CE-MRA can highlight the retrograde vertebral flow.

Scanning

A single 3D angiographic dataset is acquired of the supra-aortic vasculature, including the aortic arch, both subclavian arteries, the carotid arteries and vertebral arteries (Fig. 14.2).

- 1.5T scanners are fine, but 3.0T provides even higher contrast to noise.
- For carotid imaging, the head should be at the magnet iso-centre, and a dedicated head and neck coil provides the best signal.
- Scout images are obtained (Fig. 14.1a–c), and a fast phase-contrast MRA sequence with low spatial resolution may be used as vessel localizer for a more precise planning.
- The angiographic dataset is normally acquired in the coronal plane, to image both carotid arteries. To further characterize known carotid disease on one side, an additional sagittal acquisition can be used for optimal in-plane spatial resolution.
- In case of reverse flow in a vertebral artery due to subclavian artery occlusion or stenosis, it may be helpful to add transverse phase contrast sequences through the neck with velocity encoding in the range of 40cm/s.
- 3D contrast-enhanced MRA only displays the vessel lumen. To fully exploit MRI for the carotid vessel wall, 2D spin-echo sequences can be added to analyse the plaque composition or intima-media thickness.

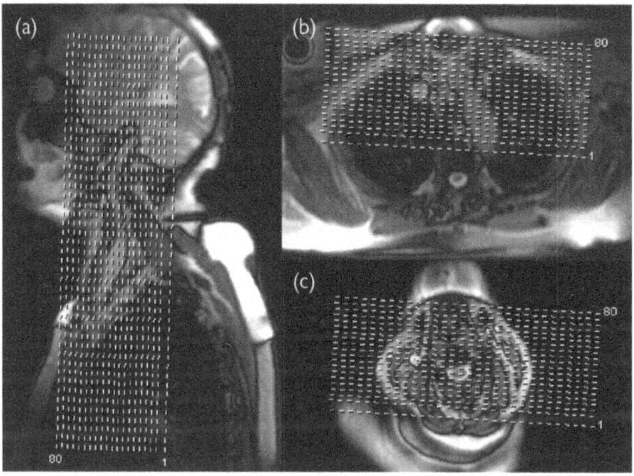

Fig. 14.1 Localizer sequence showing slice positions for the head and neck MRA data set: sagittal view (a), transverse thoracic view (b), and transverse neck (c).

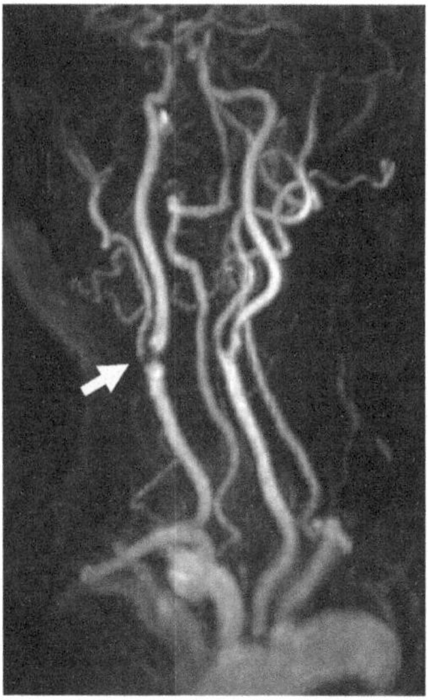

Fig. 14.2 Maximum intensity projection (MIP) in oblique sagittal view. A high-grade stenosis of the right carotid bifurcation is clearly seen (arrow).

Carotid and aortic vessel wall imaging

Atherosclerosis develops in the walls of large arteries, and thus techniques that image the vessel lumen, such as X-ray arteriography, give an incomplete picture of the distribution and quantity of atherosclerosis, and only image the silhouette of any atherosclerosis impinging on the lumen.

CMR is well-suited to both quantification and characterization of atherosclerosis in large arteries. For the moment, this is largely used in clinical research, e.g. in monitoring response to therapies, and no accepted clinical indications exist. However, in future, vessel wall imaging is likely to become clinically applicable.

Plaque anatomy and composition

- Using a combination of inherent MRI contrast generated in T1-WI, T2-WI, and proton density-weighted images (PD-WI), it is possible to determine both plaque anatomy and composition in the carotid arteries and aorta (Fig. 14.3). Atherosclerosis can also be identified in coronary arteries, but systematic evaluation of coronary artery atherosclerosis is currently difficult due to their small size and rapid motion.
- The lipid-rich plaque core appears bright (high signal) on T1-WI. It also has a shorter T2, and therefore appears dark compared with the adjacent cap and media, which appear bright on T2-weighted images.
- Calcified areas of plaque do not generate appreciable signal due to low water content, but can be detected as areas of low signal in multi-contrast images.

Scanning

The following protocol works well for vessel wall imaging:

- For quantification of aortic wall area, ECG gated double-inversion recovery (black-blood) fast spin echo images are acquired during breath-hold. (Typical parameters: FOV 200mm, TR 750ms, TE 11ms, in-plane resolution 0.8 × 0.8mm, slice thickness 5mm).
- Using an oblique sagittal image of the aorta as a pilot, serial axial images are acquired with 5mm interslice gap to cover the entire descending thoracic aorta. The mid-point of the right pulmonary artery in cross-section is used as the anatomical reference for the first slice in baseline and follow up scans.
- For the carotid arteries axial ECG-gated T2-weighted, black blood images of the neck are acquired during free breathing. Typical sequence parameters: FOV 150mm, TR 2 R–R intervals, TE 81ms, resolution 0.5 × 0.5mm in plane, slice thickness 3mm.
- Care should be taken to place aortic and carotid image slices perpendicular to the long axis of the vessel on the pilot images in order to limit partial volume effects.

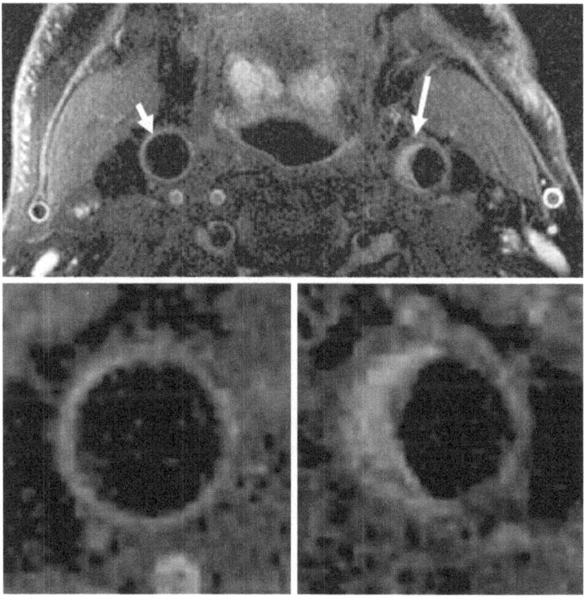

Fig. 14.3 High resolution T2-weighted transverse CMR of the neck. The upper panel demonstrates a normal smooth-walled right carotid artery (short arrow). By contrast, the left carotid (long arrow) contains a large heterogeneous eccentric atherosclerotic plaque. The lower panel shows magnified sections of each of these. Serial quantification of anatomically aligned slices can be used for studies of atherosclerosis progression and regression in humans. (Reproduced from Lee & Choudhury, 2007 with permission from BMJ Publishing Group Ltd.). Lee JM, Choudhury RP. Prospects for atherosclerosis regression through increase in high-density lipoprotein and other emerging therapeutic targets. *Heart* 2007; **93**: 559–64.

Table 14.1 MR signal characteristics of atherosclerotic plaque

	T1-WI	T2-WI	PD-WI
Fibrous cap	Intermediate SI	Intermediate SI	Intermediate SI
Lipid rich necrotic core	High SI	Low SI	High SI
Calcium	Low SI	Low SI	Low SI

Renal arteries

Background

Renovascular disease, particularly renal artery stenosis, is a cause of arterial hypertension and end-stage kidney disease. Effective treatments exist – percutaneous angioplasty/stenting and surgical repair – and renal MRA has largely replaced invasive digital subtraction angiography (DSA).

Alternative imaging includes ultrasound, but this is operator-dependent, is limited by its resolution and abdominal interfaces (e.g. bowel gas), and does not provide images for interventional planning. Computed tomography (CT) provides high resolution and is time-effective, but radiation and the use of nephrotoxic iodinated contrast hamper its widespread application in patients potentially suffering from renovascular disease.

Indications

Renal artery stenosis

Two main causes:

- Atherosclerotic disease is the most frequent. Typically eccentric narrowing at the renal artery origin, which usually involves the proximal third of the vessel and eventually progresses further.
- Fibromuscular dysplasia (FMD) produces a characteristic 'string of beads' in the mid-to distal portion of the renal artery.

Renal artery aneurysm

Most frequently results from atherosclerotic changes, but might also occur due to neurofibromatosis, polyarteriitis nodosa, or FMD.

Renal transplantation

- Before harvesting a kidney from a potential donor, anatomic variants must be identified prior to surgery. 3D CE-MRA comprehensively displays both kidneys with all variants.
- Transplant recipients can develop in-flow stenoses of the allograft artery from the iliac artery, which are an important and correctable cause of graft failure. MRA permits a multiplanar display of the postsurgical anatomy and can help identify obstacles to arterial and venous flow in the transplanted kidney.

Scanning

Both renal arteries, including major branches and accessory renal arteries, can be displayed in one MRA data set (Fig. 14.4). Functional information on flow can be acquired if required, using phase-contrast flow mapping.

- A dedicated abdominal phased array coil is best.
- The patient is placed supine with the mid-abdomen in the iso-centre.
- An oblique coronal plane, aligned with the abdominal aorta from the diaphragm to the iliac arteries, provides optimal coverage of the renal arteries and accessory vessels – acquisition time ~20s.
- Inclusion of the entire kidney parenchyma is desirable, as unsuspected renal masses or anomalies can be readily detected on the data set.
- Additional 2D sequences include T2-weighted transverse scans through the kidneys as well as a T1-weighted fat saturated scan after contrast injection.

Additional post-processing

See 📖 p.142 for general processing tips.

Calculation of cross-sectional area stenosis

Perpendicular slices through the stenotic lumen of a renal artery permit an assessment of the severity of a stenosis, comparable with intravascular ultrasound.

Reporting

See 📖 p. 386 for general MRA reporting. Additional aspects for renal arteries include:

- Fibromuscular dysplasia.
- The renal parenchyma should be checked for:
  - Cysts
  - Infarcts
  - Masses.
- Note the adrenal glands:
  - Cysts
  - Masses.

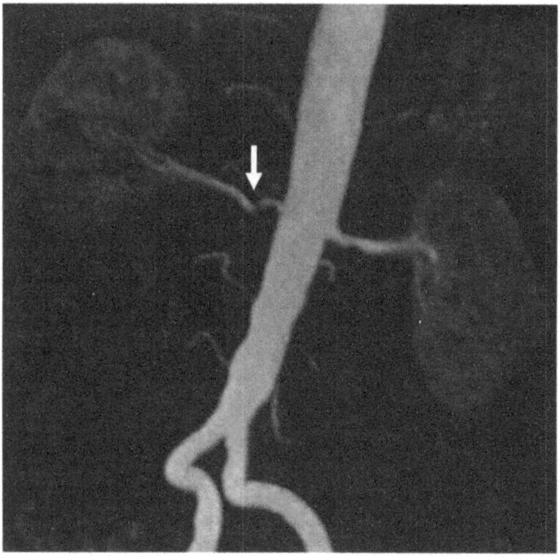

Fig. 14.4 Coronal view of a maximum intensity projection (MIP) of the renal arteries. Note the high grade stenosis of the right renal artery (arrow).

Iliac and leg arteries

Background

Peripheral vascular occlusive disease (PVOD) is due to systemic atherosclerosis, a process often simultaneously affecting other vascular beds. Atherosclerotic lesions (stenoses or aneurysms) frequently arise at sites of complex blood flow (e.g. branching points) and mechanical stress (e.g. adductor canal). 3D contrast-enhanced MRA provides a fast, comprehensive, and reliable visualization of the peripheral arterial system in patients with suspected PVOD.

Indications

- **Peripheral vascular occlusive disease:** the manifestation and extent of PVOD can be assessed accurately with 3D CE-MRA in a relatively short examination time, and those suitable for angioplasty or vascular surgery can be identified. Assessment of arterial disease in the lower leg remains challenging, however, due to substantial variations in the contrast travel-time in patients with occlusive disease. Time-resolved MRA may be an option in these cases.
- **Bypass grafts:** the patency of peripheral arterial bypass grafts can be reliably assessed and the degree of any stenosis determined.
- **Arteriovenous malformations:** arteriovenous malformations (AVM's) can cause complications due to spontaneous haemorrhage or local expansion. 3D CE-MRA can detect peripheral AVMs or fistulas, and helps distinguish feeding and draining vessels by early filling during a multi-phase examination, where both arterial and venous phases of the contrast material passage are imaged. Fast-flow AVMs can thus often be distinguished from haemangiomas or capillary malformations with slow flow.

Scanning

The peripheral arteries can be displayed in a single contrast-enhanced 3D dataset from the aortic bifurcation down to the feet (Fig. 14.5).

- Dedicated peripheral phased-array lower extremity coils guarantee optimal signal quality.
- Digital subtraction is especially helpful for the smaller vessels.
- Multi-station MRA is carried out after a single injection of contrast, using a series of 3D data acquisitions, following the bolus down to the legs (bolus chase technique). The three stations comprise the lower abdominal aorta, the iliac arteries, and the upper and lower leg arteries. While spatial resolution is lower for the upper two stations, the most distal station mandates highest spatial resolution as the diameter of the run-off arteries is small.
- The acquisition is started when the contrast reaches the infra-renal aorta. Each station is examined as fast as possible with reasonable spatial resolution in order to avoid venous overlap in the more peripheral territory.

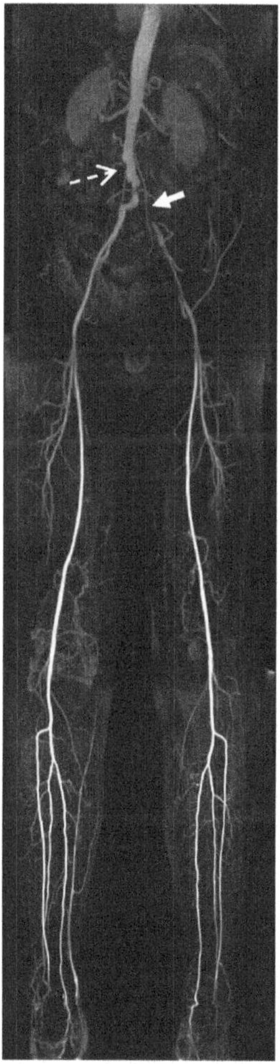

Fig. 14.5 Coronal view of a maximum intensity projection (MIP) composed of 3 multi-station MRA data sets. Note the atherosclerotic changes of the infrarenal aorta (dashed arrow) with occlusion of the left common iliac artery (thick arrow). The more distal leg vessels have no significant stenoses.

Improving the quality of very distal vessel images

- Bilateral venous compression at sub-systolic pressures over the upper thigh reduces arteriovenous recirculation time and prolongs the acquisition window for the lower leg arteries. The pressure (usually between 40–60mmHg) is kept constant from the very beginning of the examination to its end and is usually well tolerated.
- Start with a third of the volume of the contrast bolus for a single station MRA of the lower legs. After a short break (3–5min) the aorto-iliac and upper leg arteries are examined using a two-station protocol with the remaining contrast material. This technique is called hybrid-MRA.

Processing

Maximum intensity projections are generally better for smaller vessels, e.g. infra-popliteal arteries.

Future perspective

Whole-body 3D CE-MRA can provide a systemic imaging technique for this systemic disease. It involves 'chasing' the contrast bolus with 4–5 contiguous fields of view from head to toe, providing total coverage of the entire arterial tree (except for the coronary arteries) in ~1min (Fig. 14.6). This permits a comprehensive evaluation of the extent of atherosclerosis. However, whole-body 3D CE-MRA is still restricted to a few MR systems and its clinical value is currently under investigation.

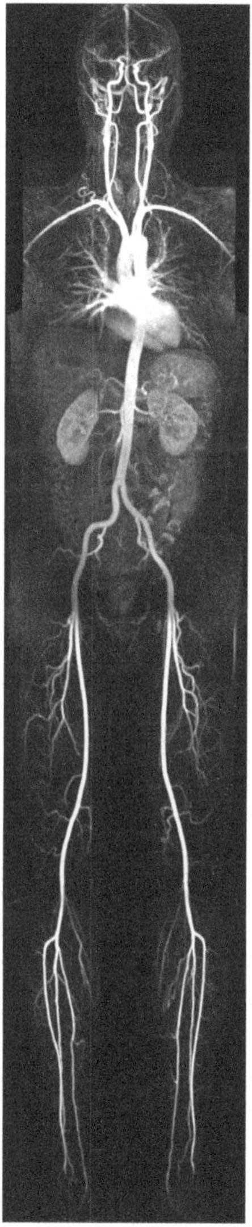

Fig. 14.6 Coronal view of a maximum intensity projection (MIP) of a whole-body MRA, compiled from 4 slightly overlapping multi-station MRA data sets. It gives an overview of the arterial vasculature from head to toe.

Coronary magnetic resonance imaging

Introduction

Imaging the coronary arteries with CMR is challenging due to their small size (2–5mm diameter), tortuous course, constant motion with both cardiac and respiratory cycles, and the variable orientation of the heart within the thorax. ECG and respiratory gating aid some of these, but the small size and tortuous course present the greatest challenges. Standard CMR slice thicknesses limit voxel resolution and accurate depiction of stenosis severity is particularly demanding. However, diagnostic images can be obtained, especially of the coronary origins, and further advances in technology will improve the robustness of MR coronary angiography for the assessment of vessel stenoses.

CMR features of coronary disease

- Origins and proximal course of the coronary arteries.
- Course and patency of coronary bypass grafts – mainly with contrast-enhanced MR angiography.
- Significant proximal and mid-vessel stenoses of the major epicardial vessels (in selected patients).

General scanning aspects

High resolution static images of the proximal coronary arteries are acquired by imaging a volume around the coronary origins. Data acquisition is limited to short periods, however, due to cardiac ± respiratory motion, and it is performed over many cardiac cycles to acquire sufficient data for image formation. This may be achieved by performing multiple breath-hold acquisitions or using respiratory gating.

Intravenous contrast

Although the addition of contrast may seem an attractive option to increase the signal/contrast to noise ratio and improve imaging, diffusion out of the arterial system during the long scans hampers image quality and contrast is not generally used. Future reductions in scan time combined with intravascular contrast agents may change this.

Fat saturation

The major coronary arteries lie within the atrioventricular and inter-ventricular grooves, surrounded by adipose tissue. Fat saturation pulses are, therefore, required to reduce the signal from the surrounding fat and highlight signal from the coronary arteries. The arteries are, however, distinguished from the myocardium and other surrounding structures.

Normal coronary artery origins

- The coronary arteries originate from the aortic root just distal to the aortic valve, in the sinuses of valsalva.
- The left main coronary artery normally originates from the left coronary sinus and varies in length before it branches into the left anterior descending (LAD) and left circumflex (LCx) arteries (Fig. 15.1).
- The right coronary normally arises from the right coronary sinus and follows the right atrioventricular (AV) groove between the right atrium and ventricle (Figs 15.1 and 15.2).

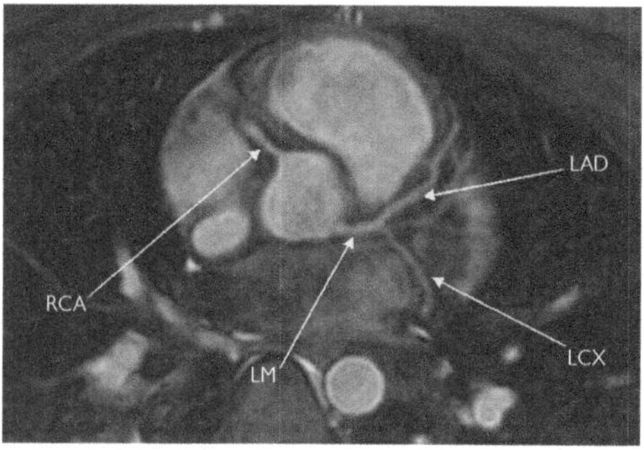

Fig. 15.1 Reformatted transverse view of the normal coronary artery origins. The left main stem (LM) branches into the left anterior descending LAD and left circumflex (LCx) arteries. The right coronary artery (RCA) enters the right atrioventricular groove and leaves the imaging plane.

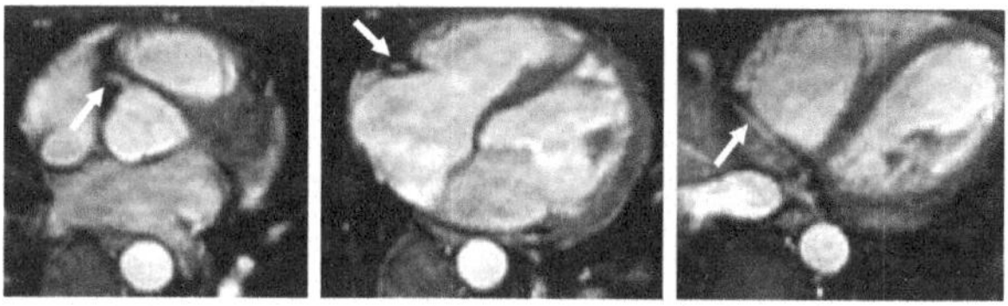

Fig. 15.2 Three unformatted transaxial slices from top (left) to bottom (right) demonstrating the right coronary artery as it courses along the right AV groove in its normal position.

Cardiac motion compensation

The motion of the coronary arteries during the cardiac cycle greatly exceeds the dimension of the vessels being imaged. The patterns of motion are predictable, however, and the timing and duration of image acquisition during the cardiac cycle can be optimized:

When to collect coronary image data

Two periods normally exist during the cardiac cycle when the coronary arteries are relatively motionless for a short while. A trigger delay is required to ensure image acquisition during this coronary 'rest' period:

- At the end of systole during iso-volumetric relaxation.
- During mid-diastole before atrial contraction.

The latter is normally used due to its longer duration, although its timing varies with heart rate. In patients with very high heart rates, a mid-diastolic rest period may not be identifiable. In these cases, imaging during the end systolic rest period is often a better choice, though it is very short, typically < 75ms.

Acquisition length

The acquisition time must be short enough to collect data during the above time periods. The number of segments (lines of k-space) acquired during each cardiac cycle normally requires individual adjustment.

Technique

Identification of the timing and duration of the rest period is accomplished with a cine acquisition.

- Acquire a single transverse SSFP cine image in the mid-upper RV, perpendicular to the right coronary artery in the AV groove. This allows observation of RCA motion through the cardiac cycle (Fig. 15.3).
- From the cine acquisition, identify the beginning, end, and duration of the rest period (Fig. 15.4).
- Adjust the trigger delay and acquisition time so image acquisition fits within the rest period.

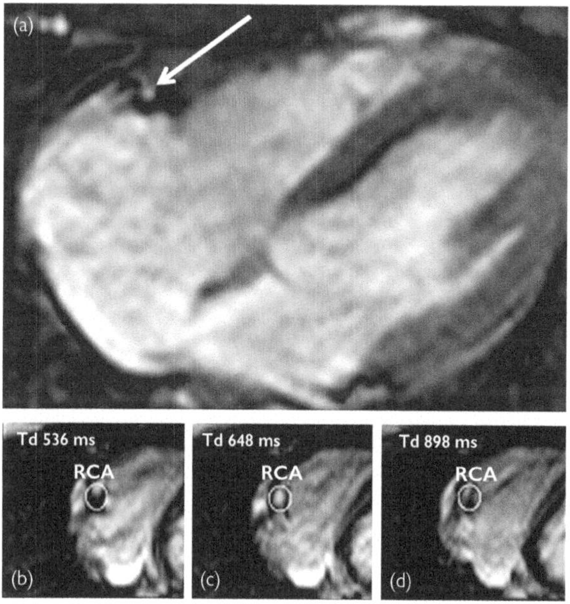

Fig. 15.3 Transverse SSFP image showing the right coronary artery in the right AV groove (a). Its position throughout the cardiac cycle can be determined, and the period of least motion identified (bottom). (b) Early diastole, still with RCA motion. The artery hasn't yet reached the optimal position (circled). (c) Mid-diastole with relatively immobile RCA (ringed) and (d) late diastole, during atrial contraction, when RCA motion occurs again and the vessel moves out of the ring.

Coronary sequences

'Coronary' sequences involve high resolution scanning of a large cuboid volume of interest containing the coronary artery/arteries (with very narrow slice thicknesses). This involves acquiring large amounts of data and is achieved by either:

- Combining 3D imaging sequences with image acceleration or partial Fourier techniques.
- Acquiring smaller 3D volumes that cover only the coronary artery of interest.

The left and right coronary systems can be imaged separately (the standard approach) or newer 'whole heart' sequences can image both coronary systems in one large image volume covering the entire heart. Both methods use multiple breath-holds/'navigator' respiratory gating, timing data acquisition to mid-diastole and fat saturation.

Individual coronary imaging

- A low resolution coronary sequence can be used as a scout to identify the area of interest, although the same trigger delay should be used for both low and high resolution images. If a large area is imaged (from the main PA to the diaphragm), it can be used to plan both left and right coronary artery positions.
- Adjusting the coverage and/or position of the imaged volume is often required as the orientation of the coronary arteries varies considerably with different orientations of the heart.
- High resolution scans can be positioned to include only the region of the proximal coronary vessels.

Left coronary artery positioning

The left coronary artery normally lies just below the main pulmonary artery, and the proximal vessels (left main stem, LAD and LCx) can be imaged in an oblique transaxial plane. Coronal scout images are good for identifying the area to be covered.

Right coronary artery positioning

- The RCA normally courses in the right AV groove and the imaging plane/slab is best positioned parallel to the basal plane. Scout images in basal short axis or transaxial planes are good for image positioning.
- Three-point planning (📖 p. 96) can be used on selected systems to indicate the course of the RCA – three points should be chosen at the ostium, in mid-vessel and a distal point.

Phase encoding direction

This must be chosen to suit the situation:

- For breath-holding techniques, the phase encode direction should be anterior-posterior (AP) to allow for a smaller AP field of view and shorter breath holds.
- For navigator sequences, phase encoding should be right-to-left in order to reduce artefacts from chest wall motion.

Whole heart imaging

Newer sequences allow high resolution imaging of the whole heart, usually with navigator respiratory compensation techniques. These take longer, but do not require locating the coronary arteries beforehand as they can be identified during post-processing. SSFP sequences are typically used for such applications.

2D or 3D sequences?

Standard 2D sequences produce image data, which can be viewed in multiple contiguous slices. These can be used to identify the coronary anatomy, but may lack the spatial resolution required to give much more information than the location of the vessels.

With the development of faster data techniques, '3D' sequences can allow 'isotropic' sub-millimeter spatial resolution (i.e. cube-shaped voxels with dimensions <1mm). The resulting image data can then be viewed from any angle (with appropriate software), which can be invaluable for coronary imaging. It can facilitate visualization of smaller vessels and stenoses, although robust quantification of stenosis severity remains a goal of many research groups around the world.

Both techniques can be used for either individual coronary imaging or whole-heart sequences.

Anomalous coronary artery origins

Anomalous coronary arteries occur in 1–2% of cases, although the incidence can be as high as 5% if separate ostia, high origins, and fistulae are included. The most common anomalies include separate ostia for LAD and circumflex arteries, a high origin of the RCA, and an aberrant circumflex artery from the right coronary sinus (coursing posteriorly round behind the aorta to join the AV groove), each with an incidence of ~0.5–1%. Defining the origin and course of anomalous coronary arteries is important as malignant and benign forms are described:

- **Malignant forms** of anomalous coronary anatomy occur when the vessel courses between the ascending aorta and the main pulmonary artery (Fig. 15.4). These are believed to be at risk of compression during systole, especially on exertion, although evidence for this mechanism is weak. There is an association between malignant forms of anomalous coronary arteries and sudden death, believed to be due to obstruction of coronary flow causing malignant ventricular arrhythmias.
- **Benign forms** include the presence of a vessel anterior to the pulmonary artery (Fig. 15.5) or posterior to the ascending aorta, where there is much lower risk of external compression.

Intervention may be necessary depending on the form of anomaly and clinical circumstances. Options include surgical re-implantation of the anomalous vessel or stenting to protect against external compression.

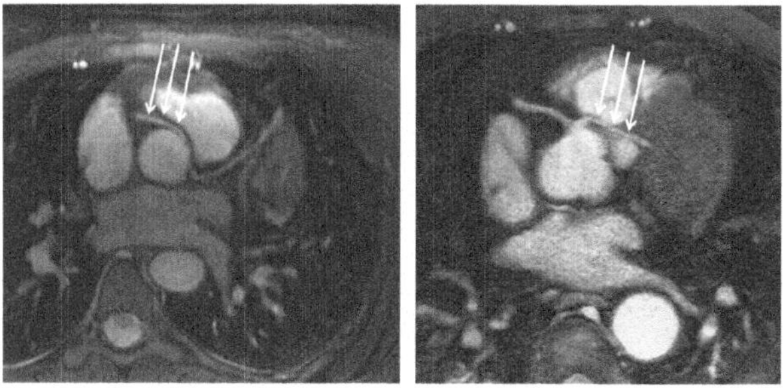

Fig. 15.4 Malignant forms of anomalous coronary arteries. (Left) An anomalous RCA originating from the left cusp and passing between the aorta and pulmonary artery (arrowed). (Right) aberrant LMS originating form the right cusp.

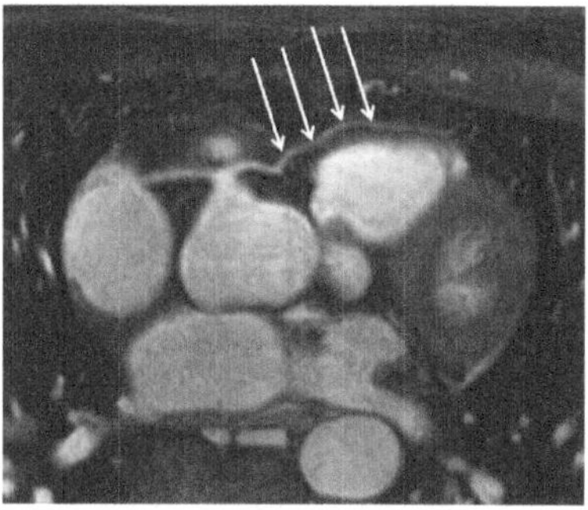

Fig. 15.5 A benign form of anomalous coronary artery origin: LAD artery arising from the right coronary cusp and coursing anterior to the pulmonary artery (arrowed).

Further reading

Angelini, P. Coronary artery anomalies. *Circulation* 2007; **115:** 1296–305.

Kim WY, Damias PG, Stuber M *et al.* Coronary magnetic resonance angiography for the detection of coronary stenoses. *N Engl J Med* 2001; **345**(26): 1863–9.

Chapter 16

Systemic and pulmonary veins

Systemic veins

The systemic veins are not routinely imaged specifically, although CMR can provide useful anatomical information when required. Common reasons for focused imaging include anomalous connections and stenoses/obstructions.

Scanning

Transaxial, coronal, and sagittal images

Either HASTE, turbo-spin echo or multi-slice SSFP images can be used (see Fig. 16.1) – the latter are often better for venous imaging. These are good for baseline imaging and may provide the required information, e.g. on the course of the great veins and any anomalous connection.

SSFP cine imaging through the relevant vein/connection

Although flow is slow, SSFP cines provide good contrast between the lumen and wall, and any flow disturbance or stenoses may be seen (Fig. 16.2). Use the above images in the major body planes for planning the cine image position – the baseline images may even be in an appropriate plane. There is some variation in orientation however, so flexibility is required. Thin slices may be required for smaller veins.

- The inferior vena cava (IVC) connection to the right atrium is often imaged in an oblique sagittal view (planned from the transaxial images).
- The superior vena cava (SVC) is often imaged in an oblique coronal view (again planned from the transaxial images). This plane may sometimes include the innominate vein.
- The innominate (brachiocephalic) vein normally lies in an almost coronal plane, crossing the midline from left to right in front of the aortic arch to enter the SVC.
- The subclavian veins lie in an oblique coronal plane, but are often hard to visualize with cine images due to their small size relative to the slice thickness.

Contrast angiography

Timed to the venous phase of contrast distribution, to visualize the great veins. This is useful for more tortuous or complex anatomy that cannot be visualized with cine imaging and for smaller veins, e.g. subclavian.

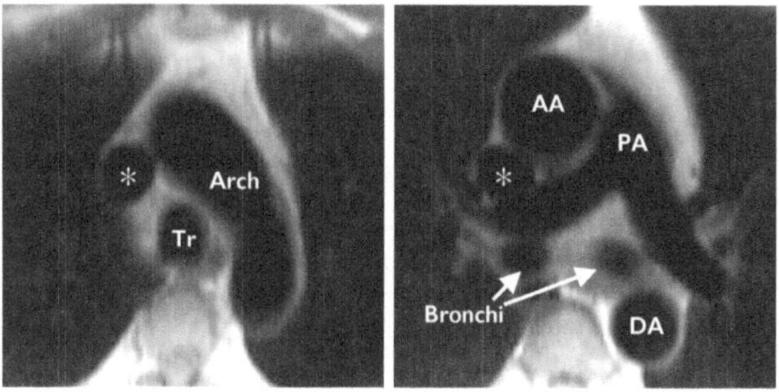

Fig. 16.1 Transaxial HASTE images in the superior mediastinum showing the SVC (*) as it descends from superior (left) to inferior (right). Tr = trachea; AA = ascending aorta; PA = pulmonary artery; DA = descending aorta.

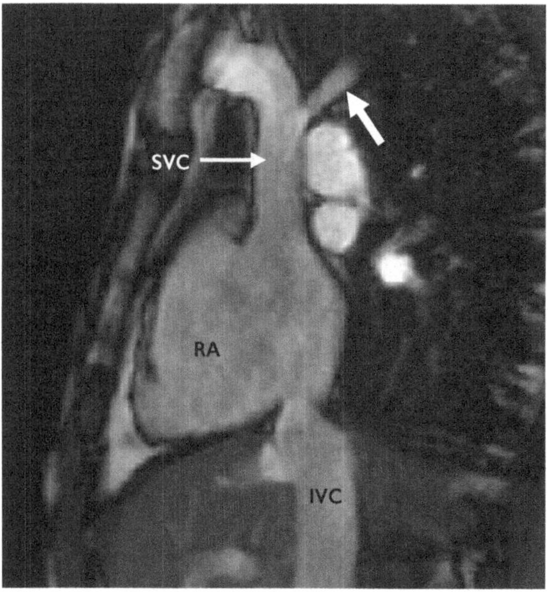

Fig. 16.2 Oblique sagittal SSFP image showing systemic venous drainage into the right atrium (RA). Note the azygous vein draining into the posterior aspect of the SVC (thick arrow) and the IVC coursing through the liver before entering the right atrium just above the diaphragm.

Left superior vena cava

Background

- Prevalence: 0.3% of the population (~3% if other congenital heart disease present).
- 90% have bilateral SVC's; a 'bridging' innominate vein is sometimes present.
- 10% have only a left SVC, with an innominate vein draining the right subclavian and jugular veins from right to left across the midline.
- The left SVC drains into an enlarged coronary sinus before entering the right atrium.
- Occurs due to persistence of the left anterior cardinal vein *in utero*, forming the left SVC, with or without regression of the right anterior cardinal vein (which forms the normal right-sided SVC).

Associated abnormalities

A left SVC can be an isolated finding, but the rarer variant (with absent right SVC) is also associated with other anatomical conditions (from Bartram *et al.*, 1997):

- Left azygous vein joining the left SVC (44%).
- ASD (16%).
- VSD (5%).
- Coarctation of the aorta (7%).
- Tetralogy of Fallot (7%).
- A-V canal defects (11%).
- Coronary sinus 'unroofing'. A connection to the left atrium (which lies above the coronary sinus) is formed by an absence of the superior section (or 'roof') of the coronary sinus, causing a right-to-left shunt (7%).

It can also be associated with rhythm abnormalities – AF, AV re-entry tachycardias, and SA and AV nodal problems.

Clinical significance

As an isolated finding, a left SVC is of no functional significance as venous drainage occurs to the appropriate cardiac chamber without shunting.

Pacemaker/ICD insertion

A left SVC can cause significant problems when inserting a transvenous pacing or ICD lead. Commonly, this is performed via the left subclavian vein and would follow the course of the left SVC into the coronary sinus before entering the right atrium. Pacing can be achieved via this route but is much more complex. Alternatives include pacing via the right subclavian vein, or if a bridging innominate vein is present, to guide the lead across this into the normal right SVC.

Scanning

- Normally easily identified on transaxial (Fig. 16.3) or coronal imaging.
- Cine imaging in a modified LV vertical long axis (VLA) view can sometimes visualize the vein running behind the left atrium (Fig. 16.4).
- A basal short axis view can identify the dilated coronary sinus (Fig. 16.3).

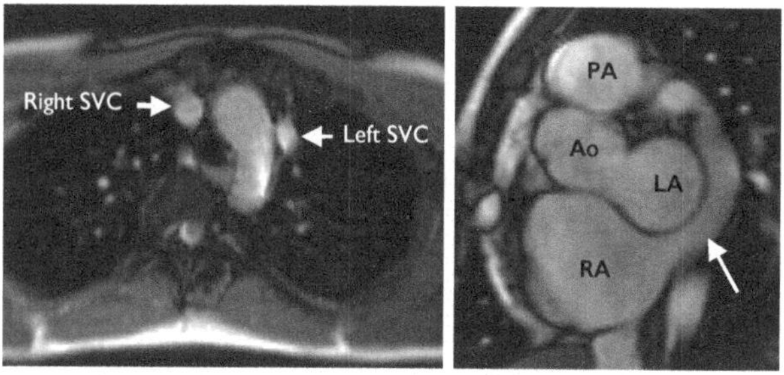

Fig. 16.3 Bilateral SVC's. (Left) Transaxial SSFP image showing both right and left SVC's either side of the aortic arch. (Right) Dilated coronary sinus (arrowed) in a short axis basal slice. PA = pulmonary artery; Ao = aorta; RA = right atrium; LA = left atrium.

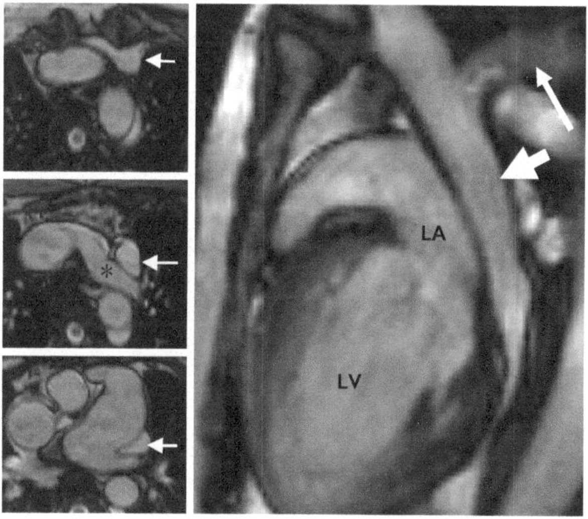

Fig. 16.4 Left SVC without right SVC. (Left) Transaxial SSFP images showing the isolated SVC (arrowed) with a right innominate vein draining into it superiorly (top), the vein descending adjacent to the left pulmonary artery (asterisk, middle) and where it joins the coronary sinus inferiorly (bottom). (Right) Modified VLA view showing the left SVC running behind the left atrium (thick arrowhead), with a left azygous vein draining into it posteriorly (long arrow). LA = left atrium; LV = left ventricle.

Further reading

Bartram U, Van Praagh S, Levine JC *et al.* Absent right superior vena cava in visceroatrial situs solitus. *Am J Cardiol* 1997; **80:** 175–83.

Occluded systemic veins

Causes

SVC obstruction

- External obstruction from lymphoma or right bronchial carcinoma.
- Pacemaker leads: either their presence or recent removal of a long-standing lead, causing intravenous thrombosis.

IVC obstruction

- Thrombus: extension of iliofemoral venous thrombosis.
- Intraluminal tumours (e.g. renal cell carcinoma).
- Trauma.
- External compression (e.g. gravid uterus).
- Budd-Chiari syndrome (very rare).

CMR features

Abrupt change in lumen diameter

Best appreciated on SSFP sequences in the long axis of the vein. Ensure the vein does not move out of plane, creating an artefactual stenosis, by including a second image perpendicular to the first to check this.

Change in lumen signal characteristics

If thrombus present, signal characteristics are often altered – generally intermediate signal (compared with low signal from flowing blood on HASTE imaging, or high blood signal on SSFP imaging; see Fig. 16.5).

Altered flow

Turbulence due to a stenosis or absence of flow disturbance if occluded.

Scanning

As above, with an emphasis on obtaining long axis images of the vein.

SSFP cines and multi-slice (static) images

Ideal for identifying stenoses and occlusions. Flow disturbance can often be seen on cine imaging.

HASTE/turbo spin echo imaging

Can be helpful for identifying thrombus/other masses.

Phase velocity flow imaging

Can be useful for clarifying the nature/severity of the stenosis. Flow velocities are low, however, and it may be difficult to identify altered velocities. The absolute velocity measurement is rarely helpful – relative flow velocities are more useful.

± Contrast

- Early post-gadolinium images can be helpful for identifying thrombus (no uptake of contrast).
- MR angiography in the venous phase can visualize stenoses/occlusions.

Reporting

- Presence, location, and severity of any stenosis/occlusion.
- Any apparent cause – thrombus visible? tumour/mass seen?

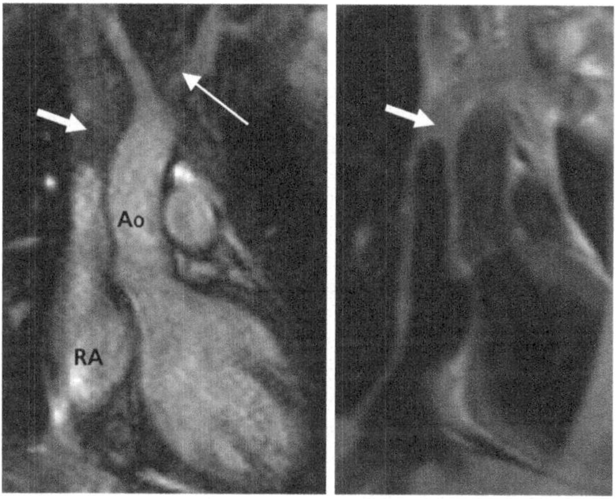

Fig. 16.5 Occluded SVC. Modified coronal views from SSFP cine (left) and turbo spin-echo sequence (right). There is thrombus in the SVC (thick arrows), caused by recent removal of a longstanding pacing wire. Extension of the thrombus into the innominate vein can be seen (thin arrow). Ao = aorta; RA = right atrium.

Pulmonary veins

Normal anatomy

The four pulmonary veins normally drain into the posterior left atrium, and are of roughly equal size (see Fig. 16.6). They have a variable orientation, but lie roughly in a coronal plane. The ostial sections are sometimes flattened, and there may be an oval or slit-like orifice in the left atrium. The left atrial appendage lies just anterior to the left upper pulmonary vein and can appear like a stump of another pulmonary vein.

Right middle accessory vein

The right middle lobe can be drained by a separate branch directly into the left atrium (the middle accessory vein) or into the right lower pulmonary vein, forming an early 'branch', rather than an accessory vein.

Common isthmus of the left pulmonary veins

The left pulmonary veins often (~50%) drain into a short common isthmus before draining into the left atrium.

Scanning

Transaxial and coronal images

Pulmonary veins can be visualized in standard planes on SSFP multi-slice (preferred) or HASTE sequences. The complex shape of the left atrium and variable orientation of each of the pulmonary veins makes this a less robust technique, however, for identifying all pulmonary veins.

Whole-heart sequences (📖 p. 405)

The high resolution can provide good visualization of the pulmonary veins, though without the surface rendered 3D views of MR angiography.

Contrast angiography (📖 p. 116)

This is the best method for imaging the pulmonary veins, particularly when planning radiofrequency ablation of the left atrium.

- Choose a coronal slab with the centre in the middle of the left atrium.
- Time the imaging to coincide the contrast bolus in the left atrium with the centre of K-space of the sequence. If the timing is correct, the left atrium and pulmonary veins can be isolated during processing using an intensity threshold technique, which removes other structures, including the pulmonary arteries. In general, it is better to have some contrast present in the aorta than significant amounts left in the pulmonary arteries (the aorta can easily be edited out in processing).
- The contrast bolus is more spread out in patients with variable heart rates or low cardiac output, and the left atrium/pulmonary veins can be harder to discriminate, with extra editing required during processing.
- The images can be processed with appropriate software, and surface rendered images are best for visualization (see Fig. 16.6). Edit out the aorta and pulmonary arteries to view the pulmonary veins easily.
- Significant left to right shunts (e.g. ASDs) can create problems with residual contrast present in the pulmonary circulation. Careful editing or visualization is required to differentiate the pulmonary veins from the arteries (see Fig. 16.7).

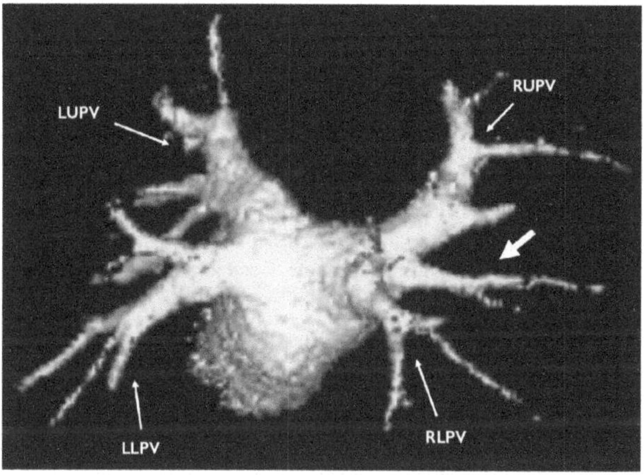

Fig. 16.6 Surface-rendered contrast angiogram of normal pulmonary veins, viewed from posteriorly. LUPV = left upper pulmonary vein; LLPV = left lower pulmonary vein; RUPV = right upper pulmonary vein; RLPV = right lower pulmonary vein. The arrow indicates an accessory right middle pulmonary vein.

Partial anomalous pulmonary venous drainage

Congenital defect with 1 or 2 pulmonary veins connecting anomalously – usually into the SVC, IVC, or innominate vein. This creates a left to right shunt of variable quantity, with potential effects including RV ± pulmonary artery dilation. May be asymptomatic, depending on the degree of shunt.

CMR features

- Abnormal connection of a pulmonary vein – unilateral mostly, bilateral partial anomalous connections are rare. Common variations:
  - Right upper and middle lobe veins drain to SVC or right atrium (most common)
  - Right pulmonary veins drain to IVC – usually entering just above the diaphragm
  - Left upper vein to innominate vein via an anomalous vertical vein
  - Left upper or lower veins to coronary sinus.
- Left to right shunt.
- Dilated RV secondary to the left to right shunt.
- Commonly associated with an ASD (especially sinus venosus type), although also associated with other congenital cardiac defects.

Scimitar syndrome

Named after the appearance of the anomalous pulmonary venous connection on CXR, which resembles a scimitar or Turkish sword. The syndrome is a combination of:

- Right anomalous pulmonary vein(s) connecting to the IVC.
- Anomalous systemic arterial supply to the right lower lung.
- Hypoplasia of the right lung ± sequestration.

There are associated lesions in 25% (ASD, VSD, PDA, coarctation).

Scanning

- ***LV and RV volumes*** To determine the effect on the RV particularly.
- ***Aortic and pulmonary flow*** For shunt calculation
- ***MR angiography*** As for standard pulmonary vein imaging. The left to right shunt will result in residual contrast in the pulmonary arteries and care is required in editing and visualization (see Fig. 16.7).

Reporting should include:

- Location and connection of anomalous pulmonary vein(s).
- Confirmation of normal connections for other pulmonary veins.
- Degree of left to right shunt: pulmonary to aortic flow volume ratio.
- LV and RV volumes and function: determines effect of shunt.
- Any other associated lesions.

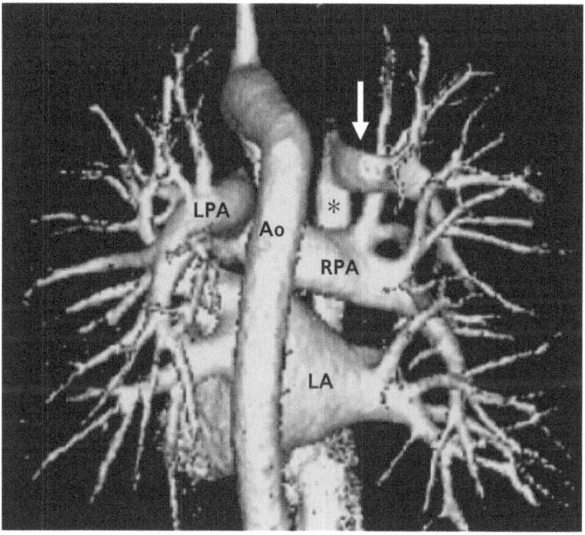

Fig. 16.7 Contrast pulmonary angiogram with surface rendering, showing partial anomalous pulmonary venous drainage from a posterior view. Three pulmonary veins drain normally into the left atrium (LA), while the right upper pulmonary vein (arrowed) is high and drains into the SVC (*). RPA = right pulmonary artery; LPA = left pulmonary artery; Ao = aorta.

Total anomalous pulmonary venous drainage

Congenital defect with all the pulmonary veins draining into the systemic venous system. The veins usually form a common trunk:

- **Supracardiac** (the most common variant): the common trunk forms an ascending vein which usually joins the innominate vein.
- **Infracardiac:** a descending vein (common trunk) drains to the IVC, portal vein, hepatic veins, or ductus venosus.
- **Cardiac:** the anomalous veins drain into the coronary sinus or directly to the right atrium. There may not be a common trunk.

Survival is dependent on mixing of the two venous systems via an ASD. Patients nearly always present as a neonate with profound cyanosis and cardiac failure, and undergo urgent corrective surgery. Adults, who form the largest group likely to undergo CMR, are usually post-surgery. This involves connection of the common trunk to the left atrium, ligation of the ascending/descending vein, and usually closure of the ASD. For the cardiac TAPVD group, the atrial septum is usually moved to include the pulmonary veins on the left atrial side.

CMR features

- Common pulmonary venous trunk, connected to the left atrium if post-repair, or systemic veins if in a rare, unoperated, patient.
- Obstruction to the pulmonary trunk or atrial connection can occur.
- Following successful repair, LV and RV volumes should be normal. Pre-surgery, RV dilatation is usual from the profound left to right shunt.
- ± Residual ASD.

Scanning

- **Standard long axis cine imaging:** may reveal the common trunk behind the left atrium (Fig. 16.8), and important for LV and RV function assessment.
- **LV and RV volumes.**
- **Additional cine imaging of the pulmonary veins:** the trunk may be viewed in a slightly oblique coronal plane, but non-standard image planes are often required. Look for stenoses in particular.
- **± Flow imaging:** if significant residual shunt suspected (e.g. from ASD).
- **± MR pulmonary angiography:** often helpful to confirm findings.

Reporting should include:

- Location and connection of common trunk/pulmonary vein(s).
- Any stenosis in the trunk or connection to the left atrium.
- Any residual ASD or shunt – quantify with flow volumes.
- LV and RV volumes and function.

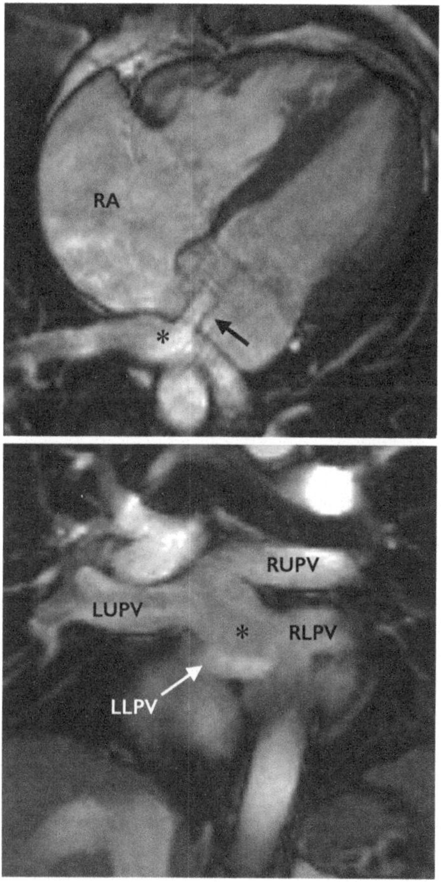

Fig. 16.8 Repaired infracardiac total anomalous pulmonary venous drainage. Top: HLA view; the pulmonary veins form a common trunk (*), which runs behind the left atrium and previously drained into the IVC. The IVC connection has been ligated and the common trunk connected to the left atrium by a 'window' in the posterior wall of the LA. With growth of the patient, this window has become relatively small and may restrict inflow (arrowed), creating an analogous haemodynamic condition to mitral stenosis. Note also the residual ASD. Bottom: coronal view through the common trunk showing the 4 pulmonary veins (the left lower pulmonary vein is slightly out of plane).

Pulmonary vein stenosis

This is mostly a recent phenomenon, caused predominantly by previous radiofrequency ablation within a pulmonary vein – a treatment for atrial fibrillation. Modern electrophysiological therapy avoids intrapulmonary ablation because of this potential problem and ablation is usually performed in a circumferential pattern in the left atrium, around the pulmonary vein ostia. However, there are still patients with previous ablation within the pulmonary veins who may require investigation. Pulmonary vein stenosis can also be congenital (rare), due to previous cardiac/thoracic surgery close to the pulmonary veins or from external compression due to tumour or other mass effect.

CMR features

- **Narrowed pulmonary vein:** this usually occurs close to the insertion into left atrium, where previous ablation therapy has taken place (see Fig. 16.9). There is no absolute cut-off for stenosis, but visual comparison to the rest of the pulmonary vein and to the other veins usually provides a good appreciation of the degree of any stenosis. Be aware of the sometimes flattened nature of the veins close to the ostium. This should not be confused with stenosis, which is usually circumferential.
- **± Adjacent mass:** if tumour/other external compression is present.

Scanning

MR pulmonary angiography (📖 p. 417) is the best method for visualizing stenosis.

Reporting should include:

- Location and severity of any stenosis.
- Any additional pathology (e.g. mass).

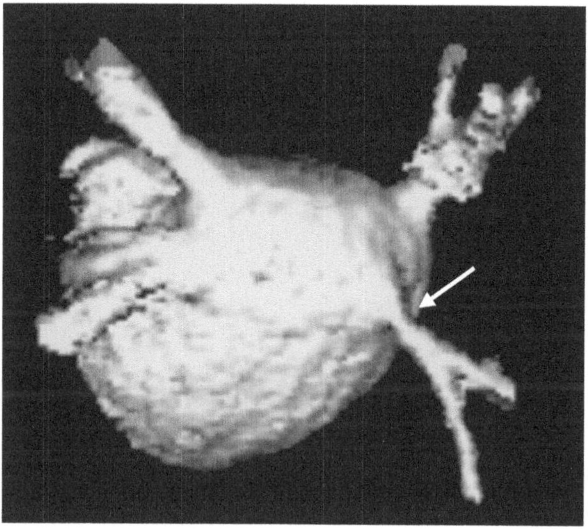

Fig. 16.9 Pulmonary MR angiogram with surface rendering viewed from the posterior. The patient had intrapulmonary vein radiofrequency ablation previously and has developed a right lower pulmonary vein stenosis (arrowed).

Chapter 17
Extracardiac findings

Background

The prevalence of significant extracardiac findings with CMR varies and is strongly influenced by patient selection. Age affects both the likelihood of cardiac-related secondary findings and incidental non-cardiac related findings. The size of the field of view (FOV) determines the coverage of the thoracic and abdominal cavities and the organs displayed.

Many additional lung parenchymal, skeletal, soft tissue and intra-abdominal abnormalities can be identified, despite the lower resolution of CMR compared to CT. The majority of these findings are not clinically important, however, e.g. simple liver cysts.

▶ It is important, whatever the coverage, that all images are reviewed, including gradient-echo localizers, to ensure relevant diagnoses are not missed.

▶ The ability to recognize abnormalities and the understanding of normal anatomy, variant anatomy, and imaging artefacts is important.

At least 4% of incidental findings have an impact on patient management and include:

- Unsuspected lung carcinoma.
- Breast carcinoma.
- Pulmonary embolism.
- Pneumonia.
- Pulmonary sarcoidosis.

The list of findings in this chapter is not exhaustive, but includes a range of common conditions and describes their typical appearance on MRI.

General approach

Baseline thoracic anatomy is commonly imaged prior to cardiac scanning in both axial and coronal planes. This is usually with single-shot fast spin echo imaging, such as HASTE, which is mostly T_2-weighted. There is often only limited gradient-echo or T_1-weighted imaging beyond the cardiac field of view.

Contrast use

An inspection of the thoracic images prior to the administration of contrast can allow additional sequences to be added pre- and post-contrast if time allows. For example, in the liver, delayed post-contrast axial T_1-weighted images can help confirm or refute the likely diagnosis of benign liver haemangiomata. The following aspects of contrast-enhanced imaging can reduce the differential:

- Lesion enhancement.
- Contrast pooling.
- Loss or increase of lesion conspicuity relative to surrounding tissues.

Tissue signal characteristics

Signal intensity in MR images depends on the pulse sequence used and the type of tissue in the image. Table 17.1 opposite is a general guide to tissue appearance on T1-WI or T2-WI.

- T_1-weighted images and gradient-echo imaging demonstrate increased signal if the following are present:
  - Fat
  - Haemorrhage (de-oxymethaemoglobin)
  - Gadolinium and other heavy metal chelates (e.g. manganese).
- Single shot fast spin echo sequences (e.g. HASTE or SS-FSE) are ultrafast, mostly T2-WI. Increased signal is demonstrated by:
  - Static fluid/water, e.g. tissue oedema
  - Proteinaceous collections
  - Fat.

Table 17.1 Signal characteristics of selected tissues on T1-WI and T2-WI

Sequence	High signal ('bright')	Low signal ('dark')
T_1-weighted	Fat Subacute haemorrhage Protein-rich fluid Slow flowing blood Calcification (rarely) Melanin Paramagnetic substances: • gadolinium • manganese • copper	Low proton density Calcification Flow void (fast moving blood) Increased water: • oedema • tumour • infarction • inflammation • infection • haemorrhage (hyperacute or chronic)
T_2-weighted	Methaemoglobin (extracellular), e.g. acute haemorrhage Increased water: • oedema • tumour • infarction • inflammation • infection • subdural collection	Low proton density Calcification Fibrous tissue Protein-rich fluid Flow void (fast moving blood) (Para)magnetic substances: • deoxyhaemoglobin • methaemoglobin (intracellular) • iron, ferritin, haemosiderin • melanin

Pulmonary/systemic disease in association with cardiac disease

Pulmonary oedema in cardiac failure

- Alveolar fluid generally has a homogeneously increased T_2 signal intensity, with a central and perihilar distribution.
- Septal lines are not normally visible on MRI.

Parenchymal lung disease in amyloidosis

- Diffuse decrease in signal on T_1- and T_2-weighted imaging.
- Parenchymal abnormalities include nodules, air space fluid, or a mass.

Pulmonary fibrosis due to amiodarone toxicity

Lung fibrosis is a spectrum from focal or diffuse alveolitis to end-stage cystic change and lung destruction. See 🕮 p. 432 for details.

- The lung changes in amiodarone toxicity reflect a pneumonitis, typically progressing to a basal lung fibrotic pattern.
- Volume changes at the bases can be appreciated if well established.
- Initially, fluid fills the air spaces with increased signal on T2-WI.

Iron-loading

E.g. multiple transfusions. Iron significantly reduces the signal from tissues.

- Diffuse low signal on T_1 and T_2 imaging (tissues appear much darker than normal). This typically occurs within the liver (see Fig. 17.1), but the myocardium may also be affected.
- T_2* measurements are useful for assessment and are currently the only non-invasive method for assessing cardiac iron (🕮 p. 208).

Sarcoidosis

For cardiac findings see Cardiac sarcoidosis, 🕮 p. 200.

- The presence of bilateral hilar and mediastinal lymphadenopathy should alert the viewer to the likelihood of the diagnosis.
- This presentation is more common in younger individuals, who can often be asymptomatic or minimally so.
- More subtle parenchymal nodularity or fissural nodularity is often beyond the capability of MRI, which requires high resolution or thin section axial CT.
- In elderly patients, the spectrum of parenchymal disease can mimic almost any lung condition. Findings include parenchymal air space change, parenchymal and fissural nodularity, interstitial disease, masses, and pleural disease. High resolution chest CT is required to confirm the diagnosis.

Other metabolic disorders

- Some inherited disorders of metabolism can be associated with myocardial disease (see Fig. 17.2), either due to abnormal accumulation within the myocardium (e.g. of proteins or carbohydrates), or due to impaired cardiac energy metabolism.
- Examples include glycogen storage diseases, mucopolysaccharidoses (e.g. Hurler's), Fabry's disease, rare disorders of fatty acid metabolism.

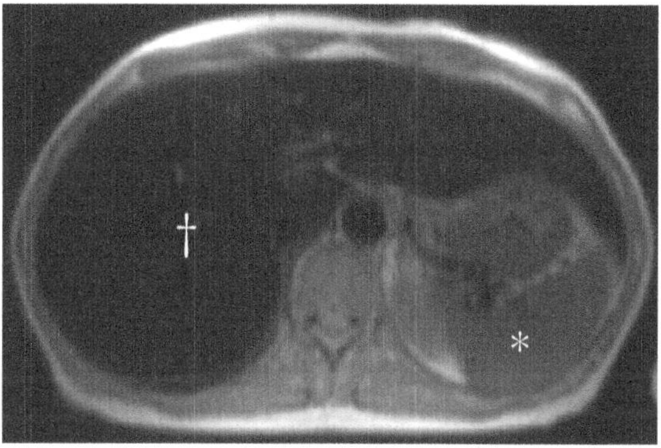

Fig. 17.1 Severe liver iron loading due to haemochromatosis. Note the lower than normal signal from the liver (†) and sparing of the spleen (*), which is of normal signal intensity on this transaxial HASTE image.

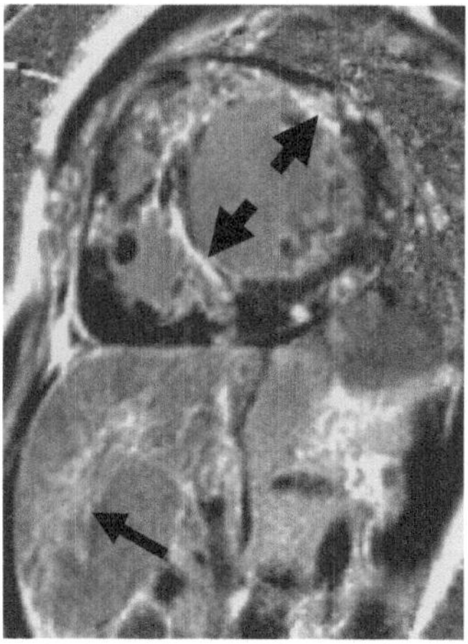

Fig. 17.2 Glycogen storage disease type III. This late enhancement image in the LV short axis plane shows significant cardiac hypertrophy with widespread fibrosis (bright signal, short arrows). Cirrhosis is also present, and the fibrous septa in the liver demonstrate similar late enhancement (long arrow).

Pulmonary disease

The ability of MRI to differentiate air space processes is often disappointing. Some abnormalities may be seen easily, however, due to the increased proton density from infiltrates and the loss of the normal air–tissue interfaces in the region of pathological infiltrates.

MRI may suggest the diagnosis in pulmonary infarction, alveolar proteinosis and lipoid pneumonia by virtue of the ferromagnetic effects of iron seen in haemorrhage, and the T_1 shortening seen in alveolar proteinosis and lipoid pneumonia. In pulmonary infarction, the loss of perfusion and increased lung signal from infiltrates in a wedge-shaped or segmental distribution may suggest the diagnosis.

Pulmonary embolism

- Pulmonary thrombo-embolism is difficult to diagnose on MRI, with an absence of parenchymal signs.
- Large thrombi may occasionally be visualized as a mass within pulmonary arteries or arterioles, with increased vascular signal distally from the slow moving blood (see Fig. 17.3).
- Pulmonary infarction, once present, may be indicated by the increased signal from the higher water content of the parenchyma, in a wedge-shaped or segmental distribution. Areas of involvement are often multiple and random in distribution. Infarction is, however, an uncommon finding.
- The use of gadolinium MR angiography can aid in the diagnosis. The ability to visualize segmental vessels is currently limited, but the sensitivity and specificity of the technique in PE continues to improve with the advent of intravascular contrast agents.

Pneumonia

- Air space signal is increased on T2-WI. As the fluid becomes consolidated (the air spaces filling with cells and bacteria), the signal increases further.
- The lobar or segmental distribution helps suggest the diagnosis.

Pneumonitis

- Increased lung signal on T_2-weighted sequences with a typically diffuse, homogeneous pattern, reflecting the process of active alveolitis.
- CT imaging provides more accurate assessment of pneumonitis and often shows a ground glass appearance of fluid density.

Lung fibrosis

- Similar imaging characteristics to pneumonitis, which is the precursor to the development of fibrosis.
- The distribution of the air space change and relative sparing of certain lung zones can aid in narrowing the differential diagnosis.
- Progression to destructive cystic change (decreased parenchymal signal) is a protracted and usually episodic process.

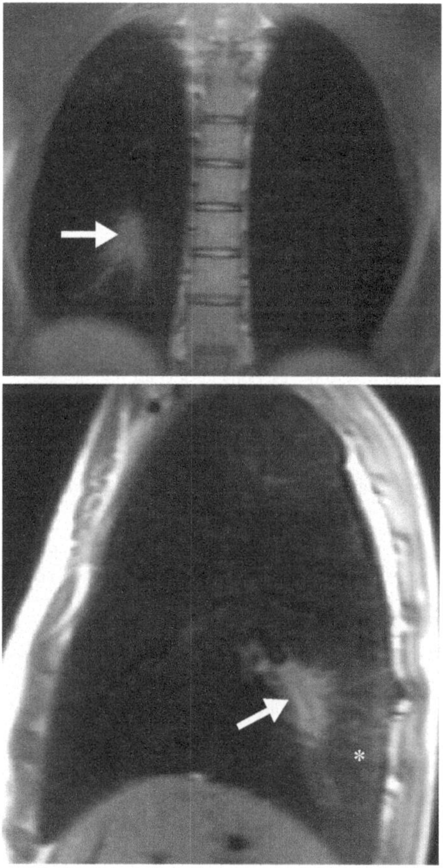

Fig. 17.3 Pulmonary embolus in the right lower lobe. Note the intermediate-high signal of thrombus within the branch pulmonary artery on coronal (top) and sagittal (bottom) HASTE imaging (arrows). A wedge-shaped increase in lung signal can also be seen distal to the thrombus on the sagittal image (bottom, *), indicating pulmonary infarction.

Carcinoma

- Generally nodules >5mm will be detected on MRI, although these commonly appear larger than would be appreciated on CT due to the reduced spatial resolution of MRI.
- Malignant tumours are usually >2cm in size and malignancy is particularly suggested if >4cm. They will usually have a spiculate and ill-defined contour, and demonstrate surrounding architectural distortion. They can cross a fissure and may have a small effusion if large enough.
- Signal intensity is generally increased on T2-WI.
- Signal voids within the lesion can be seen with focal calcification or cavitation of the lesion, especially in larger lesions.
- The presence of focal calcification with a spiculate mass would suggest carcinoma within a scar.
- MRI is well established in the assessment of apical or Pancoast tumours, to assess the vasculature and involvement/invasion of the brachial plexus.
- MRI also lends well to the assessment of chest wall disease.

Pulmonary nodules/granulomatous disease

- Single pulmonary nodules are a common and generally vexing diagnostic dilemma!
- The probability of malignancy increases with the size of the nodule:
  - Benign nodules are generally smaller than 8mm
  - Nodules that measure 8–10mm in size require evaluation of the pre-test probability of malignancy and consideration for CT-PET.
- Multiple nodules increases the likelihood of benign granulomatous disease, but also of potential metastatic disease (Fig. 17.4).
- Lesions are typically iso-intense or increased signal intensity on T2-WI.

Metastatic disease

- Typically rounded lesions and often multiple.
- Usually have a random distribution, but are invariably related to the bronchovascular bundles.
- The presence of a known previous malignancy significantly alters the pre-test probability of a malignant process with pulmonary nodules.
- Chest CT is the next imaging test of choice.

Vascular malformations

MR angiography can be used for the diagnosis of AV malformations. It is particularly useful in patients sensitive to iodinated X-ray contrast media, and in those for whom ionizing radiation needs to be reduced.

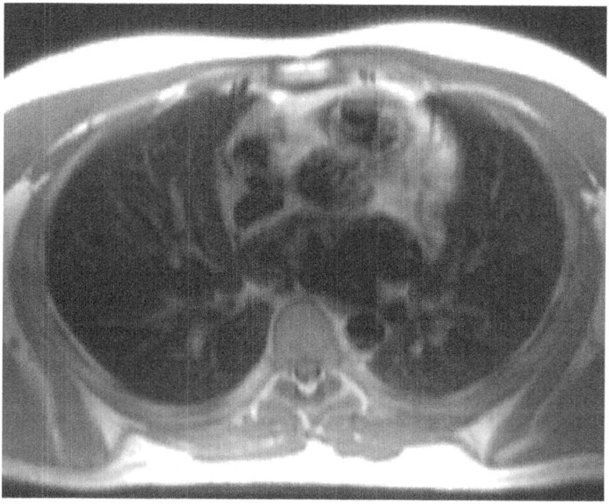

Fig. 17.4 Increased lung signal and small (<5mm) parenchymal nodules. The differential includes sarcoidosis, amiodarone-induced lung disease, and other interstitial lung disease.

Pleural disease

Pleural effusion

- Typically increased SI on T2-WI (e.g. HASTE) and SSFP cine sequences (Fig. 17.5).
- Layering of effusions, with a fluid-fluid interface indicates a complicated effusion with either infection or haemorrhage or both.

Empyema

- The presence of pleural fluid and enhancement of the pleura is suggestive of an empyema.
- The classical 'split pleural sign', where enhancement of the visceral and parietal pleura is seen (in the clinical setting of infection) is virtually diagnostic of an empyema.
- The fluid is of increased SI on T2-WI and the pleura enhances post-gadolinium on T1-WI. This is often seen on both early and delayed imaging.

Mesothelioma

- Suggested by the presence of a thick rind of soft tissue, with increased SI on T2-WI, that encases and surrounds the lung.
- Pleural effusions are nearly always present and associated rib destruction is seen in up to 12% of cases.
- On T2-WI , the fluid is of increased SI and the tumour of intermediate (iso-intense to muscle) or increased SI.
- Rib destruction and costal wall involvement is reflected by bone marrow oedema, with increased SI on T2-WI or STIR sequences.

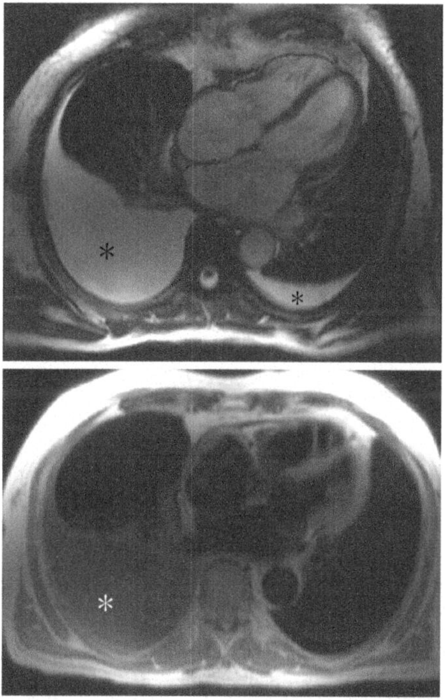

Fig. 17.5 Large right and small left pleural effusions (*). Note the homogenous high signal on SSFP imaging (top), and intermediate signal on HASTE imaging (bottom), with surrounding lung clearly seen.

The diaphragm

MRI has the ability to visualize the diaphragm in multiple planes, and good soft tissue differentiation allows accurate assessment of integrity, deformity, and function.

Traumatic rupture

Commonly missed at initial presentation and can be found as an incidental finding. The herniation of an abdominal viscous or of mesenteric fat is readily apparent.

Congenital hernias

Bochdalek

- 85–95% of diaphragmatic hernias.
- Posterolateral defect, the majority of which (90%) are left-sided. Bilateral hernias can occur rarely.
- Best imaged in the sagittal and coronal planes using breath hold sequences. These will detail the defect and its contents.

Morgagni

- 1–2% of diaphragmatic hernias.
- This is an anterior defect adjacent to the sternum, through the foramina of Morgagni.
- Imaged as Bochdalek.

Eventration

- Eventration, or laxity of the central tendinous portion of the diaphragm, can be distinguished from diaphragmatic paralysis by the motion of the remainder of the diaphragm.
- Coronal and sagittal planes are best.
- Inspiratory and expiratory sequences allow for functional assessment of the diaphragmatic movement, or this can be imaged using free-breathing cine sequences.

Diaphragmatic paralysis

- Due to phrenic nerve paralysis (Fig. 17.6).
- Common causes:
  - Idiopathic
  - Trauma
  - (Rarely) malignant.
- Previous CXR is often helpful to confirm longstanding nature.

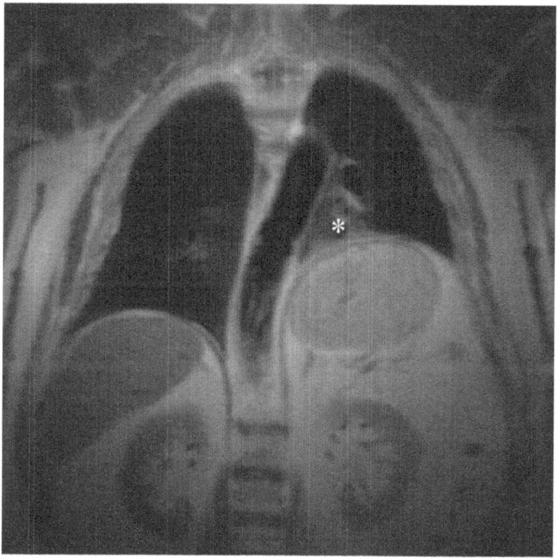

Fig. 17.6 Raised left hemi-diaphragm due to phrenic nerve paralysis, with mild atelectasis of overlying lung (*).

Mediastinal masses

Superior mediastinum

Thyroid

- The commonest masses are benign, relating to goitre from multi-cystic degeneration of the thyroid (MCDT; Figs 17.7, 17.10).
- The presence of multiple cysts with foci of fluid signal intensity, some of which can contain haemorrhage, is typical of MCDT. Foci of calcification can also be seen as signal voids.
- The thyroid generally enlarges into the anterior mediastinum, but can also involve the posterior mediastinum.

Anterior mediastinum

Lymph nodes and lymphoma

- Typically nodes are of intermediate SI on T2-WI and T1-WI (iso-intense to muscle and clearly defined by the mediastinal fat; Fig. 17.8).
- The number, size, and sites of the nodes help to distinguish the cause or likelihood of a malignant process. The presence of splenomegaly should also be noted.
- Nodes that are of increased SI may indicate a higher fluid content and can be seen in congestive cardiac failure and superimposed infection.
- **Causes of lymphadenopathy:**
  - Benign (reactive; common in COPD and lung fibrosis)
  - Lymphoma
  - Carcinoma
  - Sarcoid.

Germ cell tumours

- Teratoma, dermoid, seminoma, embryonal carcinomas (80% are benign).
- The mass may be heterogeneous with mixed SI on both T2-WI and T1-WI. The presence of calcification is reflected by signal voids, often amorphous in appearance.

Thymoma (thymolipoma)

- It is rare for the thymus to be visualized after the age of 30.
- The presence of a triangular or rounded mass should alert one to the diagnosis of a thymic abnormality.
- Commonly seen in myasthenia gravis.
- Benign and invasive thymic tumours occur.
- The presence of fat (bright SI on T1-WI) would suggest a thymolipoma, lipoma, fat pad, or hernia.

Morgagni hernia

See 📖 p. 438.

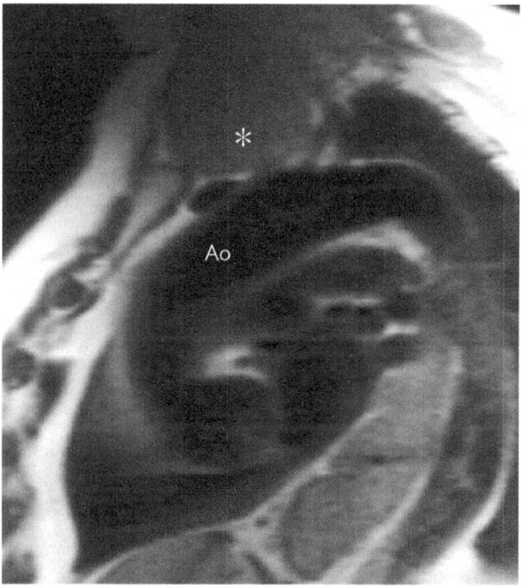

Fig. 17.7 Retrosternal goitre in the superior mediastinum on sagittal HASTE imaging (*). Note the mostly homogenous, iso-intense signal. Ao = aorta.

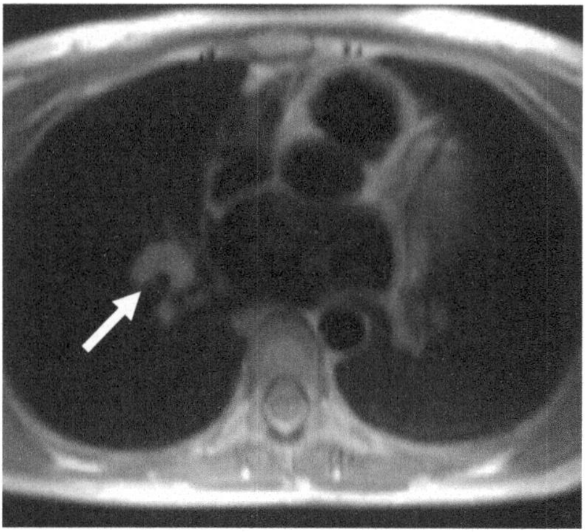

Fig. 17.8 Hilar lymphadenopathy. Note the lymph node(s) >1cm in size and iso-intense (intermediate SI) on HASTE imaging (arrowed). CT chest suggested.

Pericardial cysts

See 📖 p. 302.

Pericardial fat pad(s)

- Usually triangular shaped and lie adjacent to the pericardial sac.
- The cardiac apex is the commonest site, followed by the right cardiophrenic location.
- Readily distinguished from a 'mass' by virtue of their increased SI on T1-WI and ability to suppress the signal with fat saturation sequences.

Middle mediastinum

Lymph nodes

See 📖 p. 440.

Carcinoma (usually bronchial) 📖 p. 434

MRI can help in determining the vascular invasion of critical structures in the middle mediastinum (e.g. pulmonary artery and veins, SVC).

Bronchogenic cysts

- Congenital lesions thought to originate from the primitive ventral foregut.
- Occur within the middle and posterior mediastinum, although occasionally in the anterior mediastinum.
- Typically contain proteinaceous material and MR signal characteristics are similar to other fluids – homogenous high signal on T2-WI and low signal on T1-WI.
- Usually asymptomatic, but can compress surrounding structures or become infected.

Superior pericardial recess (part of the transverse sinus, Fig. 17.9)

An appreciation of the superior pericardial recess is important in assessing the middle mediastinum. This crescent-shaped portion of the transverse pericardial sinus lies posterior to the ascending aortic arch and often contains fluid. It may be mistaken for a mediastinal lymph node or an aortic dissection flap (see Fig. 13.16, 📖 p. 369).

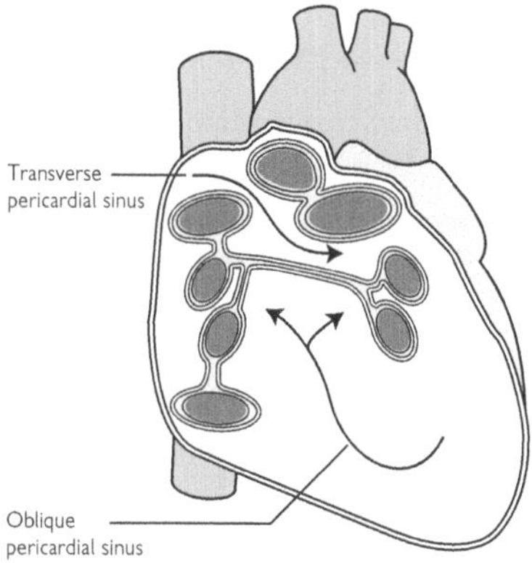

Fig. 17.9 Representation of the transverse and oblique pericardial sinuses, viewed from the front.

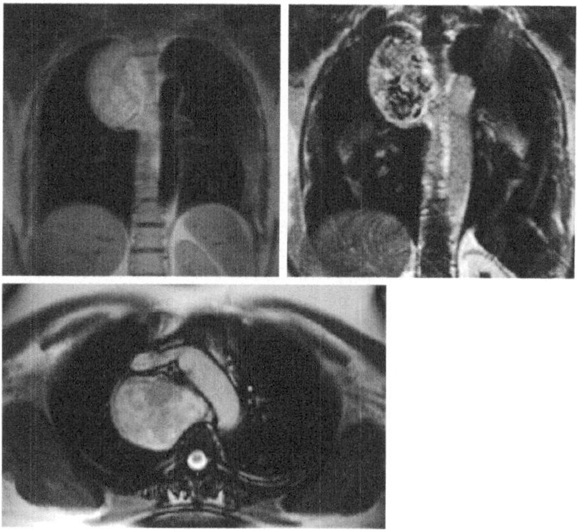

Fig. 17.10 High posterior mediastinal mass. Heterogenous signal on coronal HASTE (top left) and transaxial SSFP multislice imaging (bottom). Contrast enhancement with signal voids (top right) on late inversion recovery imaging. Likely to be a tumour; in this case an ectopic thyroid mass.

Posterior mediastinum

Oesophageal 'mass' (i.e. hiatus hernia; Fig. 17.11)

- Common.
- Air-filled mass (signal voids) communicating with the oesophagus, and containing part of the stomach (variable signal intensity from stomach contents).
- Can fool the unwary and appear as a large posterior mass. The air pockets and communication with the oesophagus/stomach are key to the correct diagnosis.

Lymph nodes

See 📖 p. 440.

Myeloma

- Two types of 'mass' seen –
  - solitary plasmacytoma of bone
  - extramedullary plasmacytoma (outside the bone marrow).
- Both are localized (isolated) forms of plasma cell dyscrasias (i.e. myeloma), compared with 'multiple' myeloma.

Solitary plasmacytoma of bone

- Has a greater tendency to progress to multiple myeloma.
- The MRI appearance is consistent with that of a focal area of bone marrow replacement; the signal intensity is similar to muscle on T1-WI and hyperintense relative to muscle on T2-WI. An extra-osseous soft-tissue component is often present
- and may impinge on the spinal cord or spinal nerve roots.
- Diffuse bony involvement is characterized by low SI on T1-WI indicating marrow replacement and increased SI on STIR imaging.

Extramedullary haemopoesis

- A compensatory process associated with chronic haemolytic anaemia. Can be seen in sickle cell disease or thallassaemia major.
- Recognized on MRI as an iso-intense epidural lesion on T_1 with intermediate to high SI on T2-WI.
- Expansion of thoracic ribs with bilateral paravertebral masses (Fig. 17.12) is characteristic. They may be seen to compress the spinal cord.
- All the vertebral bodies have low to intermediate signal intensity as a result of displacement of fatty marrow by haematopoietic marrow.
- Intermediate enhancement with gadolinium contrast.

Neurogenic tumours (neurofibroma)

- Often paravertebral tumours with homogenous SI on T2-WI.
- The key imaging sequence is post-contrast T1-WI with fat saturation - these masses 'light up' following enhancement with gadolinium.
- There may be subtle bone changes (erosion or foraminal enlargement), best appreciated on dedicated imaging.

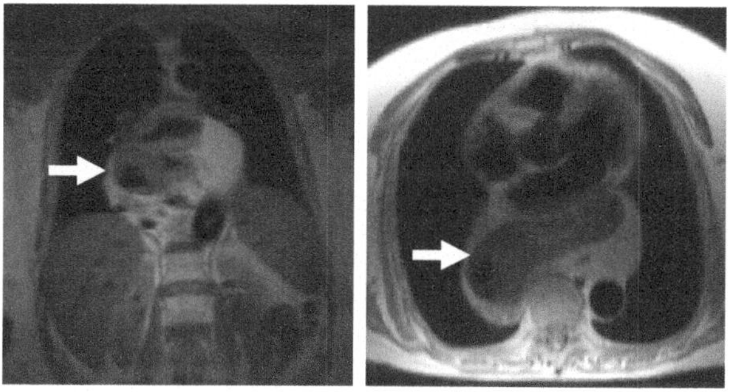

Fig. 17.11 Massive hiatus hernia, extending to the level of the great vessels. Posterior coronal HASTE image (left); transverse HASTE image (right) with 'mass' arrowed.

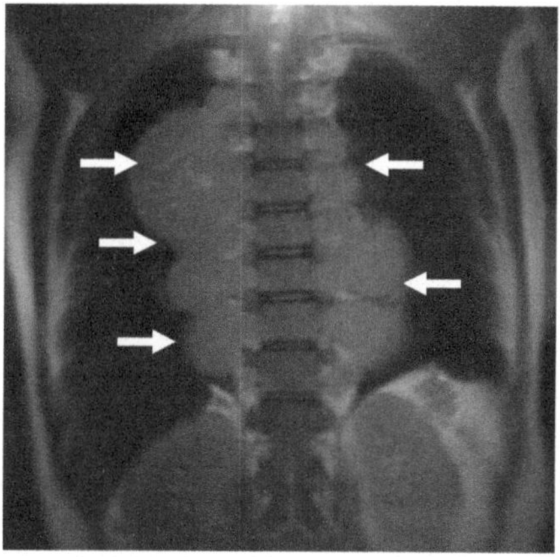

Fig. 17.12 Large paravertebral masses – this patient has thallassaemia major and the masses are extramedullary haemopoetic tissue.

Vertebral bodies

Cavernous haemangioma

- Common finding (10% of the population).
- Well circumscribed lesion, bright on both T_1- and T_2-weighted sequences, with lobular margin (Fig. 17.13).
- Generally involves the central portion of the vertebral body.
- No expansion or destruction of the vertebrae is usually seen.
- Often enhance post-contrast as they contain vascular channels within fatty matrix.
- Correlation with previous imaging can be helpful.
- Usually easily differentiated from spinal artefact (Fig. 17.14) by its well defined margin.

Metastatic disease

- Marrow replacement from tumour shows areas of reduced bone marrow signal on T1-WI, and iso-intense or subtly increased on T2-WI or STIR sequences. In general, this creates a heterogeneous marrow signal on both imaging types.
- The T_1 sequence is generally the most sensitive to the change in marrow signal from infiltration.
- A STIR sequence is recommended to identify the often minor infiltrative change.

Osteomalacia/osteoporosis

- Often difficult to distinguish from metastatic disease.
- Heterogeneous marrow signal on T1-WI and T2-WI. Marrow replacement results in reduced signal on T1-WI and increased signal on T2-WI or STIR.
- The patchy nature of the disease can be alarming!

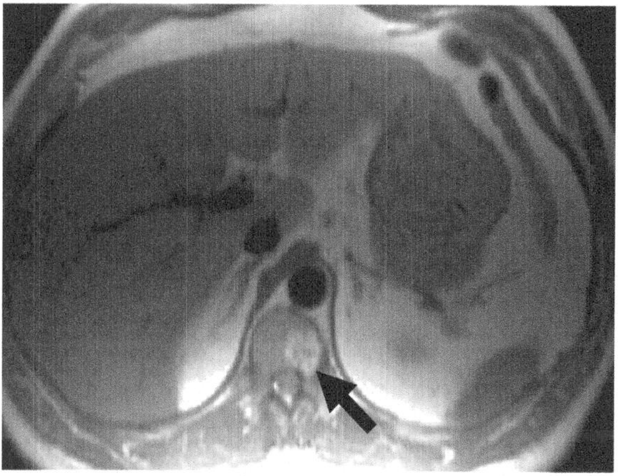

Fig. 17.13 Spinal haemangioma (arrowed) on transaxial HASTE imaging. Note the well circumscribed area with lobular margin and high signal.

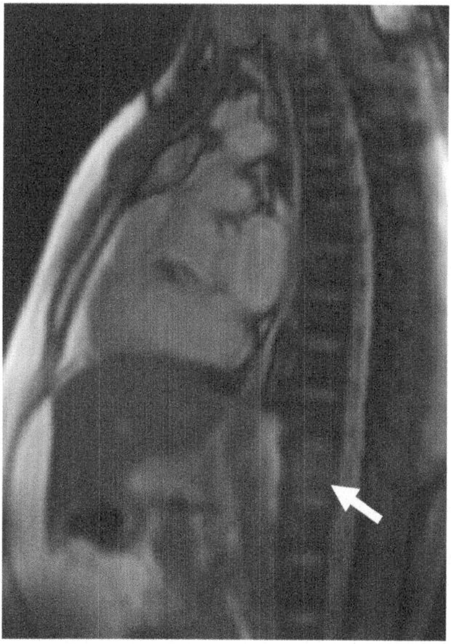

Fig. 17.14 Spinal artefact (arrowed). The high signal extends beyond the margin of the vertebral body and does not indicate marrow oedema. Moving the patient will move the artefact.

Soft tissues abnormalities

Tumours

Lipoma

- Often has a well defined capsule with fat density signal (increased on T_1, and also to a lesser degree on T_2).
- Commonly iso-intense to subcutaneous fat.
- Low grade sarcomatous change is common.

Muscle sarcoma

Often mildly heterogeneous signal within the muscle on T1-WI and T2-WI.

Haemorrhage

Heterogeneous SI depending on the stage of the breakdown of the blood products. (See Table 17.1 for specific T_1/T_2 characteristics).

Breasts

Implants

- Very well defined (encapsulated) regions of increased SI on T2-WI (Fig. 17.15).
- The periphery of the prosthetic capsule commonly calcifies with time, demonstrated by a signal void.

Fibro-adenomas

- Often small foci of increased SI on T2-WI.
- Signal voids can be seen within the lesion indicating calcification.
- No regional nodes will be seen.

Carcinoma

- Most commonly seen in the upper, outer quadrant of the breast.
- Often conspicuous in atrophic breasts with minimal glandular tissue and diffuse fatty infiltration.
- Usually have a spiculate contour and surrounding architectural distortion.

Fat necrosis

- Rounded lesions of increased signal on T1-WI.
- Uncommon.

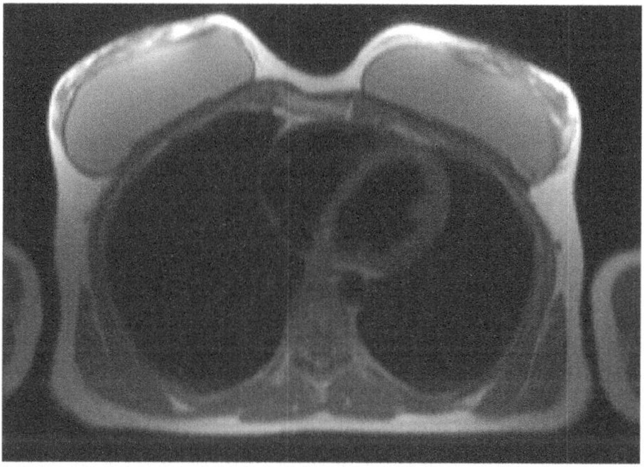

Fig. 17.15 Bilateral breast implants. Note the well defined capsule and homogenous signal.

The liver

Diffuse conditions

Fatty infiltration

Focal, diffuse or regional ↑ T_1 signal. Best appreciated on a specialized T_1 'in and out of phase' sequence, which accentuates the pattern.

Liver cirrhosis

- Small volume liver with a nodular contour.
- Heterogeneous liver texture.
- Post-contrast septa may enhance, in keeping with fibrosis.

Haemangiomata

- Benign lesions, often lobular in configuration.
- ↑ SI on T2-WI and SSFP; progressive ↑ SI on T2-WI with ↑ TR.
- Can be difficult to differentiate from simple cysts.
- Contrast can help – typically non-continuous, nodular enhancement of the wall of the lesion and pooling of the contrast with delayed imaging, resulting in characteristic late 'filling-in' of the lesion.

Simple cysts

- Well circumscribed lesions with a random distribution (Fig. 17.16).
- Usually have smooth margins with high SI on T_2 and low SI on T_1.
- Often multiple and commonly occur with renal cysts.
- Part of the fibrocystic spectrum of disease and, thus, can involve the kidneys, liver, and pancreas (see Fig. 17.18).
- Do not enhance with contrast and, thus, have increased conspicuity with better definition of the wall post-contrast. Do not show the 'filling-in' phenomenon characteristic of haemangiomata.

Tumours

Metastases

- Commonly multiple.
- Variable signal intensity. Often low SI on T1-WI and intermediate to high on T2-WI, but generally lower T_2 SI than cysts or haemangiomata, especially with longer TE (>160ms) (see Fig. 17.17).
- Features suggesting a malignant nature include irregular margins, extension beyond the liver, heterogenous signal and 'rim' effect from surrounding oedema (lower SI on T1-WI; higher signal on T2-WI).
- Post-contrast appearance depends on the vascularity – all tend to show some enhancement, differentiating them from cysts. Hyper-vascular tumours (e.g. neuroendocrine including carcinoid, renal cell, melanoma, thyroid carcinoma) show hyper-enhancement in the portal phase; hypovascular tumours (e.g. lung, breast, stomach, colorectal carcinoma) enhance less than the surrounding vascular liver (and appear hypo-intense), but the presence of some enhancement helps to distinguish from cysts.

Hepatocellular carcinoma

Generally 'ugly-looking' lesion with irregular margin and heterogenous signal ± invasion of surrounding tissues.

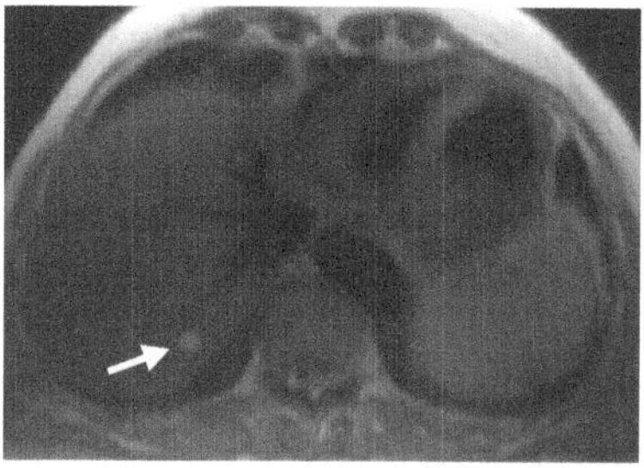

Fig. 17.16 Simple hepatic cyst. Transaxial HASTE image showing well circumscribed, homogenous spherical lesion of high signal intensity in the liver.

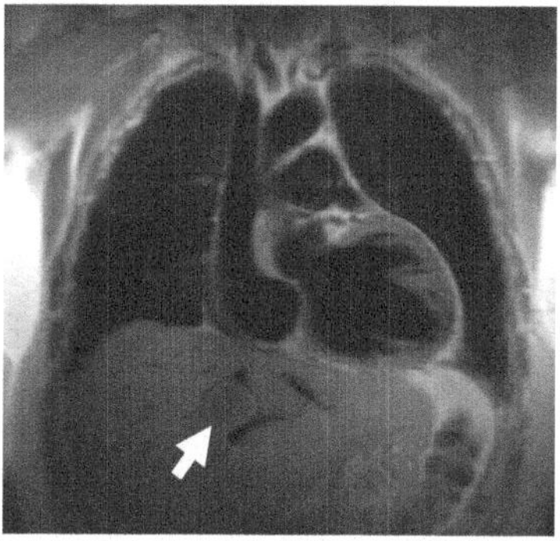

Fig. 17.17 Uncertain liver lesion (arrowed). The signal is mostly homogenous, but there is a suggestion of rim enhancement, and further imaging (e.g. CT/ultrasound) is recommended to exclude abscess or tumour.

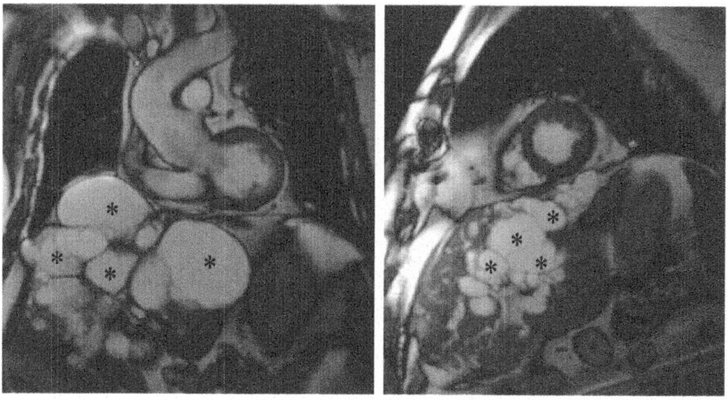

Fig. 17.18 Severe polycystic disease. Note the multiple spherical/lobular lesions in the liver with high homogenous signal intensity on SSFP images (*).

Renal masses

Benign simple cysts

Well defined contours with bright, homogenous SI on T2-WI and low-intermediate signal on T1-WI (Figs 17.19 and 17.20). The walls are smooth and thin, and the absence of nodular tissue or associated masses is important to infer the label of 'simple' cysts.

Complex cysts

- Cystic structures, which may contain haemorrhage or peripheral signal loss in keeping with rim calcification.
- Best investigated by ultrasound.

Malignant lesions

- Generally solid masses with heterogeneous SI on T2-WI and also on T1-WI as they can contain haemorrhage.
- Often distort the contour of the kidney.
- The presence of adenopathy is concerning.
- Vascular invasion can be diagnosed post-contrast in advanced tumours.

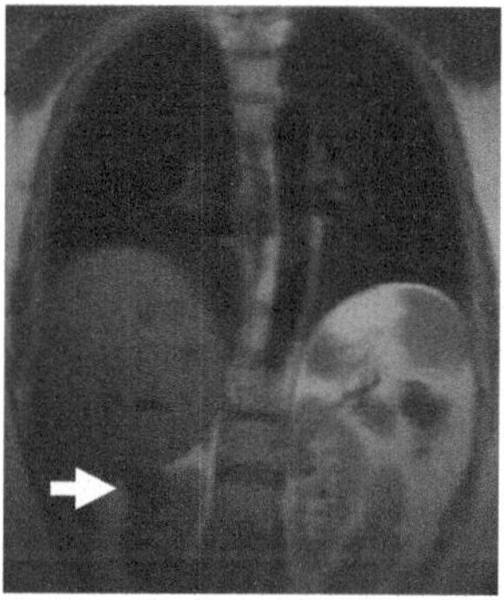

Fig. 17.19 Benign cyst in right kidney on coronal HASTE image. Note the well defined contour and homogenous signal. Ultrasound can confirm diagnosis.

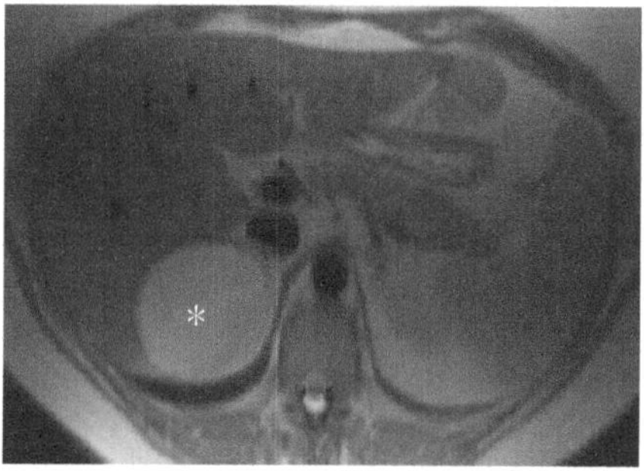

Fig. 17.20 Large cyst in right kidney (*) on transverse HASTE image. Note the well defined spherical shape and the homogenous high signal.

Pancreas

Focal masses

- Large established masses often associated with pancreatic gland atrophy, dilatation of the pancreatic duct and the common bile duct (CBD).
- The dilated pancreatic duct and CBD, when visible, is referred to as the 'double duct sign' and is strongly suspicious of malignancy.
- The presence of protein in the obstructed pancreatic duct appears as bright signal on a T2-WI sequence. The CBD also shows increased signal on T2-WI.
- When dilated secondary to a malignant neoplasm, it is commonly associated with nodal disease and vascular invasion.

Pancreatitis

Acute

- Loss of the pancreatic contour, increase in size of the pancreas (focally or diffusely) and inflammatory change within the bed of the pancreas is common.
- MRI is exquisitely sensitive for the detection of acute inflammatory change, which appears as low SI strands on T1-WI.
- Focal or generalized fluid collections are often seen as a complication of the condition and have increased SI on T2-WI.
- If further complicated by haemorrhage, T_1 images with fat saturation show increased signal due to the paramagnetic effect of the blood.
- Post-contrast, the rim may enhance in keeping with an infected phlegmon or peri-pancreatic collection.

Chronic

The gland is atrophic with ↓ SI on T_1-weighted fat suppression images and diminished heterogeneous enhancement post-contrast.

Adrenal masses

Adenoma

- Usually small masses, 1–2cm in size.
- The presence of fat within the lesion, often bilateral, indicates a functioning versus a non-functioning adenoma.
- The presence of fat signal drop-out on a specialized T_1 'out-of-phase' sequence is virtually diagnostic.

Phaeochromocytoma

- Range in size from 3 to 5cm.
- 90% are adrenal in position, 10% are malignant. 10% are bilateral.
- They have a characteristic high SI ('light-bulb') appearance on T2-WI in the vast majority of cases.

Carcinoma

- Generally >5cm in size with a mixed heterogeneous SI on T2-WI and T1-WI.
- These are aggressive tumours with haemorrhage and necrosis commonly seen.
- Calcification can be present with signal voids on T1-WI and T2-WI.
- Post-contrast there may be central areas of non-enhancement.

Other abdominal abnormalities

Spleen

- Readily measured on MRI with the multiplanar imaging giving an accurate assessment of the bipolar diameter.
- Common causes of splenic enlargement (>13cm) Fig. 17.21:
  - Generalized illness
  - Viral-related
  - Haemopoetic disease (lymphoma, leukaemia)
  - Abnormality of splenic venous drainage (portal hypertension, venous obstruction or invasion).
- Focal abnormalities of the spleen are uncommon, with benign cysts or haemangiomata the most frequently encountered findings.

Gallbladder

Gallstones are common (10–15% of the population) and can sometimes be appreciated easily on MRI (Fig. 17.22). The majority are asymptomatic, and require no investigation or treatment. Magnetic resonance cholangiopancreatography (MRCP) is a well recognized technique for assessing the biliary tract.

Free abdominal fluid

- Usually easily recognisable within the abdomen as ↑ SI on T2-WI.
- The fluid bathes the abdominal viscera, pooling in key positions as the volume of fluid increases (Morisons Pouch, paracolic gutters, pelvic Pouch of Douglas, etc.).

- If further complicated by haemorrhage, T1-WI with fat saturation shows increased signal due to the paramagnetic effect of the blood.
- Infected peritoneal fluid can also demonstrate fluid-fluid interfaces as shown by a horizontal layering of proteinaceous material with increased differential signal.
- Nodularity of the omentum or peritoneal cavity is a concerning sign, and should alert the reader as the presence of an under-lying malignancy.

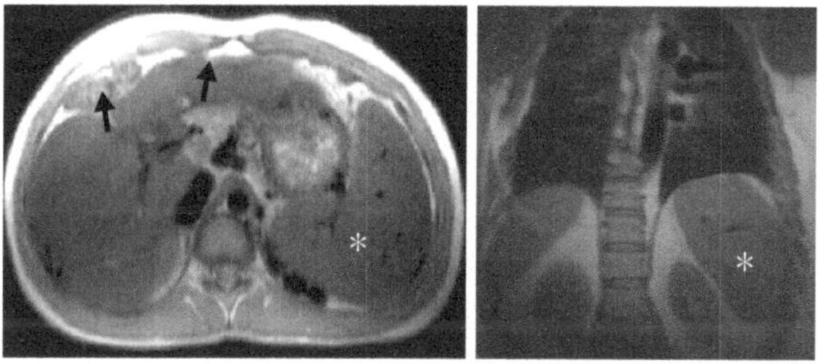

Fig. 17.21 Splenomegaly due to cirrhosis-induced portal hypertension. Note the enlarged (15cm) spleen(*), and irregular liver outline (arrowed).

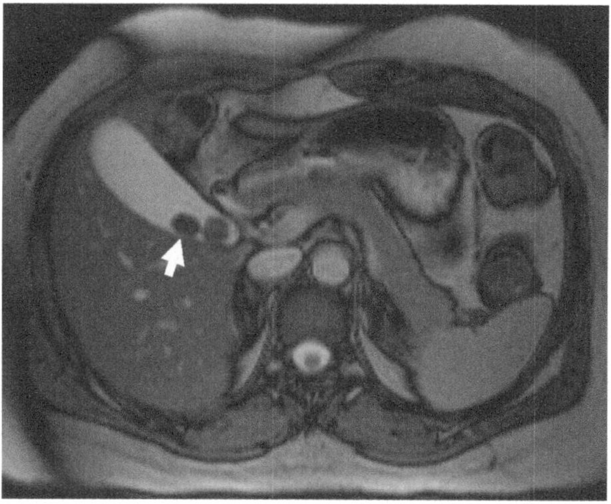

Fig. 17.22 Gallstones. Note the enlarged gallbladder with homogenous high signal from bile, and two gallstones (low intensity, arrow) in the neck of the gallbladder. SSFP image.

Chapter 18

New horizons for CMR

Introduction

CMR is the most versatile of all cardiovascular imaging techniques, and, as shown in this handbook, it can provide detailed information on cardiac anatomy, function, perfusion, tissue characteristics such as oedema and viability, and on almost all vascular territories, including vessel lumen, vessel wall, and blood flow. However, there are many additional capabilities of CMR that may well find their way into clinical practice in the coming years. Examples of these are given below.

Whole heart 4D cine CMR

Rapid acquisition of an isotropic 3D cine dataset for the heart with high temporal resolution (4D), similar to cardiac CT. With this, any imaging plane could then be re-constructed off-line during data analysis, which would greatly simplify image acquisition and enable assessment of imaging planes not planned at acquisition stage.

In future, such a dataset could also enable assessment of coronary lumen anatomy, including reliable quantification of stenosis and plaque characteristics. However, achieving the necessary spatial resolution and, at the same time, freezing cardiac and respiratory motion, remain enormous technical challenges. 1mm resolution will be sufficient for assessment of cardiac anatomy and function and is a realistic goal. At least 0.5mm will be required for coronary imaging, and whether this can be achieved is more questionable.

At present, true 4D isotropic cine CMR is not yet feasible, but this may become possible with massive parallel imaging applied at higher field strength (3T or higher). Data processing tools such as image registration may aid this approach.

Ultrashort echo time (UTE) imaging

Imaging of fibrosis and calcification is, in principle, possible using ultrashort TE sequences. These capture the rapidly decaying T_2 signal elements from tissue components with very low free water content.

Imaging cardiac and vascular fibrosis/calcification with this intrinsic MR contrast method would be of major relevance, allowing the assessment of myocardial fibrosis without the use of MR contrast agent, and, most importantly, in atherosclerosis imaging, where fibrosed/calcified plaque components could be characterized.

However, while this is already feasible in the musculoskeletal system, currently the SNR of cardiac and vascular UTE images is below the diagnostic threshold. Higher field strength, improved RF coil designs, and a better understanding of these formerly 'invisible' components may make this method clinically applicable for the heart.

Non-contrast myocardial perfusion imaging

Using arterial spin labelling methods, it may, in future, be possible to assess perfusion without the use of first-pass MR contrast techniques.

These methods already work well experimentally at high field (7–12T), but remain to be established at current, clinically used field strengths. This would allow assessment of perfusion in patients with contraindications to MR contrast agents, and provide a tool for investigating dynamic changes in perfusion.

Myocardial oxygenation

Using the blood oxygenation level dependent (BOLD) effect, CMR can potentially assess myocardial tissue oxygenation.

Deoxygenated haemoglobin in blood acts as an intrinsic contrast agent, changing proton signals in a fashion that can be imaged to reflect the level of blood oxygenation. Increases in O_2 saturation increase the BOLD imaging signal (T_2 or T_2*), whereas decreases diminish it. It is possible that, compared with perfusion, cardiac tissue de-oxygenation may be a superior parameter reflecting more directly the imbalance between oxygen demand and supply that characterizes ischaemia (Fig. 18.1).

Although the feasibility of the technique at 1.5T has been demonstrated, implementation of the cardiac BOLD approach is fundamentally limited by the relatively small difference in the signal between normal and de-oxygenated myocardial regions. Higher field strength (3T) combined with new robust steady-state free precession (SSFP) techniques that generate T_2-weighted images of the heart overcomes some of these problems.

Molecular imaging

This method has huge potential for the future. Contrast agents for molecular imaging have to be manufactured, and typically include a ligand with affinity and specificity for a molecular target (e.g. fibrin), a carrier particle and a signalling element, which for MR imaging is either gadolinium (signal increase) or iron (signal increase or decrease). Regulatory approval of such new compounds will be an additional hurdle.

In future, targeted molecular imaging may accelerate and refine diagnosis, provide more precise disease characterization, enable specific treatments to be targeted in individual patients, enable drug delivery to site of pathology, and monitor responses to treatment.

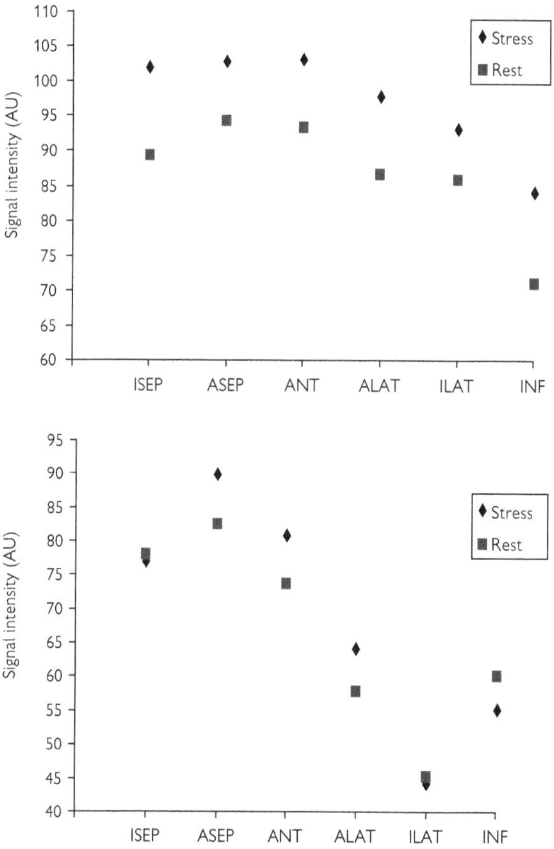

Fig. 18.1 Oxygenation imaging with BOLD. T_2-weighted signal intensity values at rest and stress. (Top panel) Normal volunteer, showing an increase in signal intensity with stress for all myocardial segments. (Bottom panel) A patient with significant stenosis of a dominant right coronary artery, showing no change or even ↓ signal with stress in the inferior septum, and inferior and inferolateral walls. ISEP = inferior septum; ASEP = anterior septum; ANT = anterior wall; ALAT = anterolateral wall; ILAT = inferolateral wall; INF = inferior wall; AU = arbitrary units.

Magnetic resonance spectroscopy

While CMR imaging uses the ^{1}H nucleus in water and fat molecules as a signal source, cardiac MR spectroscopy (MRS) allows the study of many other nuclei, such as ^{13}C, ^{23}Na, and ^{31}P, thereby allowing insights into many aspects of cardiac metabolism.

MRS is the only available method for the non-invasive assessment of cardiac metabolism without the need for external radioactive tracers and in theory, it could allow many important clinical questions to be answered. Major clinical research applications are heart failure, ischaemia, cardiomyopathies, diabetes, obesity, and valve disease.

However, the signals acquired in MRS are 100,000–1,000,000 times weaker than the signals used in MR imaging. Therefore, the temporal and spatial resolution of MRS is poor (e.g. ^{31}P MRS of the heart requires a 30ml voxel size and a 30min acquisition time).

At the moment, the method is an important research tool that can be used to detect differences between study groups, but because of its high variability, is not reliable for the assessment of individual patients.

Future developments will include:

- Improvements in coil design (phased array with optimized geometries).
- Improvements in sequence design.
- Higher field strength (7T and more).
- Hyperpolarization methods (see below).

With these improvements, cardiac MRS may eventually become a clinically valuable method.

Dynamic nuclear polarization methods

Hyperpolarization of nuclear spins can boost the MR signal by a factor of up to 100,000. The most important application for the heart is dynamic nuclear polarization (DNP) of ^{13}C. A liquid ^{13}C-containing compound, e.g. ^{13}C-pyruvate (Fig. 18.2) is frozen and irradiated by microwaves in a magnetic field. The sample is then rapidly thawed and injected quickly as the DNP state is short lived (minutes).

Potential applications

- ^{13}C-MRS of pyruvate allows analysis of various metabolic pathways (e.g. pyruvate dehydrogenase).
- ^{13}C-MRI following intracoronary bolus of ^{13}C-urea for coronary angiography.
- Tissue pH imaging using ^{13}C-bicarbonate.

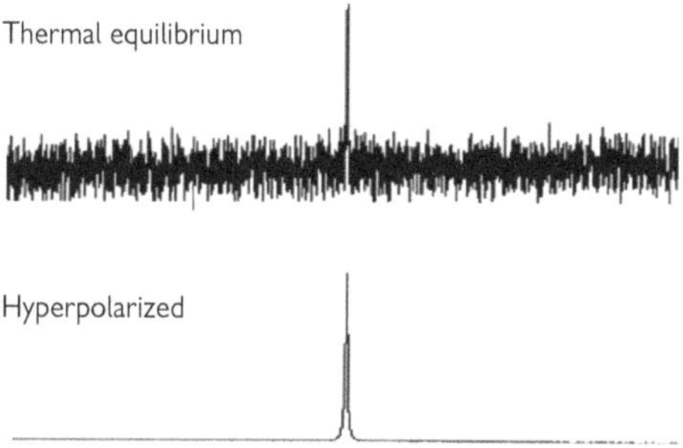

Fig. 18.2 ^{13}C-MR spectra of pyruvate at 9.4T. Compared with the normal thermal equilibrium spectrum, the hyperpolarized spectrum shows a signal increase of >22,000 times. Courtesy of Drs Damian Tyler and Lowri Cochlin, Department of Physiology, Anatomy, and Genetics, Oxford University.

Further reading

Choudhury, RP, Fuster, V, Fayad, ZA Molecular, cellular and functional imaging of atherothrombosis. *Nat Rev Drug Discov* 2004; **3**(11): 913–25.

Friedrich, MG, Niendorf, T, Schulz-Menger, J, Gross, CM, Dietz, R. Blood oxygen level-dependent magnetic resonance imaging in patients with stress-induced angina. *Circulation* 2003; **108:** 2219–23.

Kober, F, Iltis, I, Cozzone, PJ, Bernard, M. Myocardial blood flow mapping in mice using high-resolution spin labeling magnetic resonance imaging: influence of ketamine/xylazine and isoflurane anesthesia. *Magn Reson Med* 2005; **53:** 601–6.

Merritt, ME, Harrison, C, Storey, C, Jeffrey, FM, Sherry, AD, Malloy, CR Hyperpolarized 13C allows a direct measure of flux through a single enzyme-catalysed step by NMR. *PNAS* 2007; **104:** 19773–7.

Robson, MD, Tyler, DJ, Neubauer, S. Ultrashort TE chemical shift imaging (UTE-CSI). *Magn Reson Med* 2005; **53:** 267–74.

Ten Hove, M, Neubauer, S. MR spectroscopy in heart failure–clinical and experimental findings. *Heart Fail Rev* 2007; **12:** 48–57.

Index

Page numbers in *italics* refer to figures and tables.

J

K

L

M

Q

R

U

V

W